PREVENTION, POWERLESSNESS, and POLITICS

PREVENTION, POWERLESSNESS, and POLITICS

Readings on Social Change

EDITORS

George W. Albee

Justin M. Joffe

Linda A. Dusenbury

Published in cooperation with the Vermont Conference on the Primary Prevention of Psychopathology

SAGE PUBLICATIONS
The Publishers of Professional Social Science
Newbury Park   Beverly Hills   London   New Delhi

For information address:

SAGE Publications, Inc.
2111 West Hillcrest Drive
Newbury Park, California 91320

SAGE Publications Inc.
275 South Beverly Drive
Beverly Hills
California 90212

SAGE Publications Ltd.
28 Banner Street
London EC1Y 8QE
England

SAGE PUBLICATIONS India Pvt. Ltd.
M-32 Market
Greater Kailash I
New Delhi 110 048 India

Printed in the United States of America

Library of Congress Cataloging-in-Publication Data

Main entry under title:
Prevention, powerlessness, and politics.

   Edited published papers from the Vermont
Conferences on the Primary Prevention of Psychopathology
held annually since 1975.
   Bibliography: p.
   1. Deviant behavior—Prevention.   2. Social problems.
3. Victims of crimes.   4. Psychology, Pathological—
Prevention.   5. Social change.   I. Albee, George W.
II. Joffe, Justin M.   III. Dusenbury, Linda A.
IV. Vermont Conference on the Primary Prevention of
Psychopathology.
HM291.P715   1988   362.2'0425   87-20567
ISBN 0-8039-3164-6
ISBN 0-8039-3165-4 (pbk.)

FIRST PRINTING 1988

Contents

Preface

In the early 1970s, when the logical necessity of prevention efforts was beginning to permeate the consciousness of mental health professionals, the attacks of those whose vested interests were threatened by a prevention ideology were spearheaded by an argument along the following lines: "Prevention has no research base, no established methods, no demonstration programs in place, no scholarly underpinning." This was untrue, of course, but the documentation needed for rebuttal was scattered, unorganized, diffuse, and often not clearly identified as "prevention," so proponents of prevention were vulnerable to these charges.

As enthusiasm for prevention grew, various efforts were made to remedy the situation. Ours consisted of organizing in 1975 what was to be the first in a series of annual conferences—the Vermont Conference on the Primary Prevention of Psychopathology—to bring together people from a diversity of fields of present authoritative overviews of theory, research, and practice in prevention, and to discuss new directions for this approach. Articles based on the conference presentations have reached an even wider audience through their publication by the University Press of New England and now by Sage Publications. The volumes published to date constitute one of the major rebuttals of the critics' arguments that prevention has no research base.

We are, of course, delighted with the way the Vermont Conference on the Primary Prevention of Psychopathology has flourished and with the continued widespread enthusiasm for both the conference and the resulting series of books. No longer do we have to search through a dozen fields and a multitude of journals to respond to the question, "Where's the literature on primary prevention?" However, we are, in a sense, now beginning to experience some of the problems of affluence. Certainly clearly identifiable material is now available to introduce someone to the field of primary prevention, but the volumes in our series include more than 150 articles totaling nearly 4,000 pages—not too handy for people new to the field and needing a route map to find their way around.

This embarrassment of riches has led to our efforts at producing two books of readings. The first volume (*Readings in Primary Prevention of Psychopathology: Basic Concepts*, University Press of New England, 1984) used selections of published articles from the previous special topics volumes to provide a brief overview of the many facets of primary prevention, including efforts at reducing organic factors and stress, competence building, and the role of support groups. We selected a variety of articles that we felt were representative, and we cut sections of almost all those selected in order to be able to include broader coverage and to improve the book's capacity to serve as a guide to research and programs in the field.

9

This second volume of readings is a continuation of our effort to excerpt from the wide panorama of published articles those dealing specifically with the need for social change and political action to accomplish broad-based prevention efforts. In the epilogue to the first book of readings, we noted that because primary prevention efforts are proactive, and because they often require approaches that affect relatively large groups, many of these efforts involve more or less controversial attempts at modifying major sources of environmental stresses, at changing lifestyles, and even at achieving a redistribution of social power. We noted a strong tendency in our society to try to separate and isolate various social problems and stresses. We are prone to identify, for example, a social problem labeled violence against children in the family, another labeled child sexual abuse, another labeled child neglect, another labeled spouse abuse, and another problem labeled elder abuse. Each of these abuses is regarded as somehow unrelated to the others. We describe other problems and label them sexism, racism, family disruption, poverty, unemployment, the incarceration and decarceration of persons labeled mentally ill, the social isolation of the physically handicapped.

We suggest the need to ask: What do all of these problems, involving so many different groups, have in common? We suggested, at the end of the last book of readings, the best answer we could give: *powerlessness*. People without power are commonly exploited by powerful individuals, and economic groups, and the exploiters explain the resulting victims' psychopathology by pointing to some defect in those persons. Those of us interested in prevention often fail to see these relationships and even when we suspect them we hesitate to rush to the defense of the victims because we, too, are caught up in the ideology that puts "justice" in the hands of those who have power. And we are intimidated by subtle threats to our own well-being.

We believe that it makes little sense to develop separate and discrete programs directed at the prevention of child abuse, of spouse abuse, of elder abuse; or the prevention of the exploitation of women, of minority groups, of migrant farm workers, of the physically handicapped, the mentally ill, and the mentally retarded. If we view all of these groups as relatively powerless because of political and socioeconomic conditions, then a logical approach is to determine whether there might be some way to achieve an equitable redistribution of power. A slogan of the 1960s was "Power to the People!" Another piece of conventional wisdom holds that "Money Is Power." Without meaning to be simplistic, we would like to suggest that we might well examine the arguments for redistribution of power that would result from a redistribution of wealth in our society as a major form of primary prevention.

When confronted with the issue of powerlessness, many professionals tend to approach it as a question of individual aberration, or misperception of reality. The optimism of such views is commendable, but the resulting attempt to alter people's perceptions of their abilities to affect their own lives is often not only misguided, but counterproductive and ultimately damaging. In many selections in this volume, the fact is documented that many people in our society, in many situations, are victims and are powerless. If such people believe that they cannot do much to affect their life circumstances, to alleviate their misery, or to build a better world for their children, it is not because they perceive contingencies incorrectly, but because their perceptions are, in fact, accurate. They see themselves as powerless because they have no power. Without question, this perception further exacerbates their feelings of hopelessness, and further reduces the likelihood of their being able to make the necessary effort on those few occasions in their lives when they might be able to act effectively. If so, something might be said in favor of "therapy" to make them feel less powerless. But therapists are in short supply, and rarely are they available to those who concern us—and anyway, they read a different agenda.

This second volume of readings has been developed as a companion volume to the first. The present volume selects from the published articles in our series of books on prevention, some introductory orientation articles and some excerpts from others that set the stage with a description of the effects of powerlessness by describing some of the victims of our social system. This is followed by a description of primary prevention programs aimed at reducing victimization and at a redistribution of power. The articles we have chosen include programs for individuals and families, programs for larger political change affecting groups, and identification of sources of resistance and opposition from protectors of the status quo.

There is relatively little overlap between this volume and the earlier book of readings. The exception is that we have included "A Model for Classifying Prevention Programs" with some revision and elaboration, and selections from the Report of the Task Panel on Prevention to the President's Commission on Mental Health.

In preparing this book, we not only selected articles, we cut sections of almost all the ones chosen in order to be able to include more selections and to improve the book's usefulness as a guide to the field. The cuts, all of which are indicated by an asterisk (*)—so that any abruptness or lack of continuity can be blamed on us and not on the authors—were designed to help the reader not lose the forest for the trees. We have omitted those parts of articles containing lengthy presentations of experimental findings, technical details, and—dare we admit it?—repetitive or redundant material.

We have tried to preserve the logic of each article and to leave its general argument and major concepts intact. We have left most reference lists uncut: This results in the minor oddity of there now being bibliographic information on publications that are not mentioned in the text, but we felt this was a small drawback when compared to the advantage of leaving the interested reader with all the references to draw on in case she or he wishes to explore any of the topics in greater depth.

To these edited selections from our series of books on primary prevention we have added a prologue—"A Model for Classifying Prevention Programs"

(Albee)—to provide a general introduction to the entire field, brief headnotes for each section, and (in Part V) a debate between one of us (Albee) and H. Richard Lamb, a psychiatrist who raises many of the issues espoused by opponents of prevention.

The result is, we hope, an integrated set of materials suitable for introducing a student or mental health professional to the field of primary prevention or for use as a handy reference book for those involved in writing, research, or practice in the field. We hope, too, that the convenience of having two independent but related volumes will contribute to the growth of undergraduate and graduate courses in prevention (in psychology and social work departments, in education and psychiatry, and elsewhere) and that instructors will find the readings suitable as auxiliary texts to cover the prevention section of courses in community psychology, social psychiatry, community mental health, abnormal psychology, and others.

To the extent that the books of readings contribute to the development of awareness of the importance of prevention to the entire field of mental health and human development and of the urgency that attends the need to escape the straitjacket of conventional approaches to mental health problems, we will have achieved our objective.

—George W. Albee
Justin M. Joffe
Linda Dusenbury
Burlington, Vermont

Prologue: A Model for Classifying Prevention Programs

George W. Albee

The explanation most often used at present to account for mental and emotional disorders emphasizes individual defect. It says that persons exhibit abnormal behavior, or experience unusual thoughts and feelings, because there is something specific wrong inside. This defect, or illness, explanation leads to an approach to intervention that stresses individual therapy and that opposes efforts at social change. As a general rule, one-to-one therapists oriented toward individual treatment, organic or psycho-therapeutic, resist prevention efforts that stress improved social or educational experience.

One frequent criticism opponents level at advocates of primary prevention holds that their efforts are too general, too unfocused, too vague, too nonspecific. Critics of primary prevention also commonly raise one or more of the following specific objections.

It is not possible to prevent mental illness in general. There are many different specific forms of mental illness and we do not yet have clear evidence of the cause of each. Further, these critics argue, it is not possible to mount separate effective prevention programs without a knowledge of the specific cause of each specific form of mental illness.

The answers to this objection are fairly clear. Most forms of "mental illness" are not illnesses in the usual sense. Unlike genuine physical illnesses where a specific microorganism, organic defect, physical malfunction, or other objective toxic or noxious agent can be identified, most mental disorders are identified only by peculiar behavior, unusual ideation, personal report of subjective discomfort, and so forth. Most forms of "mental illness" cannot be identified by laboratory tests or other objective physical measures. Rather, the presence of a mental disorder is inferred from behavioral observation or from the report of the subject about his or her emotional discomfort. Rather than a specific condition being attributable to specific causes, it is well established that any particular stressful life experience may produce any of several different patterns of disturbance.

Thus severe marital disruption, for example, may be followed in some people by depression, in others by excessive drinking, in some by alcoholism leading to cirrhosis of the liver, in others by social withdrawal and isolation, in others by accident proneness including fatal accidents and/or suicide. Similarly, looking for a single precipitating cause leading to depression, for example, is fruitless, and leads instead to the discovery that this condition results from any of a wide variety of stress-inducing situations. In short, it is most unlikely that a specific cause will ever be identified for each of the 230 different patterns of emotional disturbance described in the American Psychiatric Association's *Diagnostic and Statistical Manual III* (DSM III). Prevention results from stress reduction, particularly those stresses arising out of difficult interpersonal relations, and from improved social coping skills and solid support systems.

In contrast to the objection that we know too little about the causation of mental illnesses to be able to prevent them, another objection argues that most forms of mental illness are a result of genetic defects and/or biochemical imbalances and, as a consequence, are not preventable through social manipulation and environmental change. This argument limits prevention efforts to genetic counseling and suggests that research money might better be spent looking for ways of correcting disturbed brain chemistry and other biological defects. Persons expressing this objection usually attempt to make a distinction between "genuine" mental illnesses, which they hold to be genetic in origin, and problems in living, which they rule out as forms of mental illness. One trouble with this position is that it is often impossible to find a clear organic cause for so-called genuine mental illnesses, like depression or schizophrenia. Further, all of the mental conditions listed in the official psychiatric nomenclature (DSM III) are officially and legally recognized as forms of mental illnesses for purposes of psychiatric treatment and for reimbursement by third-party payments. The same psychiatrists who argue that genuine mental illnesses are organic (which problems of living are not) at the same time accept reimbursement for their treatment of all DSM III conditions, including problems in living, thereby certifying them to be genuine illnesses. It follows then that efforts successful in preventing conditions like adolescent rebellion, school learning problems, tobacco addiction syndrome, and emotional disturbances resulting from marital disruption are indeed preventing conditions officially recognized as psychiatric illnesses.

Another objection cited by opponents of prevention efforts holds that research to demonstrate the effectiveness of prevention programs has not yet produced much in the way of significant positive findings, and therefore it is foolish to expend funds that are in short supply for vague and untested prevention efforts.

One answer to this objection is contained, in significant measure, in this volume, in which selected excerpts have been chosen from the first seven volumes published by the Vermont Conference on Primary Prevention of Psychopathology (VCPPP). This continuing series of books contains papers delivered at the annual Vermont Conference. Each year we have chosen a specific topical area related to primary prevention of psychopathology and have invited distinguished contributors to theory and research to present papers. The resulting annual volume is a record of what is known about prevention in that particular area. It is interesting that critics of prevention apply a distinctly higher standard of evaluation to research in this field than is applied to research in psychiatric treatment. The history of psychiatric treatment is replete with examples of poor research efforts that have been hailed as important breakthroughs and which, after a few years, turn out to be relatively ineffective or even damaging.

Critics of prevention efforts are often disdainful of programs attempting to effect positive social change, to build a more humane and secure society, efforts to make parents more loving and nurturant, schools more supportive and rewarding, work more challenging and interesting, employment more certain, etc. They regard all of these efforts in social change engineering as unrelated to mental health and mental illness. While it may be admirable, they argue, to do our best to improve the lot of humankind, this is really not the major business of workers in the field of mental health who have no special talent or knowledge about political and economic issues.

The answers to this objection, of course, are contained, in part, in this volume. Social stress will be shown to increase emotional disturbance and distress, and the reduction in stress will be followed by a reduced disturbance. Instilling rational attitudes toward sexuality, and providing accurate sexual knowledge, will be shown to be associated with mature sexual behavior, while sexual ignorance and misunderstanding will be shown to be associated with anxiety and pathological sexual disturbances. These and other findings reported in this volume underscore the importance of social change aimed at the reduction of unnecessary stress, at more rational sex education, and toward the fostering of mutual support groups and positive self-esteem. It is the responsibility of the mental health worker continuously to interpret to society, and especially to legislators and persons responsible for social policy and educational programs, the relationship between these societal variables and resulting distress or lack of distress.

Another related objection from those who oppose an environmental model argues that efforts at strengthening mental health, at improving the adaptive skills and potentials of persons by enhancing their coping skills, are really not relevant to the prevention of mental illness. This argument fails to take into account the traditional public health model for disease prevention that has an important lesson for those interested in the prevention of psychopathology. Traditionally public health efforts at the prevention of diseases have involved three strategies: (1) removing or neutralizing the noxious agent, (2) strengthening the resistance of the host, and (3) preventing transmission of the noxious agent to the host. This model has been remarkably successful in reducing or eliminating many of the great plagues that have afflicted humankind in the past. Efforts at removing or neutralizing noxious agents in the water supply have reduced or eliminated diseases such as typhoid fever and cholera. Strengthening the resistance of the host, through vaccination for example, has eliminated smallpox. And preventing transmission, by eliminating mosquitoes that transmit yellow fever or malaria, is a third example of effective prevention. In the field of psychopathology, the noxious agent often is uncontrolled stress. Strengthening the host includes the teaching of coping skills, the enhancement of self-esteem, and the provision of support groups. Preventing transmission may be accomplished by eliminating messages that lead to sexist, racist, ageist, and other pathological attitudes. Illustrations of all of these approaches are contained in the pages that follow.

One of the most common objections to prevention efforts holds that because there is such a limited amount of tax money available for the field of mental health and mental illness it is important to use these scarce funds for the treatment of persons who are currently suffering, rather than diverting money into uncertain and unproven prevention efforts that could have effects only many years later. This objection raises the question of whether the mental health professions now are seeing the persons most in need of help. Let us consider this issue in some detail.

A major (1984) epidemiological study of adult emotional disturbances, supported by the National Institute of Mental Health (NIMH), involved interviews with a selected sample of thousands of adults in New Haven, Baltimore, and St. Louis. Extrapolating from the results of these interviews, NIMH estimated that at least 19% of the adult population of the United States (43 million people) has a diagnosable mental disorder! This study did *not* include homeless persons, institutionalized persons, children and adolescents, and did not inquire of the sample about their possible sexual disorders. All of these latter groups would be expected to add many millions more to the number of affected adults. Clearly, these numbers become so large as to be almost meaningless when considered against the very small number of mental health professionals engaged in individual treatment or therapy (probably no more than 50,000). In recent years in the United States there have been, annually, approximately one million divorces, shown by Bloom (1978) to be a significant source of stress leading to any of several different damaging emotional reactions; in addition the stress of the loss of loved ones through death frequently results in severe emotional distress and/or reactive depression. Large numbers of other persons experience emotional crises. Involuntary unemployment, for example, has been shown (Brenner, 1973, 1977) to produce any of several severe consequences including a rise in admissions to mental health clinics and mental health hospitals, an increased incidence of cirrhosis of the liver, alcoholism, fatal accidents, suicide, and an excess of deaths from all causes.

In 1978 the President's Commission on Mental Health reported on the frightening number of underserved and unserved persons in the field of mental health. Part of the problem results from the maldistribution of professionals who tend to be concentrated in the affluent suburbs of populous states.

Who are these underserved and unserved? They are described in several different places in the commission's report. They include children, adolescents and the elderly—all of whom are identified repeatedly as underserved by mental health professionals. These three groups together represent "more than half" of the nation's population. Then there are the minority groups that include 22 million black Americans, 12 million Hispanic Americans, 3 million Asian and Pacific Island Americans, and one million American Indians and Alaska natives. All of these groups are underserved or, in many instances, inappropriately served by persons insensitive to cultural differences or incompetent in appropriate languages. While these identified groups of 38 million persons clearly overlap somewhat with other groups identified as underserved, we are not yet at the end of the statistical complexities. Five million seasonal and migrant farm workers are largely excluded from mental health care. Moreover, we discover that often women do not receive appropriate care in the mental health system. Neither do persons who live in rural America, or in small towns, or in the poor sections of American cities. Neither do 10 million persons with alcohol-related problems, nor an unspecified but growing number of persons who misuse psychoactive drugs, nor the very large number of children and parents involved in child abuse, nor 5 million children with learning disabilities, nor millions of physically handicapped Americans, nor 6 million persons who are mentally retarded.

The Future Is Worse!

Kramer (1981) has raised some important and alarming questions about what he refers to as "the rising pandemic of mental disorders" throughout the world. He points out that the United States faces, in the decades immediately ahead, a steadily increasing prevalence rate of serious mental disorders, as well as medical diseases involving hypertension and cerebro-vascular accidents. The growth in frequency of these conditions will result from the large increase in the number of persons in those age groups who are at higher risk for their development, as well as the steadily increasing *duration* of such chronic conditions directly resulting from the develop-ment of effective techniques for prolonging the lives of affected individ-uals. In brief, more people, throughout the world, are living into middle age and old age and the chronic mental and physical conditions that are more likely to occur with advancing years are not only occurring but are being treated in ways that prolong their duration.

In a paper entitled *Failures of Success*, Gruenberg (1977) talks about the increase in prevalence rates of conditions that are age specific:

It is obvious that, with increasing duration, we would expect the proportion of the population at any given age group suffering from these conditions to rise. And, in fact, as a result of advances in medical care, we are seeing a rising prevalence of certain chronic conditions which previously led to early terminal infections, but whose victims now suffer from them for a longer period. The goal of medical research work is to "diminish disease and enrich life" (Gregg, 1941), but it produced tools which prolong diseased, diminished lives, and so increased the proportion of people who have a disabling or chronic disease.

That is a major but unintended effect of many technological improvements stemming from health research. These increasingly chronic conditions represent the failures of success. Their growing prevalence and longer duration are a product of progress in health technology.

Among the other "failures of success" we should take note of effective medical techniques for prolonging the lives of the severely retarded, for intervening successfully with severely premature and underweight infants, infants with severe perinatal handicaps and complications, all resulting in a subsequent increase in the prevalence of mentally and physically handi-capped persons. Before the development of antibiotics, the life expec-tancy of severely retarded "crib cases" and other institutionalized retard-ates was fairly short because of the prevalence of infectious diseases in institutions. Now with antibiotics, and de-institutionalization, many severely handicapped individuals have a much expanded life expectancy. The de-institutionalization of persons labeled schizophrenic has increased the number of pregnancies in schizophrenic women, for example, and therefore the number of children born with the risk of being reared with an alleged genetic handicap and/or with a schizophrenic mother. Infants born with phenylketonuria (PKU) are being identified through routine lab tests and are being treated with a special diet, allowing them to live into adult childbearing years with the resulting increase in genetic carriers.

Kramer is not suggesting that we turn back the clock on all of these medical advances, but that we be aware of the serious problems these changes promise to cause in our future. The mechanisms he discusses are occurring world wide, including the less developed regions. Indeed, as Kramer points out, there will be further aggravation of the problem of chronic conditions as developing countries industrialize, as their populations move from rural agrarian to urban industrial areas, and as the pattern of living in extended families shifts to a more nuclear family structure. Kramer sees one of the few hopes to be effective research emphasizing *the prevention of chronic disease.* He points to the current increases in the prevalence rate of schizophrenia, the growing rate of admission to mental health facilities and prisons, to homes for the aged and to nursing homes and suggests that prevention is the only logical solution.

If the prevalence rate of mental and emotional disorders in the United States is about 15 percent then with a population increase of more than 20 percent expected over the next 25 years we will have more than 40 million persons with "hard core" mental disorders by the year 2005. Inasmuch as the prevalence of disorders is a function of both incidence and duration, advances in treatment methods for mental disorders can only have the effect of increasing their prevalence. The proportion of the population over 65 will continue to increase rapidly for both white and nonwhite groups. The increase in the rate of the latter will be more dramatic because of remarkable progress in improving life expectancy for nonwhites in recent decades. The proportion of older persons is not only increasing but the number of them who live alone is also increasing, particularly among females. And, as we know from other studies, the rate of mental and emotional disorders among single (including separated, divorced, and widowed) elderly persons is high and increasing.

It is also worth noting that because of differential birth rates, we can expect a 40 percent increase in new cases of schizophrenia among non-whites because of the increase in the number of 15 to 34 year olds, the group at highest risk.

Kramer (1981) concludes his frightening analysis with the following:

Although there are many shortcomings and gaps in currently available morbidity and mortality statistics, those that are available are sufficient to illustrate the extraordinary increases that can be expected in the number of persons who will be affected by major problems of disease and disability that are of concern to mental health. This includes persons in every age group, from the youngest to the oldest. Prevalence rates of mental disorders, Down's Syndrome, hypertensive disease, cerebrovascular disease, cirrhosis of the liver, diabetes, visual and hearing impairments, and other chronic conditions are increasing throughout the world. This worldwide increase in the prevalence of mental disorders and chronic disease may be best characterized as a rising chronic disease pandemic....

The number of cases of mental disorder will continue to increase *until effective methods are discovered for preventing their occurrence and equally effective and practical methods are found for their application. It is, therefore, particularly important that our policy makers give the highest priority to the support of research and research training directed toward discovering the preventable causes of those conditions that are increasing in prevalence.* (pp. 27, 28, 31, emphasis added)

We have identified a number of factors associated with increased incidence of mental disorders, and we have also found ways to intervene proactively with groups, especially those at high risk for later psychopathology, to reduce the subsequent incidence. Some of these preventive strategies involve the reduction of noxious agents, and some involve strengthening the resistance of the host. These strategies can be related to incidence according to the following model.

$$\text{Incidence} = \frac{\text{Organic Factors} + \text{Stress} + \text{Exploitation}}{\text{Coping Skills} + \text{Self-esteem} + \text{Support Groups}}$$

To succeed in preventive efforts is to reduce the incidence (the number of new cases) of the various emotional disturbances. There are several strategies for accomplishing such a reduction.

Organic factors. The first strategy is to minimize, or to reduce, the number of the various organic factors that sometimes play a role in causation. The more the negative organic factors can be reduced or eliminated, the lower will be the resulting incidence. Several sections in this volume consider genetic, prenatal, postpartum, and later childhood experiences. We also have included material on the preventive value of working with cardiac patients to prevent or reduce sexual dysfunction, and on the benefits of promoting positive health behaviors.

Stress. A second strategy that is obvious from the formula involves the reduction of unnecessary or avoidable stress. As we move into this area, we discover that relationships become more complex. No longer are there such simple cause and effect relationships as we observed in organic factors. Stress takes many forms. Reducing stress may require changes in the physical and social environment. Environmental stress situations involve a whole complex of interacting variables. Some forms of social stress are a product of deeply engrained cultural values and ways of life that are not easily susceptible to change. Readings are included that deal with stress in general, and with particular, and common, sources of stress.

Exploitation. This factor differs from the others in the formula in an important way. Variations in the degree or type of exploitation affect all the other variables in the model—stress, coping skills, self-esteem, the nature and type of support groups available, and even the incidence of organic factors. For example, in a society in which a power elite exploits the environment for personal profit without regard to the social costs and consequences of their greed, the incidence of birth defects may be increased by environmental contamination or malnutrition, physical health of workers may be damaged, and so on. Since exploitation encompasses all the other variables, as well as being something that itself, with its many faces, contributes to psychopathology, it needs to be considered in both its larger and its smaller sense.

Persons who are victims of exploitation in any of its myriad forms suffer serious emotional damage. The exploitation often involves the use of excessive power by the exploiter to force the victims to conform or to behave in ways that are degrading, demeaning, dehumanizing and/or dangerous. While the experience may well be both stressful and damaging to self-esteem, there is a qualitative difference that justifies separate analysis of this factor. In many societies and throughout the history of many cultures, women and children have been exploited by powerful male patriarchal elites. Rape and the sexual abuse of children are obvious examples of exploitation. But there are many other more subtle ways that people can be subject to daily humiliations.

It is important that we try to learn about a society, or any other group sharing a common culture, those things (like sex roles and class position) taken for granted. What are the unquestioned assumptions, the accepted ways of understanding reality, that never rise above the threshold of conscious awareness because no one feels they can question or examine them?

Damage done through *exploitation*—economic, sexual, through the media, causes increased incidence of emotional pathology. The exploited groups are not responsive to exhortations or to other quick-fix solutions. Certain kinds of exploitation result in low self-esteem and become a kind of self-fulfilling prophecy. Members of ethnic minorities and women, who learn from earliest childhood that their race or sex is regarded as inferior by the white patriarchal culture grow up with lower self-esteem that may be exceedingly difficult to change. Feelings of powerlessness are a major form of stress. Preventive efforts may have to take the form of laws to ensure equal opportunity, public education, changes in the way the mass media portrays these groups, and in pervasive value system changes. Clearly, such efforts often encounter the angry resistance of the power forces that get real benefit from the values being criticized.

A reduction in incidence also may be accomplished by developing feelings of competence—better social coping skills, improved self-esteem, and solid support networks. Each section deals with one of these factors. Wherever possible this material is organized in a developmental sequence within sections.

Overall, the readings that follow should give flesh to the bare bones of the formula outlined. In addition, we hope they will provide a starting point enabling those who see that prevention is our only hope to approach the task with the confidence that comes from being aware of these numerous examples of both the promise and the efficacy of programs to prevent psychopathology and promote human competence. This body of knowledge, of which the present volume is only a sampling, should also help to give the lie to those who would cling to outmoded, ineffective, and, in the long run, inhumane attempts to comfort the victims instead of preventing the casualties.

In the present volume, we have attempted to select from material presented in all of the previous volumes that reflects social forces leading to stress, exploitation and powerlessness. We also have selected some illustrative examples of the plight of the victims, and then we proceed to present a range of proposed prevention programs for dealing with the problems of exploitation and powerlessness.

References

Albee, G. Preventing psychopathology and promoting human potential. *American Psychologist,* 1982, 37, 9, 1043–1050.

American Psychiatric Association. *Diagnostic and Statistical Manual of Mental Disorders* (Third Edition). Washington, D.C.: APA, 1980.

Bloom, B. Marital disruption as a stressor. Chapter 6. In Forgays, D.G. (ed.) *Environmental influences and strategies in primary prevention.* Hanover, N.H.: University Press of New England, 1978.

Brenner, M.H. *Mental illness and the economy.* Cambridge, Mass.: Harvard University Press, 1973.

Gruenberg, E. M. Failures of success. Health and society. *The Milbank Memorial Fund Quarterly,* Winter, 1977.

Klerman, G. Speech at the University of Vermont, March 13, 1980. *Faculty symposium on the social and biological origins of mental illness.*

Kramer, M. The increasing prevalence of mental disorders: Implications for the future. Paper presented at the National Conference on the Elderly Deinstitutionalized Patient in the Community. May 28, 1981.

President's Commission on Mental Health. *Report to the President.* Washington, D.C.: U.S. Government Printing Office, 1978.

Ryan, W. *Distress in the city.* Cleveland, Ohio: The Press of Western Reserve University, 1969.

I.   Introduction to Primary Prevention

As in the earlier volume of readings concerned with basic issues, we begin this volume with a selection of material from the Report of the Task Panel on Prevention to the President's (Carter) Commission on Mental Health.

This commission, whose honorary chair was Rosalynn Carter, was composed of 20 people, the majority of whom were not members of the traditional mental health professions, but who represented a wide range of backgrounds and perspectives. Each of the task panels reporting to the commission dealt with some specific aspect of mental health, and each was composed of persons with special competency in the subject area. The Task Panel on Prevention included persons from social work, psychology, psychiatry, genetics, the law, and education—as well as from lay groups and consumers. The definition of prevention adopted by the task panel included both attempts at reducing stresses and efforts at improving the competence of people for handling life's stresses. Selections from the report include, in addition to definitions, an examination of barriers to prevention efforts, a consideration of priorities, and a series of examples of existing research on competency training, the impact of social systems, and stress reduction. The final report of the commission led to the passage of the Mental Health Systems Act in 1980, which recommended establishment of a Center on Prevention at the National Institute of Mental Health.

Following the report of the Task Panel on Prevention, we have included excerpts that focus on the issue of powerlessness and psychopathology (Joffe and Albee), and on the basic underlying "causes of the causes" (an article in which Joffe identifies broad demographic variables, such as poverty, poor education, and low social class, as causal variables). Then follows the late Burton Blatt's incisive indictment of American business values that cause human damage. These values are well reflected in the cynical use of the media to sell consumer goods, and we have included White's demonstration of the role of the mass media in fostering psychopathology and in exploiting the *anomie* and boredom that affects so many millions of Americans.

M. Brewster Smith's excerpt summarizes themes that emerged from our Conference on Social Change and Political Action and we have included his identification of these themes as a sort of agenda for action.

Report of the Task Panel on Prevention

❖ *SUMMARY*

Western society's approach to persons with mental disorders has progressed in a series of steps. Each step has been characterized by increasingly humanitarian concern. For thousands of years the insane were reviled, feared, and rejected. Two hundred years ago, in the first mental health "revolution," they were led by Pinel out of the fetid dungeons, up into the light and into more humane treatment. A second revolution, led by Freud, greatly increased our understanding of the continuity between the insane and the sane. Half a century later, a third revolution was dedicated to providing care in a single comprehensive center accessible to all those at high risk. Now, less than a quarter century later, we are on the threshold of a fourth and most exciting mental health revolution. Its goal is to prevent emotional disorders.

Although each revolution has drawn strength from, and built on, earlier ones, we have come more and more to recognize that widespread human distress can never be eliminated by attempts—however successful—to treat afflicted individuals. We shall continue to do everything we can for persons in pain. But we are also determined to take action to reduce the identifiable causes of later distress, and thereby decrease the incidence of emotional disturbance and disorder.

Primary prevention means lowering the incidence of emotional disorder (1) by reducing stress and (2) by promoting conditions that increase competence and coping skills. Primary prevention is concerned with populations not yet affected by individual breakdown, especially with groups at high risk. It is proactive: it

❖ This symbol throughout the text indicates the cutting of original material for the purposes of this volume.

From "Report of the Task Panel on Prevention," in Justin M. Joffe, George W. Albee, and Linda D. Kelly (eds.) *Readings in Primary Prevention of Psychopathology: Basic Concepts.* Copyright © 1984 by the Vermont Conference on the Primary Prevention of Psychopathology. Reprinted by permission.

often seeks to build adaptive strengths through education and reduce stress through social engineering.

An important "paradigm shift" must be considered in focusing attention on research in primary prevention. There are good reasons to believe that just as an emotional disorder may result from any of several background factors and life crises, so can any specific intense stressful event precipitate any of a variety of mental and emotional disorders. Different life histories and different patterns of strengths and weaknesses among different individuals can and do lead to different reactions to stress. This new paradigm requires that we recognize the futility of searching for a unique cause for every emotional disorder. It accepts the likelihood that many disorders can come about as a consequence of many of the varieties of causes. This paradigm leads to the acceptance of the argument that successful efforts at the prevention of a wide variety of disorders can occur without a theory of disorder-specific positive causal mechanisms.

Our recommendations include a focus on a coordinated national effort toward the prevention of emotional disorder with a Center for Primary Prevention within the National Institute of Mental Health, with primary prevention specialists deployed in each of the ten USPHS Regional Offices, with the establishment of State-level efforts, and with the creation of field stations and model demonstration centers. Because many other relevant government agencies can, and should, be concerned with prevention, we are recommending the coordination of efforts through the proposed NIMH center that is to have convening authority. We are recommending that first priority in primary prevention be directed toward work with infants and young children (and their social environments). We give a number of illustrations of the kinds of programs we have in mind. We take special note of the urgent need to reduce societal stresses produced by racism, poverty, sexism, ageism, and the decay of our cities. We make certain suggestions about funding and about a broadly competent citizen's committee to have a continuing advisory role.

PREAMBLE

The *first* revolutionary change in society's approach to the mentally ill and the emotionally disturbed was the humanitarian concern exemplified by Philippe Pinel who, in 1792, removed the chains binding the insane in the fetid dungeons of Paris. He brought those victims up into the sunlight and showed the world that kindness and concern were defensible and appropriate.

The *second* revolutionary change in our attitudes and values had its origin in Freud's work that stressed the continuities between the sane and the insane, the mind of the child and the mind of the adult, the world of dreams and the world of reality.

The *third* revolution was the development of intervention and treatment centers serving all persons needing help—comprehensive community mental health centers—where, through a single door, everyone could seek and find skilled help for the whole range of human mental and emotional problems.

Unlike political revolutions, each of these mental health revolutions drew strength and inspiration from the earlier ones.

We believe we now stand on the threshold of a *fourth* revolution. Like its predecessors, this revolution will not attempt to displace or replace progress already achieved. The new revolution will involve major societal efforts at *preventing* mental illness and emotional disturbance. It will apply the best available knowledge, derived from research and clinical experience, to prevent needless distress and psychological dysfunction. It will, in the best public health tradition, also seek to build strengths and increase competence and coping skills in populations and thereby reduce the incidence of later disturbance. This fourth revolution, if it happens, will identify our society as a *caring society*—one that both holds out its hand to its unfortunate members and does all it can to prevent misfortune for those at risk.

❖

INTRODUCTION AND RATIONALE

The development and application of primary prevention programs in the field of the emotional disorders is the great unmet mental health challenge of our time. From both a moral and ethical point of view, preventive intervention has the potential for reducing human suffering associated with emotional disorder and the impact of that suffering on family and friends. From an economic point of view, effective primary prevention programs promise to be less expensive in the long run than the direct (fiscal) and indirect (human) costs to society of not providing such services.

The term "primary prevention" refers to a group of approaches that share the common objectives of (1) lowering the incidence of emotional disorders (i.e. the rate at which new cases occur) and (2) promoting conditions that reinforce positive mental health. Primary prevention, in concentrating its efforts on promotion and maintenance of competence, is distinguished from traditional mental health services designed to identify, treat, or rehabilitate persons already disturbed (Kessler and Albee, 1975; Albee and Joffe, 1977; Cowen, 1977; Bloom, 1977; Klein and Goldston, 1977).

One way in which primary prevention works in the mental health field is to eliminate the causes of disorders of known or discoverable etiologies (e.g. cerebral syphilis). Equally or perhaps more important, primary prevention involves building the strengths, resources, and competencies in individuals, families, and communities that can reduce the flow of a variety of unfortunate outcomes—each characterized by enormous human and societal cost. Because primary prevention approaches can be applied flexibly in a variety of situations, they are an especially attractive means for reaching vulnerable, high-risk groups.

Primary prevention activities have two main justifications: (1) the body of evidence supporting the efficacy of these approaches in their own right; and (2) the growing sense of dissatisfaction, as the gap widens between demonstrated need for help and the costly, often unavailable, human resources to meet that need, with mental health's past exclusive reliance on corrective measures.

From a logistical point of view, there can never be a sufficient number of skilled health care providers to meet unchecked intervention needs. And, in any case, no major disorder in a population has ever been eliminated by providing one-to-one treatment, however comprehensive.

Historically, the mental health field has always been unswerving in its definition of mandate, i.e. to understand the complexities of psychological aberration and to contain or minimize dysfunction when called on to engage it. However constructive that mandate is, the service systems developed to meet it cannot be expected to resolve society's mental health problems. Thus, today (1) there are too few resources to deal with mental health problems as defined, (2) distribution of those limited resources is inequitable, following the ironic rule of where help is most needed it is least available, and (3) mental health energies are disproportionately allocated to the exacting and costly task of trying to overcome already rooted, crystallized, "end state" conditions— precisely those that most resist change.

The history of public health in the past century provides ample evidence that programs designed to prevent disease and disorder can be effective and reasonably economical. Infectious diseases that can now be prevented include smallpox, malaria, typhus, cholera, yellow fever, polio, and measles. An equally impressive group of nutritional disorders, including scurvy, pellagra, beri-beri, and kwashiorkor, is now also understood and preventable. Imagine what our health bill would be if those diseases were not preventable and society therefore needed to bear the costs of supporting state malaria hospitals, state pellagra hospitals, and state hospitals for polio victims.

Preventive measures have proved to be a vital extension of health care practices in physical health. The mental health field, however, has yet to use available relevant knowledge to develop comparable efforts systematically. Public health approaches offer a sound conceptual and operating framework for undertaking primary prevention in the mental health field.

Primary prevention approaches, on logical, humanitarian, and empirical grounds, thus offer an attractive, sorely needed extension of existing mental health practices that hold promise for reducing the eventual flow of emotional disorder.

In the history of medicine, the response to disease illustrates the relationship between the state of knowledge and what physicians actually do. At a time when few normal physiological processes, let alone the pathological ones, were understood, physicians had to be content with describing what they saw and paltry efforts at palliation. Only with the advance of medical knowledge was it possible to refine descriptions into diagnoses and, with an understanding of etiology, to prescribe disease-specific treatment. As we have become more sophisticated about the nature of illness, efforts to prevent illness have also increased. For diseases with specific etiologies, i.e. in which the pathogenic relationships between causative agent and disease came to be fully understood, prevention efforts were often dramatic. But as most diseases have multiple causes, they required more complex strategies for prevention as well.

Most mental conditions lack the single etiology or definitive understanding of pathogenesis needed for dramatic prevention efforts. That very fact has led many people to despair of *ever* preventing mental disturbance and to continue to advocate an exclusive emphasis on diagnosis and treatment as the only scientifically justifiable approach to mental illness. This broad kind of denial of the possibiltities of prevention has led to widespread indifference toward it both by the medical profession and within society at large. We have thus lived through an era of greater and greater expenditures for treatment and rehabilitation without a much-needed corresponding attention to existing possibilities for prevention.

Prevention in the field of mental health can properly be seen as an integrating perspective that can fuse our best understandings of the etiology of mental disorder, personal and family relationships, and individual psychodynamics on the one hand with a recognition, on the other, of the salient social forces and pressures that combine to produce the individual and collective disorganization we call emotional illness.

❖

DEFINITIONS: WHAT PRIMARY PREVENTION IS AND IS NOT

Primary prevention in mental health is a network of strategies that differ *qualitatively* from the field's past dominant approaches. Those strategies are distinguished by several essential characteristics. This brief section highlights primary prevention's essences using the direct contrast style of saying *what it is* and *what it is not*.

(1) Most fundamentally, primary prevention is *proactive* in that it seeks to build adaptive strengths, coping resources, and health in people; not to reduce or contain already manifest deficit.

(2) Primary prevention is concerned about total populations, especially including groups at high risk; it is less oriented to individuals and to the provision of services on a case-by-case basis.

(3) Primary prevention's main tools and models are those of education and social engineering, not therapy or rehabilitation, although some insights for its models and programs grow out of the wisdom derived from clinical experience.

(4) Primary prevention assumes that equipping people with personal and environmental resources for coping is the best of all ways to ward off maladaptive problems, not trying to deal (how-

ever skillfully) with problems that have already germinated and flowered.

WHAT DO WE SEEK TO PREVENT?

We believe there is sufficient evidence to encourage further development of strategies for the prevention of a wide variety of conditions, such as: the psychoses, especially organic psychoses, neuroses and other social disorders, learning disabilities, child abuse, and other behavioral, emotional, and developmental deviations that fall within the broad range of mental health problems.

One key difference between the human organism and lower animals is the much longer period of time during which the human infant and child must depend on others for survival and support. During that long growth process, successful development can be interfered with by an unusually large number of factors at any point. Thus, under certain unfortunate circumstances, all infants are at risk for subsequent emotional and developmental deviations. Scientific advances have markedly reduced the mortality and morbidity of childbirth. Never before in our history have infants had as good an opportunity as they now do to be born healthy and to thrive. Unfortunately, however, the delivery of a biologically healthy full-term infant does not guarantee smooth psychosocial development forever after. Precisely because interference with optimal development is known to occur with high frequency, and to exact a heavy toll, it is imperative that programs for primary prevention be developed. It is essential to establish priorities, to select infants and children at particularly high risk, and to develop programs to assure optimal continuing development for such target groups. We firmly believe that efforts directed toward infants and young children will provide maximum return in successful prevention.

The Task Panel advocates the establishment of programs designed to prevent persistent, destructive, maladaptive behaviors, i.e. those unfortunate "end states" that result from identifiable stresses for which the individual lacks the necessary coping skills and the adaptive competencies to handle constructively. That critical goal suggests the need to identify (1) agreed-upon behavioral conditions that pose a serious threat to others because of the damage they cause; (2) patterns of behavior that are so distasteful for the affected person that he cries out for relief; or (3) emotional states that lead to withdrawal from meaningful social partipation. Clearly, many such traits or conditions require social value judgments about what is desirable or undesirable behavior, acceptable and unacceptable styles of living. Some of these decisions, in short, may present dangers to liberty and to the freedom of people to follow their own drummers, to be unconventional, and even to be damned fools. There are many historical examples of the tyranny of the majority enforcing patterns of approved behavior and lifestyles, and too many deviants who have been punished, excommunicated, or even killed, for nonconformity. Clearly, preventive efforts must be directed toward those end states that cause either genuine harm to others or genuine unwanted suffering in affected individuals.

Attempts to classify mental conditions have turned out to be far more complex than was originally thought. The exciting successes of medicine and biology during the nineteenth century in classifying physical illnesses were viewed as models that might lead ultimately to successful classification of mental diseases. Indeed, the discovery of specific physical causes for certain mental conditions—the role of the spirochete, and the relationship of untreated syphilis to the subsequent appearance of a serious mental illness called general paresis; relationships between vitamin deficiency and pellagral psychosis; the serious social and behavioral consequences of oversecretion and undersecretion of certain endocrine glands such as the thyroid and the adrenals—each served to strengthen the belief that, eventually, all disturbed behavioral states would be found to have an underlying pathologic organic cause. That view persists even today. Some experts accept Nobel Laureate Linus Pauling's view that there can be no insanity in a healthy brain (1968). Another world famous chemist, Ralph Gerard, said much the same thing: "There can be no twisted behavior without a twisted molecule." Unfortunately, life is not so simple; indeed many everyday observations contradict that view. For example, soldiers under extreme combat stress often show serious emotional disturbances; children of disturbed parents often exhibit serious emotional problems; many persons undergoing naturally occurring life stresses, such as sudden widowhood or marital disruption, experience extreme personal anguish and depression. Yet each of these conditions is reversible. The critical point to be understood is that while all behavior has an underlying physiological *basis*, disturbed behavior need not imply an underlying pathological organic *process*. In short, people react emotionally to stress; they learn to withdraw, to attack, or to distort their relationships with others through normal physical mechanisms.

The Task Panel on Prevention thus advocates a broad-gauged effort in primary prevention directed ultimately to reducing the incidence of the major aberrant conditions and end states that have for years occupied the attention of, claimed the efforts of, and been sources of exasperation to the mental health field: the major childhood behavioral and developmental disabilities, the functional and organic psychoses, symptom and character neuroses, and profound psychosocial disorders such as delinquency and addiction. The Task Panel advocates a vigorous national effort to build health and competencies in individuals from birth, so that each person may maximize his chances for a productive, effective life.

We note especially that any serious national effort at prevention of mental disorders and promotion of mental health must also be addressed to those social-environmental stressors that significantly contribute to the pathology of prejudice. Racism is a particularly noxious influence. Likewise, bias against ethnic minorities, sexism, and ageism must be recognized as placing significant portions of the population at high risk of mental disorder merely by membership in these groups and from the environmental stress that such membership attracts. While outside the direct purview, or immediate special competence, of mental health specialists, elimination of institutionalized and other forms of racism and other biases must continue to be a priority for primary prevention as well as for other aspects of our national interest.

BARRIERS TO PRIMARY PREVENTION EFFORTS

However sensible or rational primary prevention is, however critical it is as a key future strategy for the mental health fields, it is an approach that must surmount powerful barriers, including the following:

(1) Our society is crisis-oriented; we react to here-and-now

pain, blood, and visible suffering. Because primary prevention is future-oriented, many see it as postponable—or if not that, then certainly as having low priority. Because it is oriented so heavily to strengthening people's resources and coping skills rather than addressing current casualty, it lacks a constituency and political clout.

(2) The history, traditions, and past values of the mental health professions have been built on the strategies of repairing existing dysfunction. People are attracted to mental health with that image in mind; moreover, they are trained and they practice in the same mold. That image of self and way of behaving professionally is reinforced because it serves such human needs as the need for status and economic gain and the (understandable) gratifications involved in the process of being personally helpful to distressed others. The question is whether it serves society equally well.

(3) Primary prevention in mental health is threatening to some because its very nature may raise sensitive issues of social and environmental change and/or issues about people's right to be left alone.

(4) Existing mechanisms to support certain mental health activities (e.g. funds for third-party reimbursement, treatment staff, hospital beds) are not geared to primary prevention activities. Accordingly, primary prevention proposals are viewed by some not only as threatening to rooted ways and vested interests but also as competing for resource dollars.

(5) The past lack of recognition of primary prevention as an accepted way in mental health that differs qualitatively from past approaches leaves a series of *Catch-22* residues:

   (a) Fiscal allocations for primary prevention dollars rarely exist, or are at best pitifully small.

   (b) We lack appropriate administrative structures charged with the responsibility of promoting the development of primary prevention.

   (c) Personnel trained in the ways of primary prevention are in extremely short supply. Moreover, they tend to be the last hired and the first fired.

(d) Few professionals are assigned to primary mental health activities on a sustained, full-time basis.

(e) Activities that are labeled primary prevention often, in fact, are not that at all.

(f) There has been virtually no support for research in primary prevention; yet, ironically, critics argue that the field lacks sufficient evidence to warrant programmatic action. One indication of the difference in attitudes toward treatment and prevention is that treatment efforts are mandated even without adequate effectiveness data, whereas prevention efforts are discouraged because of "lack of evidence." With respect to treatment of already identified cases, the social mandate is to "try to be helpful." No such mandate has existed for prevention efforts.

Problems such as the above cannot be engaged, much less resolved, until primary prevention is accorded a place of visibility and importance, backed by leadership with the mechanisms and resources needed to achieve true viability, rather than tokenism.

PRIORITIES

Our Task Panel was asked to order our priorities among a range of prevention interventions and among the variety of target groups for whom primary prevention efforts are possible. It is not easy to set such priorities; indeed, decisions about them could well vary as a function of the weights given to social value judgments versus scientific criteria.

We can try to illustrate the kinds of choices we considered in setting priorities among the large variety of primary prevention programs the Task Panel reviewed. We found ourselves considering:

(1) Programs with high potential for success that affect relatively few people, e.g.

(a) Genetic counseling of persons with a family history of Huntington's Disease, PKU, or Down's Syndrome;

(b) Intensive intervention with blind infants (based on the fact that such children are known to be at high risk for psychosis).

(2) Programs with significant research effectiveness demonstrated on small samples but with good prospects for reaching large numbers, e.g.

(a) Competency training in pre-school settings and early school grades;

(b) Widow-to-widow self-help counseling groups.

(3) Programs with strong *theoretical* promise for success affecting potentially large numbers of people, e.g.

(a) Helping groups for people who experience sudden or extreme stresses such as infant death, job loss, or marital disruption.

(4) Programs aimed at improving broad social situations with potentially great impact on millions of people. Because such conditions are not usually considered part of mental health's purview, considering them might give the Commission the set that the Task Panel has too wide a range of things, i.e. *everything* is primary prevention! Candidly, too, such considerations may involve sufficiently controversial social values that it would be politically wiser to avoid them. Examples include the potentially damaging mental health consequences of:

(a) Unemployment, discrimination, and lack of job security;

(b) Boring and/or dangerous work;

(c) The national epidemic of teen-age pregnancies, unwanted births, premature parenthood;

(d) Smoking and the use of drugs, including alcohol; their effects on unborn children;

(e) Ethnocentrism—racism, sexism, ageism; the damage wrought, the self-fulfilling prophecy, the damaged self-esteem of the persecutor and the persecuted.

Priority-setting may be premature. One rational, possible approach would be to base priorities on three sources of judgment:

(1)   Epidemiological information on prevalence of distress;

(2)   Value judgments solicited from affected groups, e.g. minorities, the aged, the impoverished—all at high risk; and

(3)   Research and demonstrations of effectiveness.

STRATEGIES RESTING ON A RESEARCH BASE

Members of the Task Panel, pulled between the choice of an overinclusive need to cite every relevant study done on primary prevention and the clear realization that brevity and readability were essential, opted for the latter. Somewhat self-consciously, we regarded ourselves as being among the nation's experts on primary prevention. We thus hoped that we might have enough credibility with the members of the Commission to be able to say firmly that the existing evidence indeed supports a major shift in emphasis toward primary prevention. For Commission members who already have the vision that mental health's major new thrusts must be toward the prevention of distress and the building of competence in the citizenry, we need cite only enough data to be reassuring that a broad capability for such an effort truly exists.

At the risk of sounding apocalyptic, the Task Panel believes that a firm, enthusiastic recommendation by the President's Commission for a genuinely accelerated national effort in primary prevention would be a major step forward for humankind. Symbolically, this would mark acceptance of our role as our brothers' and sisters' keepers. It would say that relevant mental health activities must go beyond the here-and-now and would thus move to center-stage a long-term view of benefiting all humankind.

Primary prevention's defining characteristics and mandates necessarily structure its main strategies. With proaction, health and competence-building, and a population orientation among its core qualities, it follows virtually automatically that primary prevention programs must be heavily oriented to the very young. Although the Panel's discussions of programs and strategies have ranged across all developmental stages, we agreed that major primary prevention efforts must be focused on the prenatal, perinatal, infancy, and childhood periods.

The National Association for Mental Health has developed a detailed program of primary prevention that guides efforts from conception through the first months of life. In our recommendations we list a number of other efforts that can be applied at prenatal, perinatal, and subsequent childhood levels. Again, we reemphasize our agreement about the importance of an approach that follows the developmental sequence. In this section, however, we will illustrate the research base with just a few brief programmatic examples.

Let us give a detailed example that involves efforts with children beginning with the pre-school years. Such an approach, consistent with the spirit of primary prevention, has yet to be harnessed systematically by the mental health fields. At the same time, a rapidly growing body of evidence demands that it be taken into serious account.

It has been known for some years that performance on an interrelated group of skills known collectively as interpersonal cognitive problem solving skills (ICPS) consistently discriminates between maladapted clinical or patient groups of children (and adults) and healthy normals (e.g. Spivack and Levine, 1963; Platt, Altmann, and Altmann, 1973; Spivack, Platt, and Shure, 1976; Spivack and Shure, 1977). Such ICPS skills as the ability to "sense" problems, to identify feelings, to use alternative-solution thinking, means-end thinking, and consequential thinking apparently provide a useful cognitive and emotional technology for engaging interpersonal problems effectively. Those who have and use those skills effectively appear to others in interpersonal relations as well adjusted behaviorally. Those who lack or are deficient in such skills are seen as maladjusted—sometimes even with clinically-significant conditions such as neuroses, psychoses, problems of delinquency, antisocial behavior, or addiction. ICPS skills can thus be thought of as mediating effective behavioral adjustment. If that is so, the challenge it presents for primary prevention is to find ways to equip children, as early and effectively as possible, with those skills. The model of ICPS skill-training well illustrates primary prevention's defining attributes: it is health-building, proactive, mass-oriented, and educational. The main theoretical constraint on the ICPS approach is the human organism's limit to

profit developmentally from such training. Once that developmental point is reached, only the formats and mechanisms of ICPS
training, not its goals, need change for different groups who can be
exposed to the approach.

Several research teams have implemented ICPS training programs directed to different target groups that are quite diverse
in terms of age, prior history, and sociocultural and ethnic
background. Their findings have been instructive—indeed, exciting.

Spivack and Shure (1974) developed one such program con-
sisting of 46 "lessons," given over a ten-week period, for four-year-
old Head-Start children. Not only did children in the program
acquire the key ICPS skills, but as that happened their behavioral
adjustment was also found to improve. Particularly interesting
was the fact that the initially most maladapted youngsters both
(1) advanced the most in ICPS skill-acquisition and (2) improved
the most behaviorally. Spivack and Shure also demonstrated direct
linkages between the amount of gain in ICPS skills—particularly
in the ability to generate alternative solutions—and improvement
in subsequent adjustment. Follow-up of program youngsters a year
later, when they had gone on to new class-settings, showed that
program improvements were maintained over time (Shure and
Spivack, 1975a). In a closely related project (Shure and Spivack,
1975b), it was shown that inner-city mothers given special training
in the ICPS method were successful in training their own children
in those skills—again with positive radiation to the adjustment
sphere. Thus, a potentially powerful primary prevention tool was
shown to have coequal applicat lity in the two settings that most
significantly shape a child's early development: home and school.

Several other groups, working within the same general framework, have provided further demonstrations of the applicability
and fruitfulness of the ICPS training model as a strategy for primary prevention (Stone, Hinds, and Schmidt, 1975; Allen et al.,
1976; Gesten et al., 1977; Elardo and Caldwell, 1976; Elardo and
Cooper, 1977). It is beyond the scope of this brief summary to
review that body of work in detail. Indeed the main reason for
providing the citations is to establish that the efficacy of the
approach is not confined to the inputs and wisdom of a single
team, working with a particular target group, in a special setting;
rather, because the approach has been shown to have generality

across diverse settings and age, sex, and ethnic and socioeconomic levels, it stands as an example of a promising generalized strategy for primary prevention.

Findings based on the ICPS approach are in the same research tradition as an earlier set of demonstrations growing out of Ralph Ojemann's pioneering programs (1961, 1969) to train children to think causally. Other workers (Bruce, 1968; Muuss, 1960; Griggs and Bonney, 1970) have shown that successful mastery of causal thinking skills is accompanied by significant gain on measures of (decreased) anxiety, (increased) security and self-concept, and improved overall adjustment status in children.

This broad competence training strategy is limited primarily by its newness and by the minimal investment that has gone into it so far. Thus, the broad range of its potential has scarcely been explored. By broad range is meant the fact that many other competencies besides those that make up the ICPS group may be clearly shown to contribute significantly to behavior adjustment. Examples might include such qualities as healthy curiosity behavior, altruism, role-taking, and the ability to set realistic goals. A promising recent study by Stamps (1975) provides evidence in support of the basic argument. Working with fourth-grade inner-city children, Stamps developed a curriculum, based on self-reinforcement techniques, designed to teach realistic goal-setting skills. Program children learned those skills readily. As their goal setting skills developed, they showed parallel improvements in achievement, in behavioral adjustment, and on personality measures. At the end of training, teachers judged them to have fewer behavior problems than demographically comparable nonprogram controls. Moreover, they showed improvement on measures of openness, awareness, and self-acceptance.

The importance of early competence acquisition can be illustrated at a somewhat different level, i.e. in relationship to a rapidly developing body of knowledge about the efficacy of enrichment stimulation programs for young disadvantaged children (Gottfried, 1973; Horowitz and Paden, 1973; Jason, 1975). Among the most impressive program efforts in the area is that of Heber (1976) and his associates, in Milwaukee—a ten-year longitudinal program with dramatic and exciting findings. Heber's program, directed to the high risk children of mothers with IQs of 75 or less, started immediately after the child was born. An intensive, saturated program emphasizing continual skill training was conducted at a day care center where the children spent all day every day for the first five years of life. Each family was also assigned a home teacher who taught mothers child-rearing and other life skills. Careful comparisons of the program children to matched nonprogram controls, over a ten-year period, have uncovered some remarkable findings. For example, this initially high-risk program sample has not only far outpaced controls, cognitively and linguistically (e.g. at age 7 they had a mean IQ of 121, versus 87 for controls), but they have also run well ahead of expectancies for a normal population of age-peers at large. The key message from this impressive demonstration is that systematic early competence acquisition seems to pave the way for effective later adaptations in key life spheres.

The main sense of the program development and research efforts we are describing here is as follows: We now know that several pivotal competencies, on the surface quite far removed from mental health's classic terrain, can be taught effectively to young children and that their acquisition radiates positively to adaptations and behaviors that are, indeed, of prime concern to mental health. Symptoms and problem behaviors are reduced after acquisition of these skills. Health has been proactively engineered, so to speak, through skill acquisition. This is a message we cannot afford to repress; it is both a paradigmatic example and further mandate for intensified primary prevention efforts.

However promising the competence training approach to date has been, it should be seen as just one model—not as a bible. We urgently need a fuller and clearer understanding of the nature of core competencies in children—how they relate to each other and, even more important, how they may radiate to interpersonal adjustment. We need to understand what changes take place with development in the nature of essential competencies. As competencies that radiate to adjustment are identified, curricula and methods for helping young children acquire them must be developed. The effectiveness of those curricula, as well as their actual behavioral and adjustive consequences, must be carefully evaluated. That is a complex and time-consuming challenge, one that must be met by a concerted effort and not by small, isolated programs or small research grants. The costs will be substantial, but so is the potential reward: a healthier, happier, more effective, better adjusted next generation, on the positive side, and a decrease in the flow of those types of emotional dysfunctions and behavioral aberrations that are at once socially draining, degrading, costly, and destructive of human beings.

Competence training, though unquestionably a powerful tool for primary prevention, is not the only one. A second strategy, also with high potential, is the analysis and modification of social systems. It can be applied at multiple levels, from broad to narrow. It rests on the view that people's (especially children's) development, adaptation, and effectiveness are significantly shaped by the qualities of a relatively few high-impact environments in which they live (e.g. families and schools and communities). Environments can be many things. One thing they cannot be is neutral. Whether planned or by default, they are factors that either facilitate or impede the growth and adaptation of their inhabitants. The following section illustrates research-based efforts to change environments, including social environments, constructively. The first and most impactful social system is the infant-caregiver relationship.

Broussard (1976) has demonstrated, under careful research conditions, negative later outcomes in first-born children whose mothers perceived them negatively shortly after birth and a month later. In those cases in which the mother reported negative attitudes toward the infant at birth and also a month later, follow-up studies through age 11 have shown a high risk of emotional disturbance in these children. Broussard is now engaged in an intervention study with a sample of these high risk infants and mothers using family interviews, home visits, and mother-infant groups up to two years following birth. Preliminary results show significantly better developmental scores for the Intervention children than for Intervention-refused and comparison groups. This set of studies again is illustrative. Viewed together with the Klaus and Kennell studies (1976) showing the critical importance of early bonding experiences between mother (and/or other caregiver) and infant, certain implications for preventive intervention emerge. Conditions designed to maximize optimal positive social perception of the infant are important to the development of a sense of self-esteem and self-worth.

The demonstration of relationships between characteristics of environments and the emotional well-being of people is not at all limited to the infancy period. Indeed, there are examples of such work involving children of all ages during the school years. Illustratively, Stallings (1975) developed a comprehensive framework for assessing class environments for young school children in Project Follow Through. She reported clear relationships between environmental properties and positive outcomes, academic as well as interpersonal (e.g. cooperativeness, curiosity, persistence). Moos and his colleagues at Stanford (Moos, 1973, 1974a, 1974b; Moos and Trickett, 1974; Insel and Moos, 1974) have pioneered the development of measures of a variety of social environments (e.g. hospital wards, schools, military companies, and work units) and have shown consistent relationships between environmental properties and how people feel and behave in those environments. Environments that score high in such relational qualities as involvement and mutual support, compared to their opposites, appear to have occupants who are less irritable and depressed, more satisfied and comfortable, and have higher self-esteem. Specifically, for high schools, Trickett and Moos (1974) demonstrated that students from classes with high perceived student involvement and close student-teacher relationships reported greater satisfaction and more positive mood states than their opposites.

Although qualities of social environments clearly affect what happens to their occupants, it oversimplifies things to assume that those effects are constant for all people. Several observers have stressed the importance of "ecological-matches," i.e. environments that are facilitative for one person can strangle another (Hunt, 1971)—a point that has been documented empirically in several studies (e.g. Grimes and Allinsmith, 1961; Reiss and Dyhdalo, 1975). Especially relevant is the extensive work reported by Kelly and his colleagues (Kelly, 1968, 1969; Kelly et al., 1971, 1977). who have examined, longitudinally, the nature of adaptive behavior in fluid (high annual pupil-turnover) and stable (low annual pupil-turnover) high school environments. Their main finding was that what is adaptive in one environment was not in the other. For example, new students integrated much more readily in fluid environments, where personal development was highly valued. By contrast, status and achievement were more important in stable environments. Insel and Moos (1974) bring the ecological-match question an important step closer to mental health's prime terrain with the following observation: "A source of distress and ill health is in the situation in which a person attempts to function within an environment with which he is basically incompatible."

The purpose of the preceding brief summary is simply to establish that there is already a body of data showing that social climate variation relates to person outcomes on variables of central interest to mental health; moreover, such outcomes may differ for different people. Although we still lack a full understanding of those complex relationships, enough is in place to pinpoint future challenges for primary prevention: What *are* the high-impact dimensions of the important social environments that shape children? How are they best *assessed*? What are the *relationships* between environmental properties and person outcomes, i.e. which qualities facilitate or impede development, and for whom? Ultimately, the goal for primary prevention is to help engineer social environments that optimize development for all people.

Research and demonstration strategies based on impactful social systems must rest on prior or concurrent efforts to provide a sound foundation of good health care and nutrition. Good health care before and at the time of birth has preventive impact. At the time of childbirth, many preventable traumata occur, both physiological and psychological, that can affect the later mental health of the child. Prolonged and difficult births often involve anoxia (lack of oxygen) for the infant. Because low birth weight is known to increase the risk of later difficulties, hospital nurseries must be available for premature infants to prevent damage. Psychologically, support from family members and others is important for the woman at the time of childbirth.

Promoting the health of the expectant mother and child during and after pregnancy, together with sound health care to avoid the complications of pregnancy, including prematurity, can materially reduce the incidence of future mental problems.

Clinical observation of many disturbed people documents the important role played by identifiable environmental social system stresses in precipitating emotional breakdown. Situations involving unusual and intense distress often serve as a kind of "natural experiment" establishing this relationship. Thus, children of parents involved in disrupted marriages, and children moved from foster home to foster home, show a high frequency of emotional disturbance. Adults who lose a job, or who experience the loss of a spouse or child, often show psychological, physiological, and psychosomatic disturbances. (See Holmes and Rahe, 1967; Dohrenwend and Dohrenwend, 1974.)

Although individuals differ in their resistance to environmental pressure, the reduction of environmental stress clearly reduces emotional disturbance. A considerable amount of recent research has related life stresses to subsequent emotional disturbances. The death of a spouse, the loss of a job, going on vacation, marriage, the birth of a child—all are environmental events that may lead to both physical and psychological disturbance.

The individual's social support system is a key factor in determining his or her response to a stressful environmental event. (Caplan and Killilea, 1976; Collins and Pancoast, 1976; Gottlieb, 1976.) We can point to members of identifiable groups and predict a higher than random chance of their later serious emotional disturbance. Children of adults labeled schizophrenic or alcoholic are more likely to be identified later as emotionally disturbed. Primary grade children who are seen by teachers or peers as having adjustment difficulties have been shown to have higher rates of later emotional problems (Cowen et al., 1974, 1975; Robins, 1966; Werner and Smith, 1977).

Research on *stress reduction* is voluminous. Interventions can range from effective sex education for school-age children to anticipatory guidance or emotional inoculation to modeling and/or abreactive approaches before predictable stresses such as elective surgery, all the way through the life cycle to widow-to-widow self-help groups during and following bereavement (Silverman, 1976, 1977). Relationships between stress and emotional disturbance are often much less visible or direct than those between environmental toxins and physical illness. But there are exceptions to this rule, one of which is documented more fully in the paragraphs to follow.

Of all social variables that have been studied in relation to the distribution of psychopathology in the population, none has been more consistently and powerfully associated with this distribution than marital status (Bloom, 1977). Persons who are divorced or separated have repeatedly been found to be overrepresented among the emotionally disturbed, while persons who are married and living with their spouses have been found to be underrepresented. In a recent review of 11 studies of marital status and the incidence of mental disorder reported during the past 35 years, Crago (1972) found that, without a single exception, admission rates into psychiatric facilities were lowest among the married, intermediate among the widowed and never-married adults, and highest among the divorced and separated. This differential appears to be stable across different age groups (Adler, 1953), reasonably stable for each sex separately considered (Thomas and Locke, 1963; Malzberg, 1964), and as true for blacks as for whites (Malzberg, 1956). Supportive evidence of these differentials was provided by Bachrach (1975), who noted that "utilization studies [of mental health services] have generally shown that married people have substantially lower utilization rates than nonmarried people and that the highest utilization rates occur among persons whose marriages have been disrupted by separation or divorce."

Not only are highest admission rates to mental hospitals reported for persons with disrupted marriages, but the differential between those rates and similarly calculated rates among the married is substantial. The ratio of admission rates for divorced and separated persons to those for married persons is on the order of 18:1 for males and about 7:1 for females for public inpatient facilities. In the case of admissions into public outpatient clinics, admission rates are again substantially higher for separated or divorced persons than for married persons. Ratios of these admission rates are nearly 7:1 for males and 5:1 for females (Bloom, 1977).

Although data documenting the adverse mental health correlates of marital disruption are especially extensive and compelling, that is by no means the only area in which linkages between life-stress and emotional upheaval have been shown. Other prominent examples include bereavement, natural disaster, loss of a child, e.g. as in the Sudden Infant Death Syndrome (Goldston, 1977), and job loss. It has been said, with good reason, that life stresses and crises involve both danger and opportunity. Such crises are frequent. They menace—often disrupt—the victim's well-being. They have potentially long-term debilitating effects. The challenge for primary prevention is to develop new program models for at-risk victims of life stresses—programs that minimize the dangers of stress situations and maximize the opportunities they offer for learning effective new ways of coping.

The Task Panel reviewed a very large number of studies of social systems and life events that produce high degrees of stress in large numbers of people. It is important, as noted above, to point out that social stress (from child abuse and marital disruption to racism, discrimination, and unemployment) increases the probability of physical and mental breakdown or disturbance. At the same time, because there are no clear-cut cause-specific connections between single identifiable stresses and a subsequent disturbance, the primary prevention strategist cannot always "produce the convincing evidence" of direct linkages of cause and effect so often demanded by research funding agencies.

It should perhaps be stated explicitly that the Panel's proposals for program development and research in primary prevention involve what philosophers of science call a major new "paradigm shift" (Kuhn, 1970; Rappaport, 1977). The area of social stress illustrates the point. The history of efforts to prevent organic disease shows that one particular research paradigm has been remarkably successful in giving us a sound research base for developing preventive methods. That traditional paradigm may be outlined as follows: (1) define a disease or condition that is judged to be in need of prevention and then develop procedures for reliably identifying persons with the condition; (2) study its distribution in terms of time, place, or person characteristics in the population in order to identify factors that appear to be causally related to it; (3) mount and evaluate experimental prevention programs to test the validity of the hypotheses generated by the previous observations.

That paradigm has been enormously successful; it was used, for example, to develop highly effective preventive programs for smallpox and cholera in the nineteenth century and for rubella and polio in the twentieth century. In the case of the emotional disorders, general paresis is now preventable, as is psychosis following pellagra—both as a result of this approach.

But there are good reasons to believe that new paradigms are now needed. One such reason is that many emotional disorders do not seem to have specific biological causal basis; indeed, most result from a multiplicity of interacting factors. Hence, a paradigm that represents a major departure from the earlier model outlined above is now having a much greater impact on our knowledge base. Its steps may be summarized as follows: (1) identify stressful life events or experiences that have undesirable consequences in a significant proportion of the population and develop procedures for reliably identifying persons who have undergone or who are undergoing such events or experiences; (2) study the consequences of those events in a population by contrasting subsequent illness experiences or emotional problems with those of a suitably selected comparison population; (3) mount and evaluate experimental prevention programs aimed at reducing the incidence of such stressful life events and/or at increasing coping skills in managing those events.

This new paradigm assumes that just as a single disorder may come about as a consequence of a variety of stressful life events, any specific stress event may precipitate a variety of disorders, as a result of differing life histories and patterns of strengths and weaknesses in individuals. For example, an unanticipated death or divorce, or a job loss, may increase the risk of alcoholism in one person, coronary artery disease in another, depression and suicide in a third, and a fatal automobile accident in a fourth. That is, this new paradigm begins by recognizing the futility of searching for a unique cause for every disorder. It accepts the likelihood that many disorders can come about as a consequence of any of a variety of causes. With this acceptance comes the realization that successful efforts at the prevention of a vast array of disorders (particularly emotional disorders) can take place without a theory of disorder-specific causative mechanisms.

This section has presented a brief distillation of some of the current knowledge base in three main areas of primary prevention in mental health: (a) competency training emphasizing developmental approaches, (b) the impact of social systems on individual development, and (c) the reduction and management of naturally occuring life development stresses. All three areas already have substantial, promising knowledge bases that not only justify accelerated primary prevention efforts for the future, but point specifically to areas in which such efforts may be most useful at once.

REFERENCES

Adler, L. M. The relationship of marital status to incidence of and recovery from mental illness. *Social Forces*, 1954, *32*, 185–194.

Albee, George W., and Joffe, Justin M. (Eds.). *Primary prevention of psychopathology. Vol. 1: The Issues.* Hanover, N.H.: The University Press of New England, 1977.

Allen, G. J., Chinsky, J. M., Larcen, S. W., Lochman, J. E., and Selinger, H. V. *Community psychology and the schools: A behaviorally oriented multilevel preventive approach.* Hillsdale, N.J.: Lawrence Erlbaum Associates, 1976.

Bachrach, L. L. *Marital status and mental disorder: An analytical review.*

Washington, D.C.: U.S. Government Printing Office, DHEW Pub. No. (ADM) 75-217, 1975.

Bloom, B. L. *Community mental health: A general introduction.* Monterey: Brooks-Cole, 1977.

Broussard, Elsie. Neonatal prediction and outcome at 10/11 years. *Child Psychiatry and Human Development,* 1976, *7.* Winter

Brown, Bertram S. Remarks to the World Federation for Mental Health, Vancouver, British Columbia, August 24, 1977.

Bruce, P. Relationship of self-acceptance to other variables with sixth-grade children oriented in self-understanding. *Journal of Educational Psychology,* 1958, *49,* 229-238.

Caplan, G., and Killilea, M. (Eds.). *Support systems and mutual help: Multidisciplinary explorations.* New York: Grune and Stratton, 1976.

Carter, Jimmy. Hospital cost containment. *National Journal,* 1977, *9,* 964-965.

Carter, Rosalynn. Remarks to the World Federation for Mental Health, Vancouver, British Columbia, August 25, 1977, p. 1.

Collins, A. H. and Pancoast, D. L. *Natural helping networks: A strategy for prevention.* Washington, D.C.: National Association of Social Workers, 1976.

Cowen, E. L., Pedersen, A., Babigian, H., Izzo, L. D., and Trost, M. A. Long-term follow-up of early detected vulnerable children. *Journal of Consulting and Clinical Psychology,* 1973, *41,* 438-446.

Cowen, E. Baby-steps toward primary prevention. *American Journal of Community Psychology,* 1977, *5,* 1-22.

Cowen, E. L., Trost, M. A., Lorion, R. P., Dorr, D., Izzo, L. D., and Isaacson, R. V. *New ways in school mental health: Early detection and prevention of school maladaptation.* New York: Human Sciences Press, Inc., 1975.

Crago, M. A. Psychopathology in married couples. *Psychological Bulletin,* 1972, *77,* 114-128.

Dohrenwend, B. S. and Dohrenwend, B. P. (Eds.). *Stressful life events.* New York: John Wiley and Sons, 1974.

Elardo, P. T., and Caldwell, B. M. The effects of an experimental social development program on children in the middle childhood period. Unpublished.

Elardo, P. T. and Cooper, M. *AWARE: Activities for social development.* Reading, Mass.: Addison-Wesley, 1977.

Gesten, E. L., Flores de Apodaca, R., Rains, M. H., Weissberg, R. P., and Cowen, E. L. Promoting peer related social competence in young children. In M. W. Kent and J. E. Rolf (Eds.), *Primary prevention of psychopathology. Vol. 3: Promoting social competence and coping in children.* Hanover, N.H.: University Press of New England, 1978.

Goldston, S. E. An overview of primary prevention programming. In D. C. Klein and S. E. Goldston (Eds.), *Primary prevention: An idea whose time has come.* Washington, D.C.: U.S. Government Printing Office, DHEW Pub. No. (ADM) 77-447, 1977, pp. 23-40.

Gottfried, N. W. Effects of early intervention programs. In K. S. Miller and

R. M. Dreger (Eds.), *Comparative studies of Blacks and Whites in the United States: Quantitative studies in social relations.* New York: Seminar Press, 1973.

Gottlieb, B. H. Lay influences on the utilization and provision of health services: A review. *Canadian Psychological Review,* 1976, *17,* 126–136.

Griggs, J. W., and Bonney, M. E. Relationship between "causal" orientation and acceptance of others, "self-ideal self" congruence, and mental health changes for fourth- and fifth-grade children. *Journal of Educational Research,* 1970, *63,* 471–477.

Grimes, J. W. and Allinsmith, W. Compulsivity, anxiety, and school achievement. *Merrill-Palmer Quarterly,* 1961, *7,* 247–261.

Heber, R. Research in prevention of socio-cultural mental retardation. Address presented at the 2nd Vermont Conference on the Primary Prevention of Psychopathology. Burlington, Vt., 1976.

Holmes, T. H., and Rahe, R. H. The social readjustment rating scale. *Journal of Psychosomatic Research,* 1967, *11,* 213–218.

Horowitz, F. D., and Paden, L. Y. The effectiveness of environmental intervention programs. In B. M. Caldwell and H. Ricciuti (Eds.), *Review of child development research.* Vol. 3. New York: Russell Sage Foundation, 1973.

Insel, P. M., and Moos, R. H. The social environment. In P. M. Insel and R. H. Moos (Eds.), *Health and social environment.* Lexington, Mass.: Lexington Books, 1974.

Jason, L. Early secondary prevention with disadvantaged preschool children. *American Journal of Community Psychology,* 1975, *3,* 33–46.

Joint Commission on Mental Illness and Health. *Action for Mental Health.* New York: Basic Books, 1961.

Kelly, J. G. Towards an ecological conception of preventive interventions. In J. W. Carter (Ed.), *Research contributions from psychology to community mental health.* New York: Behavioral Publications, 1968.

Kelly, J. G. Naturalistic observations in contrasting social environments. In E. P. Willems and H. L. Raush (Eds.), *Naturalistic viewpoints in psychological research.* New York: Holt, Rinehart, and Winston, 1969.

Kelly, J. G., et al. The coping process in varied high school environments. In M. J. Feldman (Ed.), *Studies in psychotherapy and behavior change.* No. 2: *Theory and research in community mental health.* Buffalo: State University of New York, 1971.

Kelly, J. G., et al. *The high school: Students and social contexts in two midwestern communities.* Community Psychology Series, No. 4. New York: Behavioral Publications, Inc., 1977.

Kessler, M., and Albee, G. W. Primary prevention. *Annual Review of Psychology,* 1975, *26,* 557–591.

Klaus, M. H., and Kennell, J. H. Maternal-infant bonding. St. Louis: C. V. Mosby Co., 1976.

Klein, D. C., and Goldston, S. E. *Primary prevention: An idea whose time has come.* Washington, D.C.: U.S. Government Printing Office, DHEW Pub. No. (ADM) 77-447, 1977.

Kuhn, T. S. *The structure of scientific revolutions.* 2nd ed. Chicago: University of Chicago Press, 1970.

Malzberg, B. Marital status and mental disease among Negroes in New York State. *Journal of Nervous and Mental Disease,* 1956, *123,* 457-465.

Malzberg, B. Marital status and incidence of mental disease. *International Journal of Social Psychiatry,* 1964, *10,* 19-26.

Mead, Margaret. Conversation with Mrs. Rosalynn Carter, The White House, June 28, 1977, as reported by Mrs. Carter, remarks to the World Federation for Mental Health, Vancouver, British Columbia (August 25, 1977), p. 1.

Moore, Barrington, Jr. *Reflection on the causes of human misery and upon certain proposals to eliminate them.* Boston: Beacon Press, 1970.

Moos, R. H. Conceptualizations of human environments. *American Psychologist,* 1973, *28,* 652-665.

Moos, R. H. *The social climate scales: An overview.* Palo Alto: Consulting Psychologists Press, Inc., 1974. (a)

Moos, R. H. *Evaluating treatment environments: A social ecological approach.* New York: John Wiley and Sons, 1974. (b)

Moos, R. H., and Trickett, E. J. *Manual: Classroom Environment Scale.* Palo Alto: Consulting Psychologists Press, Inc., 1974.

Muuss, R. E. The effects of a one and two year causal learning program. *Journal of Personality,* 1960, *28,* 479-491.

National Association for Mental Health. Primary prevention of mental disorders with emphasis on prenatal and perinatal periods. Action Guidelines. Mimeographed, undated.

Ojemann, R. H. Investigations on the effects of teacher understanding and appreciation of behavior dynamics. In G. Caplan (Ed.), *Prevention of mental disorders in children.* New York: Basic Books, 1961.

Ojemann, R. H. Incorporating psychological concepts in the school curriculum. In H. P. Clarizio (Ed.), *Mental health and the educative process.* Chicago: Rand-McNally, 1969.

Pauling, Linus. Orthomolecular psychiatry. *Science,* 1968, *160,* 265-271.

Platt, J. J., Altman, N., and Altman, D. Dimensions of real-life problem-solving thinking in adolescent psychiatric patients. Paper presented at Eastern Psychological Association Meetings, Washington, D.C., 1973.

Rappaport, J. *Community psychology: Values, research and action.* New York: Holt, Rinehart, and Winston, 1977.

Reiss, S., and Dyhdalo, N. Persistence, achievement and open-space environments. *Journal of Educational Psychology,* 1975, *67,* 506-513.

Richmond, Julius. Remarks made at his swearing-in ceremony as Assistant Secretary of Health, Department of Health, Education, and Welfare, Washington, D.C., July 13, 1977.

Robins, L. *Deviant children grown up.* Baltimore: Williams and Wilkins Co., 1966.

Shattuck. L., et al. Report of the sanitary commission of Massachusetts. Quoted by Jonathan E. Fielding, in Health promotion: Some notions in search of a constituency. *American Journal of Public Health,* 1977, *67,* 1082.

Shure, M. B., and Spivack, G. *A preventive mental health program for young "inner city" children: The second (kindergarten) year.* Paper presented at the American Psychological Association, Chicago, 1975. (a)

Shure, M. B., and Spivack, G. *Training mothers to help their children solve real-life problems.* Paper presented at the Society for Research in Child Development, Denver, 1975. (b)

Silverman, P. R. The widow as a caregiver in a program of preventive intervention with other widows. In G. Caplan and M. Killilea (Eds.), *Support systems and mutual help: Multidisciplinary explorations.* New York: Grune and Stratton, 1976, pp. 233–244.

Silverman, P. R. Mutual help groups for the widowed. In D. C. Klein and S. E. Goldston (Eds.), *Primary prevention: An idea whose time has come.* Washington, D.C.: U.S. Government Printing Office, DHEW Pub. No. (ADM) 77–447, 1977, pp. 76–79.

Spivack, G., and Levine, M. Self-regulation in acting-out and normal adolescents. Report M–4531, National Institutes of Health, 1963.

Spivack, G., Platt, J. J., and Shure, M. B. *The problem-solving approach to adjustment.* San Francisco: Jossey-Bass, 1976.

Spivack, G., and Shure, M. B. *Social adjustment of young children.* San Francisco: Jossey-Bass, 1974.

Spivack, G., and Shure, M. B. Preventively oriented cognitive education of preschoolers. In D. C. Klein and S. E. Goldston (Eds.), *Primary prevention: An idea whose time has come.* Washington, D.C.: U.S. Government Printing Office, DHEW Pub. No. (ADM) 77–447, 1977.

Stallings, J. Implementation and child effects of teaching practices on follow-through classrooms. *Monographs of the Society for Research on Child Development,* 1975, *40* (Serial No. 163).

Stamps, L. W. *Enhancing success in school for deprived children by teaching realistic goal setting.* Paper presented at Society for Research in Child Development, Denver, 1975.

Stone, G. L., Hinds, W. C., and Schmidt, G. W. Teaching mental health behaviors to elementary school children. *Professional Psychology,* 1975, *6,* 34–40.

Thomas, D. S., and Locke, B. Z. Marital status, education and occupational differentials in mental disease. *Milbank Memorial Fund Quarterly,* 1963, *41,* 145–160.

Trickett, E. J., and Moos, R. H. Personal correlates of contrasting environments: Student satisfaction in high school classrooms. *American Journal of Community Psychology,* 1974, *2,* 1–12.

Werner, E. E., and Smith, R. S. *Kauai's children come of age.* Honolulu: University of Hawaii Press, 1977.

Powerlessness and Psychopathology

Justin M. Joffe and George W. Albee

❖   There is a strong tendency in our society to separate and isolate social problems. We have a social problem labeled violence against children in the family, and others labeled battered wives, sexism, racism, abuse of elderly persons, family disruption, poverty and unemployment, the incarceration and decarceration of persons we call mentally ill, the neglect of the mentally retarded, and the isolation of the physically handicapped, to name just a few.

What do all these problems involving different groups have in common? We have suggested, for your consideration, the best answer we can come up with. It is their powerlessness. People without power are commonly exploited by powerful economic groups who explain the resulting psychopathology by pointing to the defectiveness of the victims. The rest of us do not rush to the defense of the victims because we are caught up in the ideology that puts "justice" in the hands of those with power. We join the groups "blaming the victims."

If the foregoing analysis is accurate, it makes little sense to develop separate programs for the prevention of child abuse, spouse abuse, elder abuse, the exploitation of women, minority group members, migrant farmworkers, the handicapped, the mentally ill, and the mentally retarded. If we see all these groups as powerless because of socioeconomic conditions, then a logical approach is to determine whether there might be an equitable redistribution of power. One of the slogans of the 60s was "Power to the people." Another piece of conventional wisdom is that "Money is power." Without meaning to be simplistic, we would like to suggest that we examine the arguments in the papers for a redistribution of power through a redistribution of wealth in our society.

Two further comments on the relationship between power and psychopathology seem to be needed to round out the picture. The first has to do with objective and subjective realities, the second with the complexity of factors that are associated with psychopathology.

From Justin M. Joffe and George W. Albee, "Powerlessness and Psychopathology," in Justin M. Joffe and George W. Albee (eds.) *Prevention Through Political Action and Social Change.* Copyright © 1981 by the Vermont Conference on the Primary Prevention of Psychopathology. Reprinted by permission.

When confronted with the issue of powerlessness, many psychologists tend to approach it as a question of individual aberration or misperception of reality. The optimism of such a view is commendable, but the resulting attempt to alter people's perceptions of their ability to affect their own lives is often, we think, not only misguided but counterproductive and ultimately damaging. So much of what the authors in this volume tell us documents the fact that many people in our society, in many situations, are powerless. If they believe that they cannot do much to affect their circumstances, alleviate their misery, or build a better world for their children it is not because they perceive contingencies incorrectly, but because their perceptions are accurate. They see themselves as powerless because they have no power. No doubt this perception itself further exacerbates their feelings of hopelessness and further reduces the likelihood of their making the necessary effort on those few occasions in their lives when they might be able to act effectively. If so, something might be said in favor of "therapy" to make them feel less powerless. But therapists are in short supply and rarely available to those who concern us—and anyway they read a different agenda.

In any case, what do we know about the effects of feeling that one is in control of a world where, in fact, one is not? It seems that either our "therapy" has to create a very powerful delusional system so that the powerless never notice that their actions are not efficacious, or we have to run the risk of those who have *feelings* of control being even more frustrated when they encounter reality. We think that the analyses in this volume suggest that to prevent psychopathology we should not alleviate feelings of powerlessness by altering perceptions but by altering reality. We realize that this is not as straightforward as we may be implying. A key question—to which we have not found an easy answer—is how to make those who feel powerless take action to alter the distribution of power. Perhaps an answer is to be found in the process of helping people understand why they feel powerless and helping them to attribute that feeling to the socioeconomic system rather than to personal inadequacy. This obviously harks back to the condemnation of the defect model of psychopathology and to Ryan's idea of blaming the victim. The problem of powerlessness is exacerbated by the victims, in fact, blaming themselves, as they accept society's assessment of their plight. The rationalization at once excuses the rest of us from working for social change (instead we can do individual therapy with chemicals or couches) and keeps the victims from blaming anyone but themselves. The message we see in all this is that our role is to assure those who feel helpless that their feeling is due to their in fact being powerless—perhaps only then will they attack the system that has made them so.

Binstock suggests that we will not have significant social changes until a national political crisis has been precipitated by "coalitions of the severely deprived." He suggests that we "undertake direct militant action in our local communities." The tactics of Saul Alinsky and of Martin Luther King were effective, he notes, in provoking social change. Indeed, during the early history of social work, effective organizing of rent strikes, sit-ins, and welfare demonstrations by coalitions of have-not groups were effective in bringing about political change.

It is often said that power is not given up voluntarily. Indeed, it often appears that those persons who hold power are protected by laws, by elected officials, by the police, by folkways, and, perhaps most important, by the beliefs and attitudes of the powerless! We are all encouraged to accept the superior wisdom of gurus and leaders, probably transferring our childhood reverence for parental authority onto other parentlike figures. Rebellion against authority does not come easily. But when it does come it often comes with a violence and turbulence shocking in its intensity. Once authority is challenged successfully other potential challengers take courage and continue the pressure.

Our second point about power and psychopathology has to do with the complexity of the relationship. Many of the authors have discussed political action and social change as if they took it for granted that these are the keys to reducing psychopathology and increasing human happiness. There seems to be a danger that this emphasis, appropriate enough for a volume on this topic, might imply that we and the other authors are unaware that this volume represents only one level of analysis of a complex and multi-level system. One can analyze psychopathology at various levels and in terms of various influences. Physiological and cognitive processes within the individual, the individual's interactions with a physical and psychosocial environment—including particularly the family, social institutions like schools and the workplace, political and economic systems, cultural traditions—all of these constitute relevant levels of analysis and, what is more, none is independent of the others. Not only does this imply that one can intervene at various levels to help the individual, but also that any particular intervention, if it is effective, is likely to have a great many effects, not all of which can be anticipated and some of which may be judged undesirable.

Why, then, emphasize the broader variables—neighborhoods, group prejudice, schools and prisons, economic forces, and so on—that are the focus of so much of this book? Such an emphasis seems to us to be not only appropriate but essential to primary prevention. From the field of public health we learn that those diseases that ravaged humankind for so much of its history and that have been conquered were not eliminated by interventions at the level of the individual: the greatest successes have involved approaches that reached groups of people, and often these resulted from nonspecific changes, contingent upon or associated with social, political, and economic change—improved hygiene, less crowded living conditions, safer workplaces, better nutrition. Little of this advance was achieved by intervention in individual chemistry or cognitions. Laws that forced the changes that improved sanitation or provided a living wage were the levers that started the process of eliminating disease. By analogy we argue that intervention at the level of the total socioeconomic system will be the most effective approach to preventing psychopathology, though advances can be made—over less ground and with more danger of impermanence—by intervening at other levels.

Aside from seeing more clearly now that inequities in the distribution of power are at the root of the problem, we also see that the task of producing change is even greater than we imagined. Since those who are deprived of power feel powerless, they are unlikely to act; "the system" is working well, and those with power seem unlikely to want to make changes. We ourselves seem to be somewhere in the middle, neither the most powerful nor entirely powerless, able to see the psychopathogenic characteristics of the system but at the same time with a vested interest in a system that creates the victims to whom we minister. Eventually most of us become overwhelmed by the number of victims produced—they pile up faster than we can treat them—and conclude that some form of prevention is the only way of coping with the situation. Both economically and ethically, prevention has the most acceptable ratio of benefits to costs.

When we reach this point we still have various options as to the level of intervention we attempt. A major parameter of these options is the size of the group we attempt to affect: We can intervene with high-risk groups of various kinds (like pregnant teenagers or physically handicapped children), deal with institutions of many types (schools, mental hospitals, prisons), and with discriminated-against groups (the old, ethnic minorities, women), and so on. It seems that as the groups get larger the likelihood increases that political action and social change will be needed to produce real effects. When we eventually accept that such action is needed we sometimes are unnerved by the magnitude of the task: How can we patch up the casualties, improve the neighborhoods, alter the schools, redistribute power? Konopka gave us an answer, both in her example and in words: We are responsible for "helping individuals in the framework of existing conditions as well as . . . helping change social institutions. When we recognize the multiple causation of problems . . . it becomes clear that a profession which works toward social justice in a wide sense has to be responsible for amelioration and social change."

The Causes of the Causes

Justin M. Joffe

❖   In contrast to the situation of the biologically vulnerable child in the deprived environment, Ferreira suggests that the child of normal prenatal development born into the same environment will be better able to elicit a 'healthy transaction", and the impaired child in a favorable environment has a better chance of having parents who can make the necessary effort to respond to the child in a way that compensates for the initial effects of the adverse prenatal and perinatal events.

In brief, Sameroff and Chandler's (1975) transactional model of development itself suggests that adverse conditions and hazardous prenatal and perinatal events might have considerable significance for development even if the direct effects of such conditions and events were transient.

Before turning to a discussion of issues relating to prevention of adverse outcomes it should be noted that the perspective in which prenatal and perinatal factors have been viewed thus far is one of prevention of defects rather than promotion of optimal development. Much concern has focused on avoiding adverse effects, very little on whether prenatal development takes place in an environment that fosters even more favorable outcomes than usual. Should we reach a point where our "control" group is not one defined by the absence of adverse conditions during prenatal life but rather by the presence of favorable conditions—those optimizing neonatal status and functioning—it may emerge that the children who experience hazards have lost more than we thought and that the rebound that sometimes occurs in favorable postnatal environments does not bring the children to the level of functioning that we might assume them to have been capable of reaching. If such is the case we will have to give greater weight to the primary prevention of prenatal hazard than we currently do. As long as we think we can compensate postnatally for the consequences of prenatal disadvantage, there is a danger that we will not give sufficient attention to prenatal development.

Prevention

In this section some of the approaches to intervening to reduce the incidence of deviant outcomes of prenatal origin—death, malformations,

From Justin M. Joffe, "Approaches to Prevention of Adverse Developmental Consequences of Genetic and Prenatal Factors," in Lynne A. Bond and Justin M. Joffe (eds.) *Facilitating Infant and Early Childhood Development*. Copyright © 1982 by the Vermont Conference on the Primary Prevention of Psychopathology. Reprinted by permission.

stunting of growth, functional aberrations—will be considered. Issues of *what* can be done are often inseparable from questions about *how* they should be done and questions of desirability are linked with both of these, but the focus in this section is primarily on characterizing types of interventions that could reduce deviant outcomes and discussing the extent to which they can be regarded as preventive measures. Three general approaches to the task, distinguishable initially largely by the time at which they are implemented, are diagrammed in Figure 1. The first is postnatal intervention which, in principle, could be applied generally or could be restricted to groups considered to be at high risk for deviant development on the basis of measures of neonatal status or on the basis of factors (for example, socioeconomic status) that are associated with an increased probability of the child encountering circumstances that lead to less than optimal development. Depending on the nature of the risk factors the interventions might be intended to do one or both of the following:

• To interrupt the causal chain linking already encountered events to undesirable outcomes or to compensate for their effects; this might be classified as prevention of sequelae or early treatment.

• To obviate the child's encountering events that might not be conducive to optimal development, or to improve the child's ability to cope with such events in a manner that does not deflect such development.

Postnatal approaches are essential for continued optimal development in even the healthiest of neonates, and until such time as we have intervened with complete success prior to birth, postnatal measures to minimize the anticipated deleterious effects of adverse prenatal events—to treat them, to prevent their sequelae—will be essential. Since we may always have a residue of unpreventable neonatal outcomes for which we will need to implement ameliorative postnatal programs, concern for definitional purity (see Kessler and Albee, 1975; Bloom, 1980) may have to take a back seat to practical concerns. Postnatal interventions are the subject of detailed consideration elsewhere in this volume and will not be further discussed here.

In any case, intervention prior to birth is obviously more attuned to the notion that the purpose of primary prevention is to obviate negative events and promote positive ones (Bloom, 1980), *not* "to reduce or contain already manifest deficits" (Task Panel on Prevention, 1978, p. 1833).

Even limiting our concern to interventions prior to birth we are left with at least two general approaches: We can consider ways of minimizing the likelihood of adverse neonatal outcomes in the presence of threatening prenatal events—roughly characterizable as "high-risk ap-

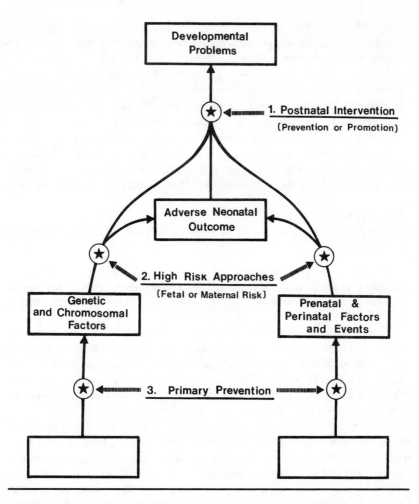

Figure 1. Approaches to prevention of adverse outcomes of prenatal and genetic factors.

proaches"—as well as ways of preventing the occurrence of such events (see Figure 1). In any case, we will see, once again, that distinctions between prevention and treatment are not straightforward. In considering each approach, three questions underlie the discussion. What kinds of techniques are available—that is, what can we do? How effective are these techniques—in particular, to what extent are they *preventive?* And how do we know when, or to whom, to apply them?

High-Risk Approaches

Similar general principles apply to prenatal intervention whether the disorders are of genetic or nongenetic origin and for this reason, and because many prenatal problems are of unknown or multifactorial origin, genetic and environmentally determined disorders will not be considered separately. Despite the risk of oversimplification, a rough distinction between the techniques and the treatments used when the concern is with identifying sick embryos or fetuses as opposed to identifying sick mothers is of some help in organizing a discussion of these approaches. In fact, of course, the two categories overlap and many of the matters discussed in the section on fetal disorders are relevant to prenatal disorders in general.

Fetal disorders.

Ingalls (1953), in discussing what he termed "preventive prenatal pediatrics", wrote:

The nearly insurmountable obstacle to clinical study of prenatal sickness arises in the fact that the patient voices no complaint, remembers nothing about his illness, hides himself from view, and puts off his visit to the doctor until the last possible moment. (p. 34)

This statement illustrates what are still unique difficulties in dealing with problems in perinatal development, although technical progress since the 1950s has made the unborn organism far less inaccessible than it was when Ingalls wrote. The development of procedures of visualizing the fetus using indirect techniques such as sonography and improved radiographic methods or direct ones such as fetoscopy, and the concurrent development of procedures of obtaining samples of fetal tissue and blood or of amniotic fluid (Golbus, 1978; Kushnick, 1979), have made it more difficult for fetuses to hide themselves from view. Advances in our ability to read the messages in amniotic and fetal fluids and cells and in maternal blood and urine have helped provide the fetus with a voice. We have, in fact, entered an era where a variety of fetal disorders, including neural tube defects and biochemical disorders of metabolism, have been, or are capable of being, diagnosed prenatally (Golbus, 1978; Kushnick, 1979; Milunsky and Atkins, 1975).

Aside from the need for technical and scientific advances to make the techniques safer, more accurate, cheaper, and capable of detecting even more disorders, we need to consider two problems of some importance. The first is the question of what is to be done when congenital disorders are detected—and is it prevention?—and the second relates to efficient and effective use of our technology. How do we know when to resort to prenatal diagnosis?

When prenatal diagnosis detects genetic or other prenatal disease, few options are available. The first, intrauterine therapy, is at present available in only a limited number of disorders. Therapy can take the form of preventing toxic changes in maternal physiology (as, for example, in dietary control in maternal phenylketonuria), of intrauterine fetal transfusion (as treatment in cases of rhesus incompatibility), and of prevention of toxic changes in the fetus (as, for example, in the use of intrauterine corticosteroids to treat congenital adrenal hyperplasia) (Hsia, 1975). Compared with postnatal treatment these approaches have the advantage of being applicable early enough to prevent changes that may be irreversible if left until after birth (Hsia, 1975). However, they are clearly no different in principle from postnatal interventions and even though they comprise earlier and potentially more effective treatment, they do not constitute prevention of the conditions themselves.

The second option in the event of prenatal diagnosis of fetal disorder is abortion. Although this is clearly primary prevention of the chronic stress that may be experienced by parents and family of an affected child, when the focus is on the condition itself, whether abortion is regarded as primary prevention or not is a matter of definition. It can reduce the prevalance of a disorder but does not affect incidence, unless one adopts birth as the point at which incidence is determined. Although it obviously prevents the birth of an infant with a given condition, it does not prevent the occurrence of the condition. Furthermore it is possible that detection and abortion of affected fetuses could result in an increase in the number of abnormal genes in the population as a whole since parents may tend to replace affected fetuses with normal infants, about two-thirds of whom will be unaffected carriers of the condition (Harris, 1975). In the case of many congenital disorders abortion is, at present, the only method available to avoid the birth of an affected child. An intriguing alternative approach is contained in the suggestion that we find ways of improving the natural mechanisms that already result in the discarding of a large proportion of damaged embryos (Fraser, 1978; Smithells, 1978), an approach that Warkany (1978) has termed "terathanasia". When prenatal diagnosis *excludes* the possibility that the fetus is defective, its findings could be said to constitute primary prevention since they eliminate a source of parental apprehension and anxiety that might affect development.

A problem that presents other kinds of difficulties for practical application of prenatal diagnosis and from the point of view of obviation or prevention of the conditions rather than their treatment is related to decisions about the circumstances in which prenatal diagnosis should be used. One possibility is to attempt to implement prenatal diagnosis universally. Such an approach would encounter formidable technical, economic, service delivery, psychological, legal, and ethical obstacles (many of which are discussed in the volume on preventing genetic disease and mental retardation edited by Milunsky, 1975a). The more practicable approach is to use prenatal diagnostic techniques only when there are a priori reasons to suspect genetic or congenital abnormalities. At present, indications for undertaking prenatal diagnosis include the following (Kushnick, 1979):

●For chromosomal abnormalities: advanced parental age, chromosomal abnormalities in a parent; previous chromosomally abnormal child or abortus

●For metabolic diseases: known maternal metabolic disorders; both parents known carriers; mother known or suspected carrier of X-linked disorder; previous affected child.

●For neural tube defects: raised maternal alpha-fetoprotein; previous affected child.

●For erythroblastosis: Rh negative mother.

The presence of indicators of these kinds defines a pregnancy in which the risk of a child with significant impairment is substantially greater than it is in the population at large. As indicated, if the aim is primary prevention, prenatal diagnosis, for whatever reason it is carried out, has limitations. Even its effective use as a method of secondary prevention is compromised as long as issues relating to the availability of adequate medical attention and the resources and knowledge to seek it remain unresolved. In addition, there are somewhat different implications for prevention depending on the kind of risk indicator which determines that diagnostic methods are invoked.

Indicators like parental age and manifest metabolic disorder offer the best possibility for prevention since they provide a way of identifying couples at risk before the birth of an affected child. Age of parents and, for some disorders, ethnicity (sickle cell anemia, Tay-Sachs disease, and so forth) can provide indications of risk before the disorders have appeared in the family. Recognized metabolic disorders in a family, although no strictly "pre-proband" indicators, at least are potentially capable of indicating risk before an affected child is born to the couple. By contrast, when risk indicators that depend on the prior birth—or miscarriage—of an affected child are relied upon, "only limited reduction in the overall postnatal incidence of the disease could be expected" (Kaback, 1975, p. 95), since the majority of cases of genetic disease tend to occur in families without a previous history of the disorder.

The final category of risk indicators includes such things as knowledge that the parents are carriers of a genetic disorder or knowledge of correlates of fetal defects, such as raised maternal serum alpha-fetoprotein. Discussion of these indicators can be recursive: unless we rely on post-proband identification of at-risk couples, with its attendant drawbacks, or screen entire populations (and this may be feasible for some disorders: see Scriver and Laberge, 1978), we need to determine on the basis of what indicators (of possible possession of deleterious genes) we will look for indicators (of prenatal disorder).

These questions as to whom to apply techniques are important not only in the context of prenatal diagnosis but also for using pre-proband identification techniques to obviate the *conception* of children with genetic disorders, a topic that will be discussed in the section on primary prevention.

Maternal risk factors.
The rationale of an approach to prevention based on maternal risk factors is that through adequate prenatal care to reduce the occurrance of disorders of pregnancy or labor or through identification and subsequent treatment or management of such disorders, adverse neonatal outcomes can be avoided or the severity of the disorders reduced. There is no shortage of risk factors that can be used to identify high-risk pregnancies: For example, McNeil and Kaij (1977) list 20 criteria used to identify obstetric risk groups in need of specialist care in the Swedish health system; Meier (1975) identifies 26 risk factors spanning maternal variables and complications during pregnancy and delivery; and Chez, Haire, Quilligan, and Wingate (1976), in the course of their comprehensive review of the relationships between prenatal and perinatal factors and adverse neonatal outcome, provide a table that contains a total of 69 pregnancy risk factors (not counting 19 fetal–maternal and neonatal factors).

A list of the categories of variables other than fetal–maternal and neonatal ones that Chez et al. (1976) present illustrates the variety of factors that can be involved in this approach:

●socioeconomic factors (for example, father's occupation, housing conditions, minority status, early prepregnancy malnutrition)
●demographic factors (for example, maternal age, weight, familial genetic disorder, poor obstetric history)
●maternal medical factors (for example, lack of prenatal care, toxemia, hypertensive disorders, mental retardation, emotional disturbance)
●placental and membrane factors (for example, vaginal bleeding, placental insufficiency, abruptio placentae)
●labor and delivery factors (for example, premature labor, prolonged labor, high mid-forceps delivery).

It seems clear that the efficacy of interventions based on the presence of risk factors of these kinds is dependent upon their being obviated entirely or treated as early as possible. This in turn depends upon the availability of prenatal care that people can afford and a recognition by consumers of the need to seek such care as early as possible. In practice it is just those groups that are at highest risk on socioeconomic criteria—the poor, the unmarried, the oppressed minorities—who are least likely to seek early care, as well as those least likely to receive adequate care when they do (Birch and Gussow, 1970). Experience in Sweden indicates that such problems may arise even when services are readily available; according to McNeil and Kaij (1977), "the women who do not take advantage of the [parent education] classes are to a large extent the very ones who need the most help—the young, the poorly informed, and foreigners" (p. 99).

In the event that risk factors are recognized, a variety of medical and "psycho-obstetric" (McNeil and Kaij, 1977) interventions are available to reduce the probability of miscarriage of embryonic or fetal damage. Depending on the nature of the condition, intervention may take the form of evaluating the condition of the embryo or fetus (perhaps followed, if indicated, by treatment or abortion) or implementing one or other form of medical management of the condition. Given the diversity of the risk factors involved, it is difficult to provide an overall characterization of the preventive status of the approach. Much depends on the nature of the risk factors.

When maternal medical or placental or membrane factors are involved, the approach can be said to constitute primary prevention insofar as the conditions can be corrected and the potential threat to the unborn child expeditiously removed; the only qualification would pertain to the question of whether the condition itself could have been prevented through earlier intervention. When the measures are palliative, as with medical or obstetric disorders that can only be ameliorated or their consequences monitored to enable treatment to be instituted expeditiously—perhaps maternal diabetes and placenta praevia constitute examples of such disorders—the approach might be termed partial prevention. When the maternal risk factors result in prenatal examination of the fetus and subsequent fetal therapy or abortion, the approach, as discussed earlier, constitutes early treatment. Similarly, when labor and delivery factors are involved, interventions will often have to be directed at neonatal amelioration of the effects on the infant.

Socioeconomic and demographic risk factors are different from the other factors considered, both in the sense of being antecedents of other risks and in being unamenable to alteration by the types of techniques used to deal with complications of pregnancy and delivery. Demographic variables may predict a greater probability that complications will occur but variables like family income, maternal age or stature, and poor obstetric history are not treatable in the same way as medical disorders. Aspects of this dilemma will be discussed later.

Primary Prevention

In discussing high-risk approaches we mostly considered methods of ameliorating or eliminating the early consequences of genetic and chromosomal factors on the one hand and prenatal and perinatal factors and events on the other. These approaches cannot be considered to be primary prevention insofar as they deal with disorders after their occurrence: in many cases the very presence of high-risk groups constitutes evidence that primary prevention measures have either not been implemented or have failed.

If we are actually to prevent risk—that is, to eliminate the occurrence of conceptuses with chromosomal and genetic disorders, women who are reproductively incompetent, the occurrence of prenatal and perinatal events that harm the unborn child—we need to identify and eradicate the factors that result in their occurrence or to alter those exposed to them in a way that makes them immune to the effects. In brief, we have to identify and control the *causes of the causes,* the events and conditions that fill the empty boxes in Figure 1. Causal chains are long and complex, and it is in the nature of scientific inquiry to be selective about which links to investigate in detail. In addition, causal chains tend to acquire more and more interlinking strands as one moves away from the effect one wishes to understand, making it less likely, and certainly more difficult to demonstrate, that earlier links constitute necessary and sufficient conditions for the occurrence of the "effect". Consequently, once important links are identified, there is a tendency to concentrate study on subsequent links rather than antecedent ones, so that the "causes of the causes" are relatively neglected.

The subsequent discussion attempts to demonstrate the greater effectiveness of directing more effort at dealing with earlier links, first briefly in considering genetic and chromosomal disorders and then at more length in considering environmentally related prenatal and perinatal factors and events.

Genetic and chromosomal disorders.

We know a considerable amount about the antecedents of chromosomal and genetic disorders. Some chromosomal abnormalities (and genetic mutations) are the result of environmental agents, which are considered in the next section. In other cases we can identify causally relevant variables, those that may not constitute immediate antecedents of chromosomal abnormalities, but that are predictive of an increased likelihood of such abnormalities. An obvious example is the relationship between maternal and paternal age and Down's syndrome (Abroms and Bennett, 1979), with considerably increased risk of chromosomal nondisjunction in older parents. Intervening to ensure that people confine child bearing to their lower risk years would presumably constitute a preventive measure although recent decreases in mean age of child-bearing women in England, Canada, the United States, and other industrialized nations (Holmes, 1978) have not, however, been accompanied by a decreased incidence of Down's syndrome, possibly indicating an improvement in ascertainment or a biological change (see Bennett and Abroms, 1979). It is interesting to note that such an approach, despite its apparent simplicity, has many ramifications. At the very least, to be maximally effective, it requires widespread educational measures and the availability (and acceptability) of contraceptive measures; it is little use telling women over 35 not to have babies unless steps have been taken to ensure that they have had the number of children they want before then (and unless they have the means of preventing further conceptions and the willingness to use them). Ensuring that a desired family size is attained during the optimal years for childbearing in turn depends in part on socioeconomic conditions and on social support services since family planning is affected by a couple's ability to afford the loss of income resulting from interruption of work and by the question of whether or not there are affordable and adequate alternatives to one member rearing the child rather than being employed outside the home.

We know enough to prevent a great many genetic disorders too. We can, as yet, do little, even if we wish to, about the ultimate causes of genetic defects, mutation, and natural selection, but we could, in many cases, take steps to deal with the proximate cause of genetically affected embryos, the mating of genetic carriers. People affected with dominant genetic disorders or X-linked ones pose a threat to their offspring regardless of the genotype of their mate, while individuals heterozygous for some autosomal recessive disorder (unaffected carriers) pose a threat only if their mate is also a carrier (Reilly, 1975). Provided such individuals can be identified, intervention to reduce the incidence of genetic disorders is possible, with the potential efficacy of intervention substantially greater in cases in which identification can be made prior to the birth of an affected child (as was discussed earlier). At present, only one preventive method is available in such cases, the prevention of reproduction—either the abortion of the conceptus or the prevention of conception. In principle, such an approach could be extremely effective: "Mass screening for genetic disease, when coupled with appropriate mating prohibitions, could permit the reduction of all identifiable disorders to mutation level in a single generation" (Reilly, 1975, pp. 430–431). Aside from technical and economic considerations (Harris, 1975), mass screening (and effective use of the information obtained) poses a variety of legal questions (Reilly, 1975). In addition, the design and implementation of programs to reduce the frequency of "deleterious" genes—negative eugenics—through voluntary or compulsory restrictions on procreation raise troubling ethical issues, the difficulties of which are exacerbated by geographic, ethnic, and class-related concentrations of certain genes and by lack of knowledge of what constitutes eugenic improvement (Lappé, 1975). Similar issues arise, though less pointedly, in attempts to apply the same preventive method on a smaller scale, through the use of genetic counseling (Milunsky, 1975b). At present, expanded availability of genetic counseling in conjunction with increased public awareness of its role probably represent the least controversial approach to the primary prevention of genetic disorders. In combination with improved techniques of identification and mass screening it has the potential to reduce markedly the incidence of such disorders.

Environmental factors and events.

In abstract terms, the process of prevention can be stated very simply: once the damaging agent is identified, any one of three actions can be taken to prevent its effects—removal of the agent, strengthening the host to increase resistance to the agent, or preventing contact between agent and host (Roberts, 1970). In the case of deleterious prenatal and perinatal environmental factors and events, we have a great deal of knowledge about the agents involved. This knowledge takes two apparently disparate forms: information about factors that cause adverse outcomes (see Table 1) and information about variables correlated with such outcomes. In neither case does the information alone seem to enable us to determine ways of removing agents, strengthening the host, or preventing contact between agent and host. In each case we seem to have to do something further with the information to design prevention programs. The remainder of this paper will briefly examine the form that these attempts take and argue that the "causes" are less relevant to prevention than the correlated variables and that the reluctance to deal directly with these variables is based on misconceptions.

First, then, we examine the prenatal "causes" of adverse development. Table 1 lists categories of causes and we can provide detailed lists of agents in each category, yet these do not, in themselves suggest what can be done. The problem seems to result from the fact that exposure to any of the agents in Table 1 could arise in many different ways, each involving multiple determinants. In practice, what we seem to do to design prevention programs is to look for these determinants—in effect, to identify the causes of the causes. We might, for example, inquire about why a pregnant woman took a prescription drug during pregnancy, and identify among the causes failures in medical education; ignorance of the patient (of the risk or of the fact that she was pregnant); too-ready reliance on chemical solutions to problems of living (in the case of a tranquilizer, say) in both doctor and patient; the overconcern of the pharmaceutical industry with profit; the unavailability, inaccessibility, or unaffordability of alternative means of dealing with problems for which the tranquilizer was resorted to; and so on. The number and scope of "prevention programs" suggested by even a casual analysis of this kind is dizzying and could involve anything from revising the medical school curriculum and increasing the number of public service messages in the media to nationalizing the pharmaceutical industry.

This kind of approach is nothing if not fruitful and does offer potential benefits, but they may be slow in coming and each program may in itself be able to show only negligible results. As Fraser (1978) suggested about the prevention of teratogenic effects, "no one preventive measure will bring about a dramatic drop in frequency. . . . We must keep on chipping away . . . ; each small decrease in the burden will be vitally important to some families, and the cumulative effect will be eventually visible" (p. 398). The practical difficulties of obtaining funding for programs that only chip away are substantial; many otherwise admirable programs will founder on the fiscal rocks given their low expectations of benefits in relation to costs. In attempting to prioritize programs we will be in danger of spending the little that is available for prevention (Albee, 1979) on pilot projects.

Parenthetically, this approach represents something of a methodological paradox. Normally, compounded variables correlated with a particular outcome are subjected to further dissection, by experimental study whenever possible, to identify "causal variables" entangled in the correlations. Yet it seems that to develop effective prevention programs we may have to go from the kinds of physical, chemical, and biological variables we have already identified to the larger network of variables that encompass them.

The second approach, which starts with the larger, correlated variables usually suggests programs that are indistinguishable from those arrived at by the first, but the process differs. In this approach, we start with the demographic variables that correlate with the outcome we wish to prevent, those variables encompassed by answers to questions about who does and does not suffer from a given condition and when and where the condition is or is not found. When we do this, we find that our best predictors are global and complex variables like ethnic group and socioeconomic status. With regard to prenatal factors, for example, the variables in the Collaborative Perinatal Project (Broman et al., 1975) with the highest correlations with IQ at age 4 were socioeconomic index and mother's education (there was also a 13 point IQ difference between black and white children) and in the Kauai study (Werner and Smith, 1977) low level of maternal education and low standard of living were among the key predictors of poor developmental outcomes at 2 years and of learning and behavior problems at 10 and 18.

What do we do with such information? The short answer is, anything but deal with the factors identified. We claim that the only proper use of such data is to look for variables within the demographic correlates that account for the effects and that it is misguided to consider that prevention might best be served by dealing with them directly. They can be unravelled in plausible ways. For example: "The poor woman having a baby may be at risk because of her age, her nutritional status, her probable poor growth, her excessive exposure to infection in the community which she inhabits, her poor housing, and her inadequate medical supervision, as well as because of complex interactions between these and other potentially adverse influences" (Birch and Gussow, 1970, p. 175). Such unravelling is useful in suggesting prevention programs: we can design programs to improve prenatal care in urban ghettos; to provide vitamin supplements for poor women; to reduce drug abuse; and so on. These are very much the kinds of programs suggested by the first approach, in which the reasons people are exposed to the proximate causes of poor developmental outcomes are analyzed.

An interesting question arises, however. Since the broad demographic variables seem to encompass something closer to ultimate causes, and since we seem to be better able to design prevention programs when we deal with causes of causes, why do we choose the middle ground? Why do we ask: What is it about poverty that produces increases in birth defects, prematurity, perinatal death, instead of designing programs to prevent poverty?[1] Why do we ask, what is it about powerlessness that produces breakdown, misery, and violence, instead of trying to redistribute power?

We seem to be given three reasons why we should leave the broader variables alone: They are not the real causes of the problems, we are not

[1] For example: "The important question . . . is: in what way do adverse socio-economic conditions produce the disorders of pregnancy and delivery?" (Joffe, 1969, p. 269). I was writing at the time about methodological issues but cannot now defend the narrowness of focus that makes analysis of the variables entwined in socioeconomic status *the* important question.

competent to deal with them, and it would not solve the problem if we did. The first reason has to do with a particular concept of what constitutes a causal relationship and implies that attempting to deal with global factors is scientifically misguided. For example:

Efforts at prevention will not succeed . . . unless we establish specific interventions that work on the causes of specific kinds of psychopathology. . . . Without an understanding of causes, we are in the position of relying on serendipity—surely a poor substitute for the solid knowledge that research can provide—or relying on vague hopes that broad, often unsubstantiated social action programs will automatically decrease the rate of mental illness by correcting social woes and increasing the general psychological well-being. Arnhoff (1975) noted, "Somewhere along the line, a problem as old as man, that of mental illness, was absorbed into the pursuit of global mental health" (p. 1281). It is this confusion of objectives that has led some workers to formulate the issue of primary prevention in terms of eliminating poverty, slums, and economic insecurity—among other commendable but nebulous proposals. (Erlenmeyer-Kimling, 1977, p. 86)

It seems that we think we have two kinds of variables: the "real causes"—things like drug abuse, marital problems, lack of parenting skills—that we can deal with as professionals, and the global and nebulous factors, like poverty, ignorance, and powerlessness that we know correlate with the causes but do not themselves constitute causes. The dichotomy is misleading in implying that the variables we can deal with have a unique scientific status—it cloaks our bias and ignorance in a scientific rationalization.

In fact, the "real causes" do not appear to be quite as different from "mere correlations" as we seem to find it convenient to believe, and if this is the case, we cannot be excused on scientific grounds from dealing with the correlated variables. This is not the place to undertake a philosophical disquisition of the nature of causation. However, it is pertinent to point out that the distinction between "genuine causes" and "merely correlated" variables is more complex than seems to be appreciated by many of those who wish to make this kind of distinction with a view to de-emphasizing the kinds of variables the importance of which I want to stress. If one takes the simplest approach, that variables have to be individually necessary and sufficient in order to be regarded as causal, one will find that very few causes have been identified in the biological and social sciences—or even in physics for that matter. In many cases we cannot claim that what we regard as a causal variable is either necessary *or* sufficient. In fact, we appear to recognize a causal relationship when we see that in the presence of a particular factor the probability of a certain outcome is increased and we have no reason to believe that both are dependent on a third variable. Given these considerations, brief as they may be, unless one has evidence that both are due to a third (genetic?) variable, there is no reason not to say that poverty and powerlessness (see Albee, 1980) cause disease—and birth defects.

Variables like age, ethnic group, socioeconomic status, education, housing conditions, and so on are not second-class scientific variables and attending to them may, in fact, enable us to design more effective prevention programs than we can when we give all our attention to *mere causes.*

The second reason we are given why we have no business with social reform is that we have no particular competence in this area and that involving ourselves in the arena of social reform detracts from our credibility and effectiveness as professionals. For example:

Instead of focusing narrowly on the environmental stressors that are likely to be amenable to the intervention of mental health specialists with community decision makers, they become preoccupied by such major and global problems as poverty and racial prejudice, and they embark themselves on quixotic remedial campaigns as revolutionaries and social agitators. Unfortunately, they are no more skilled in social action than in community mental health practice; on the one hand they make inflated rhetorical promises about putting the bad world right which eventually bring inevitable discredit, or they lead inept marches on City Hall on behalf of the downtrodden, and get repudiated both by their disappointed clients and by the municipal authorities who pay their salaries. In any event, primary prevention for which they have ostensibly been fighting, gets a bad name. (Caplan, 1978 p. 10).

Indeed we may have no special competence as professionals to solve social problems—even if we do seem to be able to identify them—but the modesty we assume when talking about poverty and injustice seems to be put aside when we attempt to influence public policy to achieve what we claim as professional goals. Do we not claim special competence in identifying needs and implementing solutions when it comes to influencing legislation or acquiring funding for prevention programs of other kinds? Is it that we define as within our professional sphere those actions and aims that we approve of, while those we disapprove of are "political"? Furthermore, with whom do we lose credibility when we attempt remedial campaigns? It seems that our inaction, rather than action, in the social arena is more likely to compromise the credibility of our efforts as professionals. Or do we believe that our efforts as professionals excuse us from working for social change? If primary prevention is to have any hope of success, it needs a more committed stance than that represented by an "I gave at the office" philosophy.

The third reason we are given why we should not attack social evils is that even if we succeeded we would not have eradicated deviance, unhappiness, or the birth of infants with impaired potential. This, too, may be true, but there are reasons to believe that this approach will achieve more than piecemeal one-small-problem-at-a-time approaches. If we are realistic, we acknowledge that each proximate cause is the outcome of complex interactions of variables and that, as Vance (1977) pointed out, "the greater the number of relevant interactions, the smaller the groupings for which a single treatment will be appropriate" (p. 208). If this is so, then either we resign ourselves to designing myriads of low-payoff prevention programs or we lay siege to the broader variables that encompass the complex interacting variables. Dealing with variables like socioeconomic status and ethnicity deals simultaneously with factors giving rise to hazardous prenatal and perinatal events, those enhancing susceptibility to such events, and those that ensure postnatal conditions that at best fail to alleviate the consequences of prenatal hazards and at worst exacerbate their efforts. In addition, the broader variables are also more promising in terms of the timing of intervention. They exert their effects earlier than the proximate causes of adverse neonatal outcomes so their eradication has a greater change of obviating problems before they occur. A further advantage to putting emphasis on prevention that can be achieved through attention to demographic variables is that the approach encompasses both prevention and promotion: Removal of the global causes of dysfunction at the very least should result in a population with the means and the desire to pursue improved function. Removing external barriers strengthens people and provides conditions in which they can direct their strength toward the removal of further barriers.

None of this is to argue that social change will solve all the problems but rather that without such change much of whatever else we do may be futile. We will have to do it over and over again. Social change may not be sufficient, but it is necessary. Even if social change brought equitable programs to prevent genetic disease, reduce reproductive incompetence, and minimize environmental hazards, we would still be left with an apparently irreducible minimum of developmental defects. The perspective of primary prevention might be defined as never concluding that the minimum has been reached.

References

Abroms, K. I., and Bennett, J. W. Parental age and Trisomy-21. *Down's Syndrome*, 1979, 2, 6–7.

Ad Hoc Committee on the Effect of Trace Anesthetics on the Health of Operating Room Personnel. Occupational disease among operating room personnel: A national study. *Anesthesiology*, 1974, *41*, 321–340.

Albee, G. W. The prevention of prevention. *Physician East*, April 1979, 28–30.

Albee, G. W. Politics, power, prevention, and social change. In J. M. Joffe and G. W. Albee (Eds.), *Prevention through political action and social change*, Vol. 5: *Primary prevention of psychopathology*. Hanover, N.H.: University Press of England, 1980.

Arnhoff, F. N. Social consequences of policy toward mental illness. *Science*, 1975, *188*, 1277–1281.

Badr, F. M., and Badr, R. S. Induction of dominant lethal mutation in male mice by ethyl alcohol. *Nature*, 1975, *253*, 134–136.

Baird, D. Social class and foetal mortality. *Lancet*, 1949, *1*, 1079–1083.

Baird, D. The epidemiology of prematurity. *Journal of Pediatrics*, 1964, *65*, 909–924.

Baird, D. Epidemiology of congenital malformations of the central nervous system in (a) Aberdeen and (b) Scotland. *Journal of Biosocial Science*, 1974, *6*, 113–137.

Baird, D., and Illsley, R. Environment and childbearing. *Proceedings of the Royal Society of Medicine*, 1953, *46*, 53–59.

Barnes, A. C. The fetal environment: Drugs and chemicals. In A. C. Barnes (Ed.), *Intrauterine development*. Philadelphia: Lea and Febiger, 1968.

Bennett, J. W., and Abroms, K. I. Changing perspectives on Down's syndrome. *Journal of the Louisiana Medical Society*, 1979, *131*, 305–307.

Bernard, R. M. The shape and size of the female pelvis. (Transactions of the Edinburgh Obstetrical Society) *Edinburgh Medical Journal*, 1952, *59*, 1–16.

Birch, H. G., and Gussow, J. D. *Disadvantaged children: Health, nutrition and school failure*. New York: Harcourt, Brace, and World, 1970.

Bloom, M. A working definition of primary prevention related to social concerns. *The Journal of Prevention*, 1980, *1*, 15–23.

Brackbill, Y. Obstetrical medication and infant behavior. In J. D. Osofsky (Ed.), *Handbook of infant behavior*. New York: Wiley, 1979.

Brady, H., Herrera, Y., and Zenick, H. Influence of parental lead exposure on subsequent learning ability of offspring. *Pharmacology, Biochemistry and Behavior*, 1975, *3*, 561–565.

Brent, R. L. Environmental factors: Miscellaneous. In R. L. Brent and M. I. Harris (Eds.), *Prevention of embryonic, fetal, and perinatal disease*. DHEW Pub. No. (NIH) 76-853. Washington, D.C., 1976.

Brent, R. L. Radiations and other physical agents. In J. G. Wilson and F. C. Fraser (Eds.), *Handbook of teratology*. Vol. 1: *General principles and etiology*. New York: Plenum, 1977.

Brent, R. L., and Harris, M. I. Summaries. In R. L. Brent and M. I. Harris (Eds.), *Prevention of embryonic, fetal, and perinatal disease*. DHEW Pub. No. (NIH) 76-853. Washington, D.C., 1976.

Broman, S. H., Nichols, P. L., and Kennedy, W. A. *Preschool IQ: Prenatal and early developmental correlates*. Hillsdale, N.J.: L. Erlbaum Associates, 1975.

Caplan, G. *The primary prevention of mental disorders in children: Developments during the period 1962–1977*. Lecture, University of Leuven, Belgium, May 26, 1978.

Carter, C. O., and Evans, K. Spina bifida and anencephalus in Greater London. *Journal of Medical Genetics*, 1973, *10*, 209–234.

Catz, C. S., and Yaffe, S. J. Environmental factors: Pharmacology. In R. L. Brent and M. I. Harris (Eds.), *Prevention of embryonic, fetal, and perinatal disease.* DHEW Pub. No. (NIH) 76-853. Washington, D.C., 1976.

Chez, R., Haire, D., Quilligan, E. J., and Wingate, M. B. High risk pregnancies: Obstetrical and perinatal factors. In R. L. Brent and M. I. Harris (Eds.), *Prevention of embryonic, fetal, and perinatal disease.* DHEW Pub. No. (NIH) 76-853 Washington, D.C., 1976.

Chyzzer, A. Des intoxications per le plumb se presentant dans le ceramique en Hongrie Budapest XLIV, Chir. Presse, 1908, 906. (Quoted by Weller, 1915).

Cohen, E. N., Brown, Jr., B. W., Bruce, D. L., Cascorbi, H. F., Corbett, T. H., Jones, T. W., and Whitcher, C. E. A survey of anesthetic health hazards among dentists. *Journal of the American Dental Association, 1975, 90,* 1291–1296.

Cole, L. J., and Bachhuber, L. J. The effect of lead on the germ cells of the male rabbit and fowl. *Proceedings of the Society for Experimental Biology and Medicine,* 1914, *12,* 24–29.

Corah, N. L., Anthony, E. J., Painter, P., Stern, J. A., and Thurston, D. L. Effects of perinatal anoxia after seven years. *Psychological Monographs,* 1965, *79,* 3 (Whole No. 596).

Cowley, J. J., and Griesel, R. D. The effect on growth and behavior of rehabilitating first and second generation low protein rats. *Animal Behaviour,* 1966, *14,* 506–517.

Durham, F. M., and Woods, H. M. Alcohol and inheritance: An experimental study. *Medical Research Council Special Report Series.* London: H.M.S.O., No. 168, 1932.

Elinson, J., and Wilson, R. W. Prevention. In *Health, United States, 1978.* U.S. Department of Health, Education and Welfare. DHEW Pub. No. (PHS) 78-1232. Hyattsville, M.D., 1978.

Emanuel, I. Problems of outcome of pregnancy: Some clues from the epidemiologic similarities and differences. In S. Kelly, E. B. Hook, D. T. Janerich, and I. H. Porter (Eds.), *Birth defects: Risks and consequences.* New York: Academic Press, 1976.

Erlenmeyer-Kimling, L. Issues pertaining to prevention and intervention of genetic disorders affecting human behavior. In G. W. Albee and J. M. Joffe (Eds.), *Primary prevention of psychopathology,* Vol. 1: *The issues.* Hanover, N.H.: University Press of New England, 1977.

Ferreira, M.C.R. Malnutrition and mother-infant asynchrony: Slow mental development. *International Journal of Behavioral Development,* 1978, *1,* 207–219.

Fraser, F. C. Interactions and multiple causes. In J. G. Wilson and F. C. Fraser (Eds.), *Handbook of teratology,* Vol. 1: *General principles and etiology.* New York: Plenum, 1977.

Fraser, F. C. Future prospects—clinical. In J. W. Littlefield, J. DeGrouchy, and F.J.G. Ebling (Eds.), *Birth defects. Proceedings of the fifth international conference, Montreal, Canada, 21–27 August 1977.* Amsterdam: Excerpta Medica, 1978.

Friedler, G. Morphine administration to male mice. Effects on subsequent progeny. *Federation Proceedings,* 1974, *33,* 515.

Golbus, M. S. Prenatal diagnosis of genetic defects—where it is and where it is going. In J. W. Littlefield, J. DeGrouchy, and F.J.G. Ebling (Eds.) *Birth defects. Proceedings of the fifth international conference, Montreal, Canada, 21–27 August 1977.* Amsterdam: Excerpta Medica, 1978.

Goldman, A. S. Critical periods of prenatal toxic insults. In R. H. Schwarz and

S. J. Yaffe (Eds.), *Drug and chemical risks to the fetus and newborn.* New York: A. R. Liss, 1980.

Graham, F. K., Ernhart, C. B., Thurston, D. L., and Craft, M. Development three years after perinatal anoxia and other potentially damaging newborn experiences. *Psychological Monographs,* 1962, *76,* 3 (Whole No. 522).

Graham, F. K., Matarazzo, R. G., and Caldwell, B. M. Behavioral differences between normal and traumatized newborns: II. Standardization, reliability, and validity. *Psychological Monographs,* 1956, *70,* 21 (Whole No. 428).

Graham, F. K., Pennoyer, M. M., Caldwell, B. M., Greenman, M., and Hartman, A. F. Relationship between clinical status and behavior test performance in a newborn group with histories suggesting anoxia. *Journal of Pediatrics,* 1957, *50,* 177–189.

Grabowski, C. T. Atmospheric gases: Variations in concentration and some common pollutants. In J. G. Wilson and F. C. Fraser (Eds.), *Handbook of teratology,* Vol. 1: *General principles and etiology.* New York: Plenum, 1977.

Harris, H. *Prenatal diagnosis and selective abortion.* Cambridge, Mass.: Harvard University Press, 1975.

Hertig, A. T., Rock, J., and Adams, E. C. A description of 34 human ova within the first 17 days of development. *American Journal of Anatomy,* 1956, *98,* 435–459.

Holmes, L. B. Genetic counseling for the older pregnant woman: New data and questions. *New England Journal of Medicine,* 1978, *298,* 1419–1421.

Hsia, Y. E. Treatment in genetic diseases. In A. Milunsky (Ed.), *The prevention of genetic disease and mental retardation.* Philadelphia: W. B. Saunders, 1975.

Ingalls, T. H. Preventive prenatal pediatrics. *Advances in Pediatrics,* 1953, *6,* 33–62.

Joffe, J. M. *Prenatal determinants of behavior.* Oxford: Pergamon, 1969.

Joffe, J. M. Influence of drug exposure of the father on perinatal outcome. In L. F. Soyka (Ed.), *Clinics in perinatology,* Vol. 6, No. 1: *Symposium on pharmacology.* Philadelphia: W. B. Saunders, 1979.

Joffe, J. M., Peterson, J. M., Smith, D. J., and Soyka, L. F. Sublethal effects on offspring of male rats treated with methadone. *Research Communications in Chemical Pathology and Pharmacology,* 1976, *13,* 611–621.

Kaback, M. M., Heterozygote screening for the control of recessive genetic disease. In A. Milunsky (Ed.), *The prevention of genetic disease and mental retardation.* Philadelphia: W. B. Saunders, 1975.

Kessler, M., and Albee, G. W. Primary prevention. *Annual Review of Psychology,* 1975, *26,* 557–591.

Klassen, R. W., and Persaud, T.V.N. Experimental studies on the influence of male alcoholism on pregnancy and progeny. *Experimental Pathology,* 1976, *12,* 38–45.

Kopp, C. B., and Parmelee, A. H. Prenatal and perinatal influences on infant behavior. In J. D. Osofsky (Ed.) *Handbook of infant development.* New York: Wiley, 1979.

Kushnick, T. Antenatal diagnosis. In H. A. Kaminetzky, L. Iffy, and J. J. Apuzzio (Eds.), *New techniques and concepts in maternal and fetal medicine.* New York: VanNostrand Reinhold, 1979.

Lappé, M. Can eugenic policy be just? In A. Milunsky (Ed.), *The prevention of genetic disease and mental retardation.* Philadelphia: W. B. Saunders, 1975.

Lutwak-Mann, C. Observations on progeny of thalidomide-treated male rabbits. *British Medical Journal,* 1964, *1,* 1090–1091.

Lutwak-Mann, C., Schmid, K., and Keberle, H. Thalidomide in rabbit semen. *Nature*, 1967, *214*, 1018–1020.

MacDowell, E. C., and Lord, E. M. Reproduction in alcoholic mice: Treated males. Study of prenatal mortality and sex ratios. *Archiv fur Entwicklungsmechanik der Organismen*, 1927, *110*, 427–449.

MacDowell, E. C., Lord, E. M., and MacDowell, C. G. Heavy alcoholization and prenatal mortality in mice. *Proceedings of the Society for Experimental Biology and Medicine*, 1926, *23*, 652–654. (a)

MacDowell, E. C., Lord, E. M., and MacDowell, C. G. Sex ratio of mice from alcoholized fathers. *Proceedings of the Society for Experimental Biology and Medicine*, 1926, *23*, 517–519. (b)

McKusick, V. A. *Mendelian inheritance in man. Catalogs of autosomal dominant, autosomal recessive, and X-linked phenotypes* (3rd ed.). Baltimore: The Johns Hopkins Press, 1971.

McNeil, T. F., and Kaij, L. Prenatal, perinatal, and post-partum factors in primary prevention of psychopathology in offspring. In G. W. Albee and J. M. Joffe (Eds.), *Primary prevention of psychopathology*, Vol. 1: *The Issues*. Hanover N.H.: University Press of New England, 1977.

Meier, J. H. Early intervention in the prevention of mental retardation. In A. Milunsky (Ed.), *The prevention of genetic disease and mental retardation*. Philadelphia: W. B. Saunders, 1975.

Milunsky, A. (Ed.). *The prevention of genetic disease and mental retardation*. Philadelphia: W. B. Saunders, 1975. (a)

Milunsky, A. Genetic counseling: Principles and practice. In A. Milunsky (Ed.), *The prevention of genetic disease and mental retardation*. Philadelphia: W. B. Saunders, 1975. (b)

Milunsky, A., and Atkins, L. Prenatal diagnosis of genetic disorders. In A. Milunsky (Ed.), *The prevention of genetic disease and mental retardation*. Philadelphia: W. B. Saunders, 1975.

Motulsky, A., Benirschke, K., Carpenter, G., Fraser, C., Epstein, C., Nyhan, W., and Jackson, L. Genetic diseases. In R. L. Brent and M. I. Harris (Eds.), *Prevention of embryonic, fetal, and perinatal disease*. DHEW Pub. No. (NIH) 76-853. Washington, D.C., 1976.

National Center for Health Statistics. *Facts of life and death*. U.S. Dept. of Health, Education and Welfare. DHEW Pub. No. (PHS) 79-1222. Hyattsville, MD., 1978.

Nitowsky, H. M. Heterozygote detection in autosomal recessive biochemical disorders associated with mental retardation. In A. Milunsky (Ed.), *The prevention of genetic disease and mental retardation*. Philadelphia: W. B. Saunders, 1975.

Nuckolls, K. B., Cassel, J., and Kaplan, B. H. Psychosocial assets, life crisis, and the prognosis of pregnancy. *American Journal of Epidemiology*, 1972, *35*, 431–441.

Pasamanick, B., Knobloch, H., and Lilienfeld, A. M. Socioeconomic status and some precursors of neuropsychiatric disorders. *American Journal of Orthopsychiatry*, 1956, *26*, 594–601.

Paul, C. Archives generales de Medecine, 1860, *1*, 513. (Quoted by Weller, 1915).

Plomin, R., DeFries, J. C., and Loehlin, J. C. Genotype-environment interaction and correlation in the analysis of human behavior. *Psychological Bulletin*, 1977, *84*, 309–322.

Redmond, G. P. Effect of drugs on intrauterine growth. In L. F. Soyka (Ed.), *Clinics in Perinatology*, Vol. 6, No. 1: *Symposium on pharmacology*. Philadelphia: W. B. Saunders, 1979.

Reid, G. Report of the Departmental Commission on the dangers attendant on the use of lead. Quoted by T. Oliver, Lecture on lead poisoning and the race. *British Medical Journal*, 1911, *1*, 1096–1098.

Reilly, P. The role of law in the prevention of genetic disease. In A. Milunsky (Ed.), *The prevention of genetic disease and mental retardation*. Philadelphia: W. B. Saunders, 1975.

Ressler, R. H. Parental handling in two strains of mice reared by foster parents. *Science*, 1962, *137*, 129–130.

Roberts, C. A. Psychiatric and mental health consultation. *Canadian Journal of Public Health*, 1970, *51*, 17–24.

Rosen, G. *Preventive medicine in the United States 1900–1975: Trends and interpretations*. New York: Science History Publications, 1975.

Rudeaux, P. La Clinique, 1910. Quoted by Thompson in *The occupational diseases*. New York: Appleton, 1914.

Sameroff, A. J. Early influences on development: Fact or fancy? *Merrill-Palmer Quarterly of Behavior and Development*, 1975, *21*, 267–294.

Sameroff, A. J. Concepts of humanity in primary prevention. In G. W. Albee and J. M. Joffe (Eds.), *Primary prevention of psychopathology*, Vol. 1: *The issues*. Hanover, N.H.: University Press of New England, 1977.

Sameroff, A. J., and Chandler, M. J. Reproductive risk and the continuum of caretaking casualty. In F. D. Horowitz, M. Hetherington, S. Scarr-Salapatek, and G. Siegel (Eds.), *Review of child development research*, Vol. 4. Chicago: University of Chicago, 1975.

Scriver, C. R., and Laberge, C. Genetic screening. An outlook en route. In J. W. Littlefield, J. DeGrouchy, and F.J.G. Ebling (Eds.), *Birth defects. Proceedings of the fifth international conference, Montreal, Canada, 21–27 August 1977*. Amsterdam: Excerpta Medica, 1978.

Slone, D., Shapiro, S., and Mitchell, A. Strategies for studying the effects of the antenatal environment on the fetus. In R. H. Schwarz and S. J. Yaffe (Eds.), *Drug and chemical risks to the fetus and newborn*. New York: A. R. Liss, 1980.

Smith, D. J., and Joffe, J. M. Increased neonatal mortality in offspring of male rats treated with methadone or morphine before mating. *Nature*, 1975, *253*, 202–203.

Smithells, R. W. Future prospects: Environmental factors. In J. W. Littlefield, J. DeGrouchy, and F.J.G. Ebling (Eds.), *Birth defects. Proceedings of the fifth international conference, Montreal, Canada, 21–27 August 1977*. Amsterdam; Excerpta Medica, 1978.

Soyka, L. F., and Joffe, J. M. Influence of concurrent testosterone on the effects of methadone on male rats and their progeny. *Developmental Pharmacology and Therapeutics*, 1980, *1*, 182–188. (a)

Soyka, L. F., and Joffe, J. M. Male mediated drug effects on offspring. In R. H. Schwarz and S. J. Yaffe (Eds.), *Drug and chemical risks to the fetus and newborn*. New York: A. R. Liss, 1980. (b)

Soyka, L. J., Joffe, J. M., Peterson, J. M., and Smith, S. M. Chronic methadone administration to male rats: Tolerance to adverse effects on sires and their progeny. *Pharmacology, Biochemistry and Behavior*, 1978, *9*, 405–409. (a)

Soyka, L. F., Peterson, J. M., and Joffe, J. M. Lethal and sublethal effects on the progeny of male rats treated with methadone. *Toxicology and Applied Pharmacology*, 1978, *45*, 797–807. (b)

Stockard, C. R. Effect on the offspring of intoxicating the male parent and transmission of the defects of subsequent generations. *American Naturalist*, 1913, *47*, 641–682.

Stowe, H. D., and Goyer, R. A. The reproductive ability and progeny of F_1 lead-toxic rats. *Fertility and Sterility*, 1971, *22*, 755–760.

Task Panel on Prevention. *President's Commission on Mental Health* (Vol. 4). Washington, D.C.: U.S. Government Printing Office, No. 040-000-00393-2, 1978.

Thomas, A., Chess, S. and Birch, H. *Temperament and behavior disorders in children*. New York: New York University, 1968.

Thomson, A. M. Maternal stature and reproductive efficiency. *Eugenics Review*, 1959, *51*, 157–162.

Thomson, A. M., and Billewicz, W. Z. Nutritional status, physique and reproductive efficiency. *Proceedings of the Nutrition Society*, 1963, *22*, 55–60.

Tizard, J.P.M. Pre-natal and perinatal factors. In J. W. Littlefield, J. DeGrouchy, and F.J.G. Ebling (Eds.), *Birth defects. Proceedings of the fifth international conference, Montreal, Canada, 21–27 August 1977*. Amsterdam: Excerpta Medica, 1978.

Vance, E. T. A typology of risks and the disabilities of low status. In G. W. Albee and J. M. Joffe (Eds.), *Primary prevention of psychopathology*, Vol. 1: *The issues*. Hanover, N.H.: University Press of New England, 1977.

Warkany, J. Terathanasia. *Teratology*, 1978, *17*, 187–192.

Weathersbee, P. S., Ax, R. L., and Lodge, J. R. Caffeine-mediated changes of sex ratio in Chinese hamsters, *Cricetulus griseus*. *Journal of Reproduction and Fertility*, 1975, *43*, 141–143.

Weathersbee, P. S., Olsen, L. K., and Lodge, J. R. Caffeine and pregnancy: A retrospective study. *Postgraduate Medicine*, 1977, *62*, 64–69.

Weller, C. V. The blastophthoric effect of chronic lead poisoning. *Journal of Medical Research*, 1915, *33*, 271–293.

Werner, E. E., Bierman, J., and French, F. *The children of Kauai: A longitudinal study from the prenatal period to age ten*. Honolulu: University Press of Hawaii, 1971.

Werner, E. E., Bierman, J. M., French, F., Simonian, K., Connor, A., Smith, R., and Campbell, M. Reproductive and environmental casualties: A report on the 10 year follow-up of the children of the Kauai pregnancy study. *Pediatrics*, 1968, *42*, 112–127.

Werner, E. E., Simonian, K., Bierman, J. M., and French, F. Cumulative effect of perinatal complications and deprived environment on physical, intellectual and social development of preschool children. *Pediatrics*, 1967, *39*, 490–505.

Werner, E. E., and Smith, R. S. *Kauai's children come of age*. Honolulu: University Press of Hawaii, 1977.

Wilson, J. G. Embryological considerations in teratology. *Annals of the New York Academy of Sciences*, 1965, *123*, 219–227.

Wilson, J. G. Embryotoxicity of drugs in man. In J. G. Wilson and F. C. Fraser (Eds.), *Handbook of teratology*, Vol. 1: *General principles and etiology*. New York: Plenum, 1977. (a)

Wilson, J. G. Environmental chemicals. In J. G. Wilson and F. C. Fraser (Eds.), *Handbook of teratology*, Vol. 1: *General principles and etiology*. New York: Plenum, 1977. (b)

Winick, M. Maternal nutrition. In R. L. Brent and M. I. Harris (Eds.), *Prevention of embryonic, fetal, and perinatal disease.* DHEW Pub. No. (NIH) 76-853. Washington, D.C., 1976.

Yerushalmy, J. Biostatistical methods in investigations of child health. *American Journal of Diseases of Children,* 1967, *114,* 470–476.

Yerushalmy, J. Relationship of parents' cigarette smoking to outcome of pregnancy—implications as to the problem of inferring causation from observed observations. *American Journal of Epidemiology,* 1971, *93,* 443–456.

Young, R. D. Influence of neonatal treatment on maternal behavior: A confounding variable. *Psychonomic Science,* 1965, *3,* 295–296.

Bureaucratizing Values

Burton Blatt

What Is a Least Restrictive Environment?

What is going on in the United States? How free are we? Never mind the mentally retarded—how free are you? Let us take a look at a few aspects of life in the United States today. The Talmudists have the luxury—indeed, the divine responsibility—to read word by word, letter by letter, and to compare a tiny mark to an even tinier mark. Because they no longer have legal power over the people, they can be legalists of the narrowest variety. Contrast them with the founding fathers of this country who needed a Supreme Court to interpret the law in the context of the times. To appreciate the concept of "least restrictiveness" requires, I think, an overview of a couple of society's institutions and not the Talmudist's, nor the scientist's nor the compulsive's special talents. That is, I think that "least restrictiveness" should be understood as a whole and not by its parts. Of course, the catch is that the concept is too complex to be understood that way. And, of course, there is too much to know about all of those institutions to get it all down here. But you live in our society as well as I do, and you know what is happening as well as I do. Consequently, these remarks are intended to do no more than to make us want to think about what we already know.

First of all, it seems to be as true today as it was when Calvin Coolidge said it years ago, that "the business of America is business." That is why we need stock exchanges and antitrust laws. That is why we need law schools, corporations, and Madison Avenue, and much of what is on television, and much of what is on people's minds. That is why General Electric claims "Progress is our most important product," though nobody believes them. And it is in the name of business that DuPont can bellow from today to doomsday that chemistry makes better things for better living, but nobody will believe DuPont. Because it is good for business, Nestlés can get away with promoting in Third World countries powdered milk that may be as lethal to babies there as uncontrolled asbestos plants are here.

It seems impossible to conjure up the march of American business without its accompaniment of nonsense and outright hazard. Our sys-

From Burton Blatt, "Bureaucratizing Values," in Justin M. Joffe and George W. Albee (eds.) *Prevention Through Political Action and Social Change.* Copyright © 1981 by the Vermont Conference on the Primary Prevention of Psychopathology. Reprinted by permission.

tem and its freedoms have been designed to foster the creation of wealth and power, not to control them when they are used or pursued irresponsibly. That is why Ralph Nader is now inevitable and necessary, though terribly wrong. He is incontestably right that "they" are bastards. "They" could not be anything else because the profit motive and the free market are utterly indifferent to human values—unless those values affect sales. However, Nader is mistaken when he suggests that what "they" are doing, from price-fixing to manufacturing gas tanks that explode, represents some sort of aberration that could be corrected without attacking the business of America at its heart. And Nader is quite wrong in his avalanche of proposed laws for us to control the bastards. The effect of those regulations is likely to be as destructive as "their" lawlessness. We betray the human race and, in the final accounting, the individual as well, when we deny that the world must necessarily be a dangerous place. Most of us would pay high prices for our freedom; I am claiming now that Nader wants to exact a higher price for my safety than I am willing to pay.

American business has given us the possibility of the four-day work week and the two-home and three-car family at the same time that it has given us the choice of destroying either our health or our freedoms. Seizing upon the wonders of American technology, big business has made us free, but within narrower confines than ever before. It has given us the time to pursue virtually any hobby or interest we have, but it has also enticed us to sit in drugged stupors watching a lighted box. In America, only the truly brave, strong-willed, innovative person can exploit the genius of the American system and reject the damaging side-effects that accompany progress and that make us less well off than our grandparents.

"Mediacracy": Mass Media and Psychopathology

David Manning White

Philosophers apply the term sickness to all disturbances of the soul, and they say that no foolish person is free from such sickness; sufferers from disease are not sound, and the souls of all unwise persons are sick.

Cicero *Tusculanarum Disputatium III.iv.9*

❖ Corporate amorality can injure individuals. For example: On September 10, 1974, NBC broadcast a two-hour movie for television called *Born Innocent*, starring Linda Blair as a runaway adolescent committed by her parents to a detention center. During the course of the film Blair is "initiated" into the center's way of life by a gang-rape in a communal shower. The scene was depicted with extremely graphic realism. Suddenly the water stops and a look of fear comes into Blair's face. Four adolescent girls are standing across the shower room. One is carrying a plumber's helper, the sort of plunger that most of us use to unclog stopped-up drains. She is waving the plunger near her hips. The older girls tell Blair to get out of the shower, and she steps out fearfully. Thereupon the four girls violently attack the younger girl, wrestling her to the floor. She is shown naked from the waist up, struggling, as the older girls force her legs apart. Then, the girl with the plunger is shown making intense thrusting motions with the handle until one of the four says, "That's enough."

Four days after the broadcast a violent scuffle occurred on a beach near San Francisco, and before it was over a 9-year-old girl had been sexually assaulted with a beer bottle. The subsequent negligence suit brought by the girl's mother against NBC raises many difficult sociological as well as constitutional questions.

What was the responsibility of the network? Should it not have known that impressionable young viewers might imitate the violent dramatic scene? After legal maneuvering by the highly skillful lawyers NBC could afford to hire, the case narrowed down to whether the movie actually

From David Manning White, "'Mediacracy': Mass Media and Psychopathology," in Justin M. Joffe and George W. Albee (eds.) *Prevention Through Political Action and Social Change.* Copyright © 1981 by the Vermont Conference on the Primary Prevention of Psychopathology. Reprinted by permission.

"incited" the real-life attack. Eventually the lawsuit was dismissed when the judge ruled it was necessary to prove that NBC "intended" viewers to imitate the sexual attack depicted on *Born Innocent*. There will be future cases like this, I would venture, for sooner or later we are going to have to come to grips with the effects of TV on human conduct. It is small solace to the victim for some network apologist to express regret but temper it with the reflection there were probably hundreds of thousands of young people watching *Born Innocent* that night and only this small handful of kids in California "acted out" in this pathological manner.

One knows that the network recognized that the film might offend or disturb some viewers because it inserted the usual advisory legend at the beginning of the program: "The following program *Born Innocent* deals in a realistic and forthright manner with the confinement of juvenile offenders and its effect on their lives and personalities. We suggest that you consider whether the program should be viewed by young people or others in your family who might be disturbed by it."

As a matter of fact such disclaimers generally have the opposite effect, and I suspect that any veteran television network official would acknowledge that this is so, unless he or she were on the witness stand in a future case of the same kind. Very few parents monitor what their children are watching, and with two or three sets not uncommon in a home, one of them in the children's bedroom or den, it is becoming increasingly difficult to do so.

The question that we in the larger court of public opinion may have to answer is whether such media fare can be justified if indeed only 1 / 1000 of one percent of the youngsters who see it could be influenced in this way.

I am not implying that the producer of *Born Innocent* or the network official who scheduled it are villainous scoundrels who need to be publicly flogged. There are, indeed, some critics of the mass media who are sure that the violent, flamboyant quality of many television programs, mass magazines, Hollywood films, or rock music recordings is due to some plot on the part of the media moguls. The gatekeepers of the media, on the other hand, often rationalize such products as *Born Innocent* or *The Exorcist* by insisting that they are giving the Great American Public what it wants.

How do they know what the public wants? That is easy—the proof is in the cash box, and in a country where Mammon is a very influential god, money talks in convincing tones.

Is it spiteful to single out the mass media for their role in reinforcing an economic system that rewards it so munificently? According to Nicholas Johnson, former member of the Federal Communications Commission, the television industry averages an 82 percent return *each year* on depreciated capital. Many of us became irate when the oil industry had one of its best years in 1978, but the percentage of profit in the television industry was three times as great. Yet why pick on the mass media, when as Gossage (1961) once pointed out, the very stability of our economic system seems to rest on a magic device, the good old pyramid club. Are we not locked into a system that demands ever-expanding production, which in turn needs an ever-expanding population with a concomitant ever-expanding consumption? While respectable economists nervously watch the Gross National Product as if it were devised on Mount Sinai, most Americans play a kind of chain-letter pyramid game. There has to be a sounder approach to the economic cycle than endlessly consuming more and more, but if there is, the mass media, which rely on advertising for their life blood, do not want to discover it. In not very subtle ways the mass media continually tell us that if we want an affluent life in this country we must acquire a lot of wealth and material goods. The trouble with this message is that only a few thousand ever acquire enough money to stop the quest for it; for the rest it is an elusive, alluring brass ring that the mass media say is the alpha and omega of life.

Within a few years the Gross National Product of this country may reach two *trillion* dollars. What do we produce of such lasting value that costs 80,000 times more than the Louisiana Purchase? Even today the personal consumption expenditure by Americans is about one and a quarter trillion dollars, and if the not-very-hidden persuaders of Madison Avenue have their way we will spend more and more each year. We had better, they tell us, lest the pyramid crumble and we slide into a recession or God forbid, a repetition of the 1930s depression.

Where do we spend all that money? One major area is our mass communications system and the goods and services it produces. It is not possible to separate economic events and their impact on the mass media, nor to understand the clout of mediacracy without examining a few current trends. For example, take the record industry. Whether you bought an album of Sir Georg Solti leading the Chicago Symphony in Bruckner's Ninth Symphony or Rasputin and the Freaked-Out Monks in their last rock assault on the human ear, the list price on the albums in the last few months went up at least a dollar. That is because oil is used to make phonograph records, and as the OPEC nations dramatically raised the price of crude oil on the world market, the cost was passed on to the consumer. Despite this price increase the record industry is thriving and expects to gross more than $3 billion in 1979. Among these albums is one by a group known as the Bee Gees, the sound track for a film called *Saturday Night Fever*, which since its release in 1977 has grossed nearly $350 million.

When a motion picture such as *Star Wars* earns more than $200 million in domestic rentals alone, topping even the bonanza of a 1975 film *Jaws*, it is quite evident that the big films of the movie industry earn the much-coveted megabucks. In the world of mediacracy, the Radio Corporation of America (which owns NBC, Random House, Modern Library and Hertz Rental Cars) must be the world's leading entertainment company with over $5 billion in sales each year.

In 1896, when Adolph Ochs bought the then ailing *New York Times* for $1 million the price seemed so high that many newspaper aficionados questioned his fiscal sanity. Today the New York Times Co. has yearly sales of nearly $500 million, and in addition to the *Times* owns six dailies and four weeklies in Florida, three dailies in North Carolina, mass circulation magazines such as *Family Circle*, radio stations in New York and Memphis, and three book publishing companies.

There was a time when large newspaper chain owners such as Samuel I. Newhouse expanded their acquisitions by buying up independent newspapers, but the trend today is for the big chains to swallow up the smaller ones. Thus in 1976 Newhouse bought the eight newspapers in the Booth chain, which included *Parade*, the Sunday magazine supplement, for $300 million. An even bigger deal was consummated in June, 1979, when the Gannett chain, which already owned 77 daily newspapers and 19 weeklies in 32 states acquired the Cincinnati *Enquirer*, the Oakland (Calif.) *Tribune*, 7 television and 13 radio stations from Combined Communications Corporation. The price ticket for this merger, a mere $370 million.

In the kingdom of mediacracy the prime minister is advertising. During this decade nearly $300 billion will be spent on advertising in the United States. One is faced with the question: Why has the national yearly advertising budget risen so fast, from about $3 billion in 1945 to more than 10 times that amount today? Even allowing for inflation and a growth in our population this is an unhealthy rise.

Perhaps the consumer has reached a point of commercial saturation. What then follows is a kind of Hegelian thesis, antithesis and synthesis, with the big corporations having to spend more and more money to snag the attention of us consumers. Our antithesis is to build more immunity, and in turn, Proctor and Gamble develops newer and costlier ways to wash our rebellious minds with soap—and thus the triad begins again. I question whether it really takes a $31-billion sledgehammer to drive a 31-cent thumbtack.

But maybe even more important when I read that giant mediacrats like Newhouse or Gannett are willing to pay more than one-third of a billion dollars to augment their media empires I am deeply concerned. Let me reiterate that my concern is not that these media moguls desire to control American public opinion via news or editorials. Not since the heyday of

William Randolph Hearst has this approach been prevalent. Rather, my concern is that by the very fact of investing such vast sums of money in acquiring more newspapers, television stations, or magazines, their dominant motive is to make even more money. Thus the cycle of ever-increasing consumption grows and grows. Although I cannot substantiate my convictions with any large-scale study, I firmly believe that this false socioeconomic policy, which the media reinforce in their never-ending quest to look better to their stockholders, contributes significantly to the soil in which psychopathology thrives.

The average American adult spends nearly half of the waking hours of his or her life in some involvement with the mass media. Of the 16 waking hours, 4 are spent in front of a television set, 30 minutes or so reading a newspaper, 15 minutes with one or more of the 10,000 magazines published in this country, and about 2 and a half hours listening to radio (much of this while driving to and from work). Add an occasional excursion to a movie theater, reading a paperback thriller or mystery, playing $3 billion worth of the phonograph records or tapes Americans are buying each year, and the average is just about eight hours a day. Remember there are 60 "free" hours from Friday at 5 P.M. until 7 A.M. on Monday, when one gets ready for another working week (White, 1978).

The mass media are the primary agents of our popular culture, a multifaceted, pervasive process by which most Americans decide what they buy, what style of clothes they wear, what they eat, and certainly how they spend their leisure hours or otherwise acculturate themselves in a mass society. As Shakespeare wrote in *Antony and Cleopatra* (v, i): "When such a spacious mirror's set before him, He needs must see himself." The mass media provide this "spacious mirror," which we enter in some ineluctable way. But as the poet Rainer Marie Rilke (1923) so aptly perceived, we become a part of the mirror even as the mirror simultaneously becomes ingrained in our personal life style.

The average worker in America today has about 2,750 hours of leisure each year (after we subtract the work week, eight hours of sleep each night, eating, bathing, commuting). Why, then, are the mass media so seductive of these hardwon leisure hours? Perhaps because the seductee is getting what he or she has always yearned for, a partial, palatable answer to the questions all people ask themselves, whether they are steel workers in Dannemora or philosophers ambling down Brattle Street on their way to the Yard: Who am I, why am I here in this particular body with eyes that are too set apart and no upper lip, what is the meaning (if any) of my life vis-à-vis the universe?

Throughout recorded history most people have sought anodynes from the deepest anxieties about their existence. Without question, they did so before any aspects of mass culture pervaded their society. Karl Jaspers

(1949) quotes an Egyptian chronicler of 4,000 years ago who wrote: "Robbers abound; no one ploughs the land. People are saying: 'We do not know what will happen from day to day.' The country is spinning round and round like a potter's wheel. Great men and small agree in saying: 'Would that I had never been born.' The masses are like timid sheep without a shepherd; impudence is rife" (p. 238).

One wonders how that same Egyptian commentator would react to the national news broadcast by any of our television networks. Almost any day of the year we can hear and see some aspects of the almost insuperable problems of overpopulation, poverty, the rape of the earth's resources, not to mention the ever-present potentiality of atomic apocalypse, whether from some malfunction at another Three Mile Island plant or the paranoid miscalculation of a Dr. Strangelove in Moscow, Washington, or Tripoli. During the six decades of my life more than 50 *million fellow human beings* have died in wars, genocides, and other sundry forms of violence alone.

Most people do not want to contemplate the almost incalculable amount of violence occurring during their lifetime. They seek escape from the terrifying implications of many aspects of contemporary living, and the mass media are only too glad to accommodate them. And I do not mean to exclude myself behind some mask of elitist hauteur. I have indulged in so much media lotus-eating that any supercilious comments about the great, vulgar mass of Americans would make me an insufferable hypocrite.

In the late 1940s the mediacrats quickly surmised the seductive power of the television set. The potential profits were so staggering that they found it hard to believe. But even they could not realize that it would take only a generation to acculturate this country into a nation of videots. The 28-hour a week average that American adults (children under 12 watch a great deal more) spend inertly in front of their sets amounts to 1456 hours a year, or about a quarter of their total waking hours. This means that if the addiction to television continues unabated (and there are no signs that its popularity has waned appreciably) a one-year-old child, whose life expectancy will probably be greater than 75 years, will spend at least 110,000 total hours of his or her life willingly chained to our contemporary version of Plato's cave.

Television is a low-involvement medium that usually requires very little concentration from the viewer. It spews forth an incredible amount of what Steve Allen called "junk food for the mind." When the networks, either in a twinge of conscience, or more likely because they worry that the Federal Communications Commission may license them the way it does individual stations, air an occasional documentary, they invariably get a poor rating. Q.E.D., say the mediacrats, the audience does not care about quality programming. Perhaps they are right, but 30 years of mental pap and aesthetic mush 95 percent of the programmed time is hardly conducive to creating a climate for quality programming.

At a conference on television held at the University of Southern California, Richard Wald (1978), former head of NBC News and now senior vice president of ABC News put it very honestly. "TV harps on a very few themes," he said. "Only those eternal verities—lust, violence, sins and virtues—cut across all lines and make broad waves. These themes have always been with us, and in the past we might have confronted them on occasion, such as when we went to the theater. But now we live in a society where this is rained down upon us all the time. What is this doing to us? How is TV changing the character of modern man?"

There may be another reason for television's enormous hold on the majority of Americans, according to researchers such as Herbert Krugman, Peter Crown, and Sidney Weinstein. Utilizing brain-wave experiments over the past decade they and others have verified that television puts people into a nonthinking alpha state, the condition that occurs when someone is relaxed, passive, and unfocused (Krugman, Crown, and Weinstein, cited in Siegel, 1979).

Most of us at one time or another have slipped into a predominantly alpha state when we are day dreaming or looking at the glowing embers in our fireplace at the end of an arduous day as we start to drift off to sleep. Although our brain is always full of different types of waves, the alpha waves dominate while we watch television. We know that it is almost impossible to remain in an alpha state if one is paying visual attention or actively thinking about something. Perhaps this research only confirms what most of us knew intuitively, that TV like drugs or alcohol is a way to blot out the real world, to retreat into a nonthinking state where worry and anxieties are momentarily displaced.

As Anthony Burgess once pointed out, while hundreds of thousands die all over the world from lack of food, in this country it is a sign of poverty if one does not have a refrigerator. The poverty we individually seem most often to fall victim to is of the emotional or spiritual variety, but most Americans cannot bear to have that pointed out to them. Hence this mass escapism via the media of popular culture, especially television, which most viewers think is free. That, of course, is nonsense, for who do they think is paying the $30 billion each year in advertising but themselves? The world of television is a fantasy world.

Still, allowing a fantasy life to take a tremendous share of one's day does not seem to help those millions of Americans who are predominantly unhappy, bored with life, frustrated, frightened, or who compulsively tune in such programs as "The Price is Right," indulging some obsessive dream that they will win a new car or a trip to Las Vegas. Perhaps they use the fantasy world of the media to compensate for disappointments in their daily lives.

Day after day, year after year of this plastic view of life, of being the ultimate consumer, the sweet target of the Big Sell eventually breaks down the will of millions of Americans to live in any kind of creative way. They turn to the mass media as a magic mirror to tell them, "Oh, yes, you're the fairest one of all (or will be if you use enough Oil of Olay). You're John Travolta and Sophia Loren and tomorrow you'll win $1 million in the lottery." And I say that this is a cruel exploitation of the *anomie* that afflicts millions upon millions of Americans.

Granted that though very few of us go through life without some anxieties, low periods, and a variety of inner struggles, somehow, after a while, most of us manage to "hang in tough" and make a rational detente with the problems that are bothering us. Not so fortunate is that 15 percent of our population whose internal conflicts cause them so overwhelming a sense of turmoil that pathological behavior is almost inevitable, particularly when the source of the difficulty is often quite obscure and the symptoms that help is needed extremely hard to identify.

How do we spot one of the walking wounded who spends his lunch hour at an adult book store perusing the latest shipment of child pornography? The human scum who produce and distribute this particularly noxious form of mass medium are sometimes punished with a misdemeanor fine. But in a lawyer-wise society in which smoke screens about the First Amendment are bandied about with solemn protestations, it should not be forgotten that the $100 million spent on kiddie-porn contributes to our vaunted Gross National Product. This helps to pay the wages of a lot of people who work in paper mills or on the assembly lines of a factory that makes offset presses.

Whether the mediacracy is only the mirror for hundreds of thousands of acts each day that are violent, cruel, or pathological enough to interest or titillate the public, or whether they actually instigate such behavior begs the question. That the mass media, particularly television, are a major agent of socialization in the lives of children is beyond debate; that they become a fantasy substitute for reality by these same children when they grow into adulthood must also be considered.

As George Gerbner has shown in his long-range studies at the University of Pennsylvania, the content of television reinforces various cultural beliefs, and, likewise, the social realities of life are modified in the mind of the viewer by the image portrayed on the screen. Thus, Gerbner and Gross (1976) found that heavy viewers see the world in a much more sinister light than individuals who do not watch much television.

It is time now to offer some solutions rather than add detail upon detail to what may already seem too gloomy a jeremiad. Yet, we should recall that more than 50 years ago H. L. Mencken said essentially the same thing and this before radio and television became major factors in our mediacracy. "What ails the newspapers of the United States primarily," he said, "is the fact that their gigantic commercial development compels them to appeal to larger and larger masses of undifferentiated men, and that the truth is a commodity that the masses of undifferentiated men cannot be induced to buy" (Mencken, 1919, p. 104). This pessimistic evaluation of mediacracy was echoed by later critics such as Walter Lippmann and contemporary press critics such as Ben Bagdikian and Edward J. Epstein. If I concur, it is because the future indicates expansion of the basic corporate nature of the mass media with increasing conformity and depersonalization.

What can we do about the negative aspects of mediacracy? One thing seems certain to me: Any major solution will need to involve individuals and small groups, rather than for us to expect meaningful legislative action at the state or federal level. The most significant action would be to educate our citizenry about the patterns and practices of mediacracy. This educational process must begin very early in the child's acculturation, and I propose that the first or second grade in our public schools is not too soon. By the time the student has graduated from high school and watched 15,000 hours of television (as opposed to 12,000 hours total in his or her formal education) the narcotizing pattern of videocy is too well engrained; the mediacrats have them for the rest of their lives. Not every student, of course, but 80 to 90 percent of them.

We need to explore the ways that children can learn to be "critics" of the mass media, so that they can discern the banal and deleterious from those aspects of the media that indeed can be vivifying. With the help of some colleagues from the School of Education at my university who have expertise in primary grade curricula, I am trying to formulate this challenge into a plan of action. The best way not to be "hooked" on television, indiscriminately micturating away the days and nights of your life trying to escape from reality in tubal vassalage is to have a balanced concept of leisure.

There are other, more immediate, ways that we as individuals can show our distaste for mediacratic power. From the National Citizens' Council for Broadcasting in Washington, D.C., one can get the names of local groups in one's area who are equally concerned with the mediocre quality of television, as well as information on how to protest to a sponsor who endorses gratuitously violent programs. A small group of concerned viewers in Newton, Massachusetts, started Action for Children's

Television a decade or so ago, and it has become a strong, articulate foe of some of the more amoral practices of the television industry vis-à-vis children. The PTA Action Center in Chicago will send information about its successful campaign for less violence on television programs, and it also maintains a national toll-free hot line to answer questions about the television industry.

The Communications Act of 1934, which created the Federal Communications Commission, empowered the commission to grant licenses to serve the "public convenience, interest, or necessity." A television channel is an enormously lucrative prize worth millions of dollars in profit each year in scores of cities throughout this country. Those who are lucky enough to have secured such a license ought to be regarded not solely as owners of private property with which they can do what they want, but rather as trustees of public property, that is, the air waves, and they should be called on to meet the obligations of public trust.

The Federal Communications Commission is currently engaged in hearings relative to an updating of the 1934 act, which has been obsolescent for years. Some of the questions that might be considered but probably will not be because of the powerful lobby by the three major networks are:

1. Why not license networks as well as individual stations?
2. Why do the networks allow the sponsors and advertising agencies to influence the content of their programs? Should there not be a major stipulation in the networks' license renewal that they must pledge themselves to maintain full control over their programming? There are other media which live off advertisements but do not allow advertising agencies or sponsors to dictate or censor content, but not television. As long as television permits this practice we can expect its mediocre quality to continue.
3. Should not television licenses come up for annual renewal, instead of every three years? Those stations that fail to meet their obligations should have their licenses revoked, but in an agency, which for decades has been the preserve of political hacks, the FCC has, to my knowledge, only revoked one television license in its nearly 50 years of existence.

Do the people of this country want a better system than the present mediacracy? As long as the system relies on mass circulation figures, Nielsen ratings, or corporate earnings as the dominant criteria of success, the great majority of Americans will never know what a better system could be, any more than the people in Plato's cave knew the external realities of the world in which they lived.

It is good to remember that the meaning of the word *psyche* in its

Greek origin meant *soul* or *life* itself. So in a larger sense *psychopathology* signifies those elements in modern life which contaminate our spirit, as well as the more scientific meaning of mental illness. And yet that is exactly my point, even though I cannot muster a single chi-square or factor analysis to prove it. I believe that mediacracy in the United States by its lucrative pandering to the escapist tastes of Mencken's "undifferentiated masses" is, in this larger sense, responsible for much of the psychopathology that abounds. Perhaps you recall the myth about Psyche and the god Eros who fell in love with her. Despite the many ordeals inflicted by jealous Aphrodite, Zeus married the two lovers on Mount Olympus amidst great rejoicing. The day when the great power of the mass media is used for something beyond the glorification of Preparation H will be another occasion for joyous dancing on Mount Olympus.

References

Gerbner, G., and Gross, L. The scary world of TV's heavy viewers. *Psychology Today*, April, 1976, 42–43.

Gossage, H. The gilded bough: Magic and advertising. *Harper's Magazine*, May, 1961, 71–75.

Halberstam, D. *The powers that be.* New York: Random House, 1979.

Jaspers, K. *Vöm ursprung und ziel der geschichte.* Munich: R. Piper, 1949.

Mencken, H. L. *Prejudices: First series.* New York: A. A. Knopf, 1919.

Rilke, R. M. Spiegel: Noch nie hat man wissend beschrieben. From *Die sonnette am Orpheus.* Hamburg: Insel Verlag, 1923.

Siegel, B. T.V.'s effect from Alpha to Z-z-z. *Los Angeles Times*, March 11, 1979.

Wald, R. Speech at conference on "Television and Society," University of Southern California, November, 1978.

White, D. M. Popular culture: The multifaceted mirror. In D. M. White and J. Pendleton (Eds.), *Popular culture: Mirror of American life.* Del Mar, Calif.: Publishers Inc., 1978.

Themes and Variations

M. Brewster Smith

❖   First, our consensus, then, about the objectives of primary prevention in relation to political action and social change. I think we are very strongly agreed on this point. Slightly different language is used but the ideas seem to be synonymous. We are talking about the objective of *empowering* people, increasing people's options, giving them the potential to live their own lives to a fuller extent. So it is a matter of *quality of life*, but, as Betty Friedan puts it in the context of women's issues, it is not just a matter of *quality*: It is a matter of the extent to which people are really living. This goal is clearly related to how people handle their problems in living, although it may not be so directly related to some of the conventionally conceived mental illnesses. One set of related ideas that we did not talk about at the conference, which is closely related to our goals, is Seligman's increasingly rich conception of learned helplessness and the strategies for dealing with it, initiated in relation to animal models for the study of depression (see Seligman, 1968; Abramson, Seligman, and Teasdale, 1978). He has carried these ideas forward to become much more relevant to the challenge of empowering people to be "unhelpless" in their own lives.

A second consensus concerned the major locus of the problems of psychopathology, the place where prevention is most urgently needed. Here, we clearly agreed with the major thrust of the President's Commission on Mental Health: The problems of psychopathology are heavily concentrated among the poor, the oppressed, the powerless, the dehumanized, the stigmatized. Like the first consensus, this one involves our values but I think the facts here are quite incontrovertible. By whatever criterion of psychopathology you use, the powerless, oppressed segments of the population are where the most problems emerge and where typically the least service has been given.

The third area of consensus concerns the major obstacles in institutions and attitudes. Here we have three familiar labels, plus some parallel matters of concern: *racism*, which we have learned about from various angles in the papers by Hilliard, O'Gorman, and Clark; *sexism*, which Friedan has been calling to our attention; and *ageism*, as evoked in Robert Bin-

From M. Brewster Smith, "Themes and Variations," in Justin M. Joffe and George W. Albee (eds.) *Prevention Through Political Action and Social Change*. Copyright © 1981 by the Vermont Conference on the Primary Prevention of Psychopathology. Reprinted by permission.

stock's paper. But parallel with racism, sexism, and ageism, are, of course, the similar institutional and attitudinal barriers stigmatizing and ostracizing the handicapped, which Blatt has cataloged, and the class exploitation and economic oppression that many of the writers saw as underlying or related to other forms of oppression.

References

Abramson, L. Y., Seligman, M. E. P., and Teasdale, J. D. Learned helplessness in humans: Critique and reformation. *Journal of Abnormal Psychology*, 1978, *87*, 49−74.

Seligman, M. E. *Helplessness: On depression, development, and death.* San Francisco: W. H. Freeman & Co., 1968.

Tyler, L. *Individuality: Human possibilities and personal choice in the psychological development of men and women.* San Francisco: Jossey-Bass, 1978.

II. Effects of Powerlessness: The Victims

This section presents a series of illustrative excerpts describing the victims of our social system—including children (particularly those growing up in the ghettos of the inner city), people living in a sea of deprivation, people who are called retarded, and prison inmates. We include portraits of powerless mothers, and powerless women and children, who are victims of sexual abuse. Women and children are at high risk for many forms of psychopathology because of dependence; children react with emotional disturbance to multiple family stresses, as do children about whom society cares little (the retarded, the handicapped, the minorities, the sexually abused and exploited); also at risk are women who are targets of mass media messages suggesting that people get married and live happily ever after. We also present excerpts from descriptions of the adult sexual problems endemic in our society. This section on victims concludes with a major article by Elizabeth Taylor Vance, who examines the factors associated with high risk for low-status groups: women and inner-city minority groups.

The Education of the Oppressed Child in a Democracy

Ned O'Gorman

I remember, with a considerable chill, one summer I spent at the Aspen Institute of Humanistic Studies. I had been invited there to join in a seminar on the humanities with a rather awesome array of very powerful gentlemen. They were, nearly every one of them, but for a few like myself called to enlighten them in the way of the humanities, in "control" of something—conglomerates, universities, governments—here and abroad. They held certain of the world's secrets in their hands, they knew how to control oil, governments, land, power—physical and corporate—arms, the press. The corridors and plateaus of power were the loci of work for them as my nursery school in Harlem is for me. They lived in those charged and teeming landscapes with complete security but for one intrusion of the serpent.

The seminars in Aspen, for those of you who have not been there—I have been twice and I think I shall not be asked again—are microcosms of what must be the Platonic ideal of that universal gymnasium in the sky, where men meditate on the nature of man in the order of creation. During my visits there I was astonished to find how Aristotle and the Stock Exchange found themselves for moments in an easy, if idiotic, dialogue.

But the serpent intruded and the serpent was a word. The word was oppression. There in Aspen, in that idyllic landscape, the word was avoided, explained away, shunted into the Platonic shadows as if it were an obscenity. I spoke in that seminar and in the seminars that followed of the reality of oppression. But when I mentioned that word it drove my fellow seminarians into fits of rage, the moderators of the seminars into silence, and me into a quite ungentlemanly petulance and at one moment tears. From the most misty-eyed liberal it brought glances of suspicion and hostility. When I asked that the word be studied as we read, say, Machiavelli's *Prince*, it had to be watered down to a mild rhetoric: alienated,

From Ned O'Gorman, "The Education of the Oppressed Child in a Democracy," in Justin M. Joffe and George W. Albee (eds.) *Prevention Through Political Action and Social Change.* Copyright © 1981 by the Vermont Conference on the Primary Prevention of Psychopathology. Reprinted by permission.

marginated, poor, but never, never, never, oppressed peoples. If we agreed that the oppressed did exist, it meant that somewhere out there in the bush hid an army of discontented, angry, repressed creatures who might at any moment spring and destroy all the values the capitalist holds sacred. Somehow the democratic process, our democratic heritage—so ably (but for me simplistically) observed by Mortimer Adler there in Aspen—must have the power to cure whatever ills make a people troublesome, anxious, and marginated. The thought that the very *system itself* oppressed was an affront to the soul of capitalism and democracy.

I trust it will be clear to you now that I am using the word oppression in its most radical, simple sense: It is that process within a society that destroys life, inhibits life, makes growth, joy, celebration, family life, intellectual and spiritual life, physical life, impossible.

Oppression comes from many people, from many established and often trusted organizations: it comes from the churches, from the shopkeepers, from the government, from the courts, from the citizens, from the schools, from the very people oppressed. Oppression is in every society, somewhere in its fabric, a malignant power that must be destroyed. We ought now to reflect, perhaps, those of us for whom the liberation of our brothers and sisters caught in the embrace of death-in-life is the reason for our being, perhaps on those in our society who are the most oppressed of all: the children of the oppressed.

Since 1966 I have been working with those children and in their lives I have observed oppression and its gorgon-like energy establishing the dominion of death, ignorance, hunger, sickness, despair, hopelessness, sexual and imaginative chaos, and the annihilation of creatures of incredible beauty, an annihilation as sure in its mortal, final crushing power as the ovens of the Nazis were for the Jews, the rifle of the settlers in the west for the Indians, the armies of the Colonial powers for the Africans, or the landowners and the generals for the peasants of Brazil.

So, being wiser than my co-seminarians at Aspen, we can agree that oppression of people does exist in our society, and I do not think that anyone would disagree that of all the oppressed those with the least recourse to the law, to healing, are the babes, the very young, those in utero, those whose lives in so many aspects are settled, in style and in development, during the crucial years from birth until 3 or 4.

I came to Harlem with not an idea in my mind. I came to work with God's poor and that was all. I had just returned from a tour of Chile, Argentina, and Brazil for the State Department. During that journey I discovered that my country could not judge the malaise of oppression either in its own land nor in the land of others. It was blind to oppression and nurtured it rather than destroyed it. For me it was a terrible time of the rending apart of illusions. In South America I had the first glimpse of what we are doing now in Harlem. I remember a boy in Valparaíso sucking a gasoline soaked rag to keep the hunger that gnawed at him from driving him mad. That image returns to me rather often in my dreams.

My nursery school (I call it a liberation camp) is in Harlem because I must find a place to receive the children of the oppressed in that part of our democratic society that is called the East Harlem Triangle. Places like that "triangle" exist all over this world. I must insist that you try to understand that I see all people oppressed as people *oppressed*: I do not see the color of their skin; I see their oppression. I am in Harlem because that is where I am. I trust I could work with equal energy in Calcutta, in Belfast, in a village of poor whites in Kansas. But each day into that rather rickety house we call our school come 20 little children from one particular place on this earth. The youngest is 18 months, the oldest 5. My task is to educate them but I am not so naive as to think that the main thing I must do is teach them colors, numbers, letters, shapes and so on. They are very bright children and such learning will come easily to them. I must teach them how to survive, how to understand, reflect, observe, judge, react to the forces around them that are destroying them. It is a difficult task for the world is strong and the powers of oppression powerful beyond telling and the children who come to see me are cowed by oppression, frightened by what they see, but they are powerless to understand what is taking up lodging in them. I am a great admirer of Fernand Braudel, the prodigious historian of the Mediterranean, and a thought of his about the power of individuals on the great process of time and history is one that brings me up often upon the horror of history, its mammoth, tidal energy. Braudel writes:

By stating the narrowness of the limits of action, is one denying the role of the individual in history? I think not. One may have the choice between striking two or three blows: the questions still arise: Will one be able to strike them at all? To strike them effectively? To do so in the knowledge that only this range of choices is open to one? I would conclude with the paradox that the true man of action is he who chooses to remain within them and even to take advantage of the weight of the inevitable, exerting his own pressure in the same direction. All efforts against the prevailing tide of history—which is not always obvious—are doomed to failure.

So when I think of the individual, I am always inclined to see him imprisoned within a destiny in which he himself has little hand, fixed in a landscape in which the infinite perspectives of the long term stretch into the distance both behind him and before. In historical analysis as I see it, rightly or wrongly, the long run always wins in the end. (Braudel, 1973, pp. 1243–1244)

For you see, as I work with the children and try to bring them out of silence into the light of their childhood, I work against the demons and they are powerful. I do not know even if I have any effect on anyone. I wonder if I simply thrust my vision into the darkness and bring no light to that darkness.

As I think about the form that this change must take I know that if I propose too much no one will listen; if I propose too little I do no justice to my children; and if I do not work with what there is I will make no progress at all.

The education of the oppressed child in a democracy is a notion that has not yet been thought much about in American education. Paolo Friere, in the blazing perception of his pedagogy, seems congenial to me, but I know that for the most liberal of educators in this country he is remote and too difficult. The problem is "difficult," quite simply that. The depth of it is troublesome to the most optimistic of teachers. What must be formulated is a language, a science, a method. We are strangers in a landscape teeming with death and incredible forces of life.

How then do I see this problem of educating the oppressed child in a democracy? I can write only about what I have seen. I am not a teacher by training. I am a poet and that gives me perhaps one talent that all teachers ought to have: I have been taught to observe the world closely. The four children I shall describe now, very briefly, are typical of those who come to us. What I have seen is the basis for what I envision our task to be, as teachers of the oppressed.

Monica is 18 months old. When she came to us she could not smile. She could not respond to affection. She could not eat. She screamed and slept. Her parents are alcoholics. She is plagued with a perpetual cold, is in and out of hospitals with severe bronchitis. She is very beautiful and very intelligent. But the life she leads, is *forced* to lead, has damaged the core of her spirit.

Jerry is two. Twice he has come close to death. He is starved by his mother, beaten, abandoned. In his eyes there is the waste spaces of a shattered spirit. He is covered with burns and when he was once admitted to the hospital for an asthma attack he was infested with lice.

Lucy is four. She has been raped once and is now infected with gonorrhea.

John has seen his aunt shoot dope, observed an uncle attempt to murder his wife. He is one of the wisest children I have ever known. His ability, at age six, to hold a coherent conversation, to ask precise questions, and to take instruction is formidable. But already at this early year of his life I see his face change, his spirit wither.

Somehow I must heal him, all the children, as I teach them. So after 13 years of observation and work I began to see the beginnings of a method of healing. I will tell you of it, though it might anger some of you. It has angered my most liberal friends. But it has in it I think the germ of an approach to liberation of our oppressed children, though it must offend our most cherished democratic principles of privacy, individualism, and the sacredness of family, for it begins with the simple, universal premise that in all children if there is no opening to the world during the early years of childhood the future is doomed to tragedy. For the children of the oppressed the opening to the world is, I think, at once political, historical, imaginative, and rooted in the nature of oppression.

When John came to me at three years old he was an enraged child. I could not touch him, hold him, talk to him. I knew as I have suggested that he was a child of startling intelligence. I had to enter into his spirit somehow, so that I could free him into peace and a lucid intercourse with his own life and the life around him. I decided one day that I would talk to him about his life. I began each morning, when the memory of the past night was fresh, to question him about what had happened to him since he left our liberation camp the day before. I asked him what he had eaten, what he had heard. I asked him about his guardians, their friends, and what had occurred during meal time and afterwards. I asked him when he went to sleep, when he got up, what time he had breakfast, what television programs he had watched. I asked him what state his flat was in when he had gotten home. I asked him who stayed with him during the night (often he was left alone with his 2-year-old brother). At first he would say nothing. Then, slowly, he would tell me of beatings, drugs, sexual brutality among his kin, attacks by rats, overflowing toilets, midnight arrivals of police, sudden bizarre trips through the street with his mother in the dark of a storm.

What was happening to him? I was not ever really quite sure. I stood on shaky grounds. I was worried that perhaps I was harming him, forcing him to be disloyal to his family, perhaps forcing him to confront events that he could not properly understand. My coworkers were furious at me as I went about this search for John's response to his life. But I had to continue for I knew that I was on the right track. I knew that the brilliant child had to begin now to face head on the life he led. There was no time to waste. If I stopped what I was doing for fear that I was causing him harm, I would have had to wait until that time that would never come, when he would be "ready" to face the powers of darkness that possessed him and his life. No, I knew, I was certain, that now was the time to begin breaking down the fear, the terror, breaking them down by making him face them no matter how hard it was for him. I knew unless he began then to come up out of the depths of his oppression that he never would survive. He had to begin a process of learning that would bring him knowledge about the state of his life.

He had then, to begin then to understand his oppression. He lived in a world where *nothing was ever questioned, where nothing, no matter how brutal, how inhuman it might be, was ever judged*. No one he knew ever came to his defense, no one ever explained to him that what was happening to him was wrong. No one had ever told him that he was a creature with the right to survive, to grow, to endure, to be happy. He had no way to form a moral stance before evil and oppression. So I had, as I provoked him to talk, to create in him a larger view of the world; that is, I had to teach him to extend his understanding of himself to others. I thought that such an act from a 6-year-old would be impossible. I knew that I did not want him to hate those around him, though probably hating them would have been better than tolerating them. We were undergoing, the two of us, a process of enlightenment that had to transcend mere consciousness; that had to transform itself into an act of charity, self-awareness.

I waited. I had faith in that child. And one morning that faith bore fruit. It was perhaps the happiest day for me in the past year. John walked in and began, as he usually did, to tell me of the events that had happened to him during the night. He was filled that day with grisly tales. As he finished talking to me Lilly brought in her daughter. The child seemed especially still and sad. John looked at her, and after the mother had gone, sat beside her, and with the most extreme gentleness asked her if she were hungry. He asked her what had happened that made her seem sad. He asked her questions that brought him out of himself, into the presence of another.

I account that somehow a triumph. He began to communicate to another a sense of the world that he had gained for himself. He became lucid. He became a judge of what he saw and heard. He speculated. He wondered. He knew that what had happened to him might have happened to another. He entered into the world of other people. I think of Piaget's (1948) warning: "If there were not other people, the disappointments of experience would lead to overcompensation and dementia" (p. 206).

It is that regression into a spiritual and intellectual universe of mute and unintelligible signs and events that render our children at an early age paralyzed in spirit.

What I had worked toward with John was a radicalization of his being at those twin wellsprings of intellect and imagination. I moved him out of the darkness of a blind acceptance of what *was* into the light of a kind of verification of being, his being, at its most profound, at its holiest.

I must move John, and all the children, toward a revolutionary act of life amidst death. We must teach our children, those of us who teach the oppressed child, that they have not inherited the earth and that there are reasons why they have not inherited the earth. We must establish schools where the oppressed child is liberated. And this next year for John is one of eternal importance for him; his survival depends upon what happens to him next September. If that brilliant and good child enters the public schools he will either be judged unruly and/or retarded, or he will be ignored, or he will manage to rise above it all and triumph, or he will simply decline into sullen despair and fail.

Where then do we begin to change the schools that receive children like John? The challenge is so vast, so terrible in its consequences. I am quite ignorant of where one does begin. I would suggest perhaps we begin with the teachers. The schools do not yet have teachers trained in the psychology, history, and quality of oppression. We have good teachers in the public schools but there are not enough of them for whom liberation and learning is one act in any pedagogy of the oppressed. A teacher of oppressed children must receive them with the knowledge that they *are* oppressed, that each one's *life*, in all its variety, *is* in mortal danger: that liberation is the goal of teaching and that no matter how brilliant, well-intentioned and dedicated a teacher might be, to teach John must be to liberate him. I am not certain how I would train a teacher but I do know that John needs that teacher desperately.

The texts must be revised; the food the children eat in the schools must be prepared with the understanding that the children who come to the schools from the communities of the dispossessed are usually malnourished. The classrooms, the materials used in them, the whole shape and strategy of the day must be reviewed and fundamentally recharged with the goal of healing, radicalizing, and liberating the oppressed child from bondage.

I watch the children and until last spring I despaired of their life but now I think we are ready to take another step to assure them the possibility of survival. So we begin this fall, if all goes well, our own school, certified by the city, with a qualified day care teacher (I do not qualify since I did my studies in 16th century English literature) in a building on 129th Street in Harlem, a building now undergoing a renovation into a simple but beautiful space. I can see nothing else for me to do. If I am serious about the children who come to me, sometimes for four years, I must do more for their survival than cast them out into the public schools. If I do not build this school, this liberation camp, then I betray John and all the others, especially little Juliette who is 19 months.

With the help of our educational consultants, Bettye Caldwell and

Rosmary Lea from St. Bernard's school, we are now beginning the planning of our curriculum, or rather we are beginning our strategy of liberation for that is what we must do—liberate, strengthen, train our children, so that they can "overcome." As we teach them how to read we must do it so that they can read in a real and vibrant way the world around them. We must—as we teach them to spell, add, subtract, play—teach them to go deeply into their own lives and find there the forces that are poised ready to destroy them; go deeply into their lives, into their individual, solitary, private selves and find the strength to fight the oppression around them. I must teach them to believe in themselves, to question what is happening to them, judge what is happening to them often through the despair and oppression of their very kin.

But we are working in the dark for I do not think that what we intend to do has ever been done in quite this way before. To think that Paolo Friere, the phenomenal teacher of the oppressed decade will be of much help to the educational establishment in this land, even to its most liberal membership, is, as I have suggested, a dream. He is far too daring, far too dangerous. But we must talk to our children about the historical moment in which they live, as Friere does to the peasants of Pernambuco. We must talk to them of housing, crime, liquor, dope, anger, violence; we must make them ready to affirm life over death, hope over despair, joy over misery, family over sexuality, love over violence. Everything we do must be focused in an act of liberation. Nothing must be done in secret. Nothing must be done for window dressing to please parents, the government, foundations. Everything must be done to instruct our children in the methodology of survival. We will use what the world had to offer us: Mao, Mozart, Martin Luther King, César Chavez, Camus, Kant, Montessori, flowers, fish, blocks, the ballet, languages, maps, good food, paints. But we will use them all to create within the child the liberated spirit of the conqueror of oppression.

I trust that I have not offended anyone by suggesting that the education of our children must be different from any education given the middle class and by suggesting that in the suffering of the oppressed child is the seed of our methodology of liberation. Their imprisonment in a racist world is the first landscape of their freedom. It is there that they take their first step toward liberation. We must enter, with science and compassion, into the act of oppression in all its simmering horror. Only then will we understand.

I will conclude this meditation, this very tentative meditation, on the education of the oppressed with the stories of two women. They are intended to be parables.

Evelyn worked for me for one year. She was 20 years old then. One day I asked her to quarter and peel a dozen or so apples. I left her to do it and went out into the playground with the children. When I returned I saw that she had not gone far with her work but was struggling with a knife to dislodge something in the apple. I could not understand what she was trying to do. Perhaps I thought, there was a nail in it for I could think of nothing else that made sense. "There's something in there Ned, something hard." I took the apple and cut through it easily, and realized as I was doing it that she had hit the core with her knife and did not know what it was. She had never quartered an apple before, never gotten out the core and pits.

Lillian is a dope addict, a whore, a rotten mother, and all around, a very unpleasant woman. But she is brilliant, cagey and well spoken. I met her once walking down Madison Avenue. She was in bad shape and carried a notebook under her arm. I asked her what the book was and she said it was nothing, just something she had been doing for years. I asked if I could see it. She gave it to me and on the first page she had written: "Lillian's Knowledge Book." She told me that when she could not bear life any longer she would go to the public library and outline articles in the Encyclopedia that interested her. I left her and felt very rudimentary awe in my heart. I was furious at the schools, at the world, at her kin, for allowing that extraordinary desire for knowledge to rot so that all that was left was a notebook: Lillian, on the brink of the abyss and her note-book. Likewise, Evelyn and her muddle with the apple.

The work in our school is a parable, for we observe day in and day out, every season, in every kind of calamity, the holy signs of greatness, smoldering beneath the wrecked spirit. For Lillian and Evelyn, in their youth, the healing and the learning that they sought was denied them. To the world they brought not the power of their humanity, but silence and wasted glory. They were once the children of the oppressed. Now, their children come to me and leave me to enter the schools, the same ones their parents entered. But no, they will not fail for we have determined in our small and weak vision of our life that our children at 57 East 129th Street in Harlem, U.S.A. will be the healing and the healed of the oppressed, the revolutionaries, the heroes, the heroines, the liberated.

References

Braudel, I. *The Mediterranean and the Mediterranean world in the age of Philip II.* Vol. 2. New York: Harper & Row, 1973.

Piaget, J. *Judgment and reasoning in the child.* Totowa, N.J.: Littlefield, Adams & Co., 1948.

Talking to Your Children's Souls: Portraits of Deprivation

Thomas J. Cottle

One could very appropriately call the last few decades in America the period of self-consciousness. The term, of course, is a complicated, almost mischievous one. To be self-conscious can connote self-interest to the point of wasteful vanity. On the other hand, it may connote a careful, cautious, discerning approach to all matters, private as well as public. Surely the last years have revealed Americans—or some of them—reveling in excessive, narcissistic behavior. Self-interest has been glorified, and whether or not we admit to it, there is not a great deal of incentive across the society for generous, much less openly altruistic, behavior.

Consonant with this philosophy, or overriding life style, the most needy people in our country have seen very little progress in the state of their well-being. Governmental policies at state and federal levels come and go, but whatever the effects, planned or unplanned, of these programs, a sizable group of poor people remains. Moreover, given the way contemporary programs are run, a sizable population of poor people will continue to exist. There is no longer need to recapitulate the familiar statistics nor human scenes of poverty. Indeed even as I write these words I recognize their familiar ring and the normal response made to them. Yet, a rather intriguing aspect of America's so-called needy classes now presents itself. For if one looks across the social and economic boundaries of the culture, one finds a truly extraordinary panoply of variegated peoples, all of them having one thing in common: The belief that their respective group, if not they themselves as individuals, has been deprived. Surely the very poor of the land feel this, but quite remarkably, one hears the same refrains of deprivation among families of all social classes. They have been excluded from some prized resource or something. They are out of touch with some liberal agency or seat of power, or they feel, somehow, separated from mystical, magical powers. Again, people of all

From Thomas J. Cottle, "Talking to Your Children's Souls: Portraits of Deprivation," in Justin M. Joffe and George W. Albee (eds.) *Prevention Through Political Action and Social Change.* Copyright © 1981 by the Vermont Conference on the Primary Prevention of Psychopathology. Reprinted by permission.

classes and circumstances seem to feel they have lost out, or are lost in the pursuit of their real and imagined life goals. Or perhaps they harbor some actual or primitive competitive sense and have determined that given the society's standards of accomplishment or worth, they have lost. The loss, moreover, is irrevocable and puts them in the difficult position of being separated from successful people, truly affluent or comfortable people.

Driving this sense of loss and separation is the belief that one is legitimately entitled to, well, something, or more than one has. Politics, social history, one's origins, the degree of one's loyalty to country, years of hard and thankless work, anything and everything may be invoked to justify one's sense of entitlement, a sense not so incidentally, born from the public virtue of individualism or individually based achievement. One man, one vote, quickly becomes transliterated to: I am, therefore I am entitled. As a result of this clamoring for what one believes one is entitled to, the entire structure of political action, seemingly, has been transformed. National mass movements of a voluntary nature are far more difficult and treacherous to establish than they were even a decade or so ago. Now, as Theodore Roszak (1978) points out, we seem to have an endless chain of voluntary associates, each with his or her own special political concern and focus, each feeling his or her rights have been jeopardized or compromised, and each feeling his or her own political claim is utterly legitimate, whether or not it touches upon the political legitimacy or claims of the next in line.

To be sure, many of these political associates transact their business as if they were merely calling attention to themselves, which, I suppose, is a first step of political reform. Some, moreover, act as if the look-at-me aspect of their work constituted the entirety of their politics. But whatever their claims and strategies, it cannot be denied that they all are claiming they have been victimized by large-scale, planned, and systematic deprivation. In a word, they lack something, usually some fundamental right, and in many cases, when one examines their situation, one can feel sympathetic to their cause. In many cases, furthermore, one is impressed by the leaders of these voluntary associates, whose number and variety would have surprised even Alexis de Tocqueville, who saw in America's voluntary associations the genuine strength of America's political energy. Indeed, the string of voluntary associations is extraordinarily impressive, despite the selfish, or highly self-interested, or even solipsistic nature of individual political struggles.

No one, clearly, can set forth with objectivity and disinterest, a hierarchy of America's political needs or list America's most deprived populations. Self-interest dominates our culture to uncontrollable degrees. We are, in many respects, a culture reeling out of control, partly because of the irreconcilable nature of our excesses and deprivations. We reel from the bureaucratic neutrality foisted upon us, from institutions that literally revel in dehumanizing processes and policies, and from still unsolved matters of racism, poverty, and colonialism. In a sense, America has not found itself and has not yet determined just what age it would like to be, much less what it believes it ought to be when it grows up.

Still, on the subject of deprivation, it is my impression that the various political voluntary associations, or even the innumerable political and social groupings, have recently tended to act much like siblings competing with each other for some real or imagined parental attention. No, this is not precisely the case. In fact, the very poor of the country and a certain portion of the country's minority families have now passed through an era—as short lived as most American eras—where it seemed as if they were receiving, not only the attention, but the benefits all people covet. Against the background of an omnipresent racism and a generalized disgust for and with poverty, most Americans could tolerate popular political movements aimed at redressing the inequities of poor and minority people. But only up to a point. After a time, the country responded in a sense to the antipoverty and black movements with a resounding "We want it, too." A reaction to the poverty programs was set in motion. If some groups were getting special attention and additional resources, then why could other groups not enjoy a commensurate amount of attention and resources. The majority of Americans resented poor and minority populations before our brief period of attention to these families, and they resented them even more intensely as they saw them actually having some of their demands met. Compounding the problem was the belief, sometimes legitimate, sometimes invalid, that benefits were accruing to some populations at the direct expense to other populations. In many cases, however, the resentment of another person receiving some minimal attention only exacerbated many people's contention that they were the truly overlooked souls of the earth, the genuinely dispossessed people.

❖   The first life study is that of a young American boy and it addresses the matter, the business really, of medical care, or the lack of it.

The second story is of a young West Indian girl who lives in London. Though some might automatically assume that we perhaps "contaminate" our data and exegesis by focusing on a foreign case, I think in fact just the opposite holds true: The account of Doreen Grainger just may sum up the spiritual pain of economic deprivation in the most universal of terms. Besides, an occasional glance at Europe, a glance that may burgeon into what we call cross-cultural research, can only inform us and give us a perspective on our own lives, as well as provide us with a sense of how extensive and rapacious is this thing called poverty.

❖   Wilson Diver is the smallest, thinnest, and most frail-looking of the nine Diver children. At 12, he looks younger than his 11-year-old sister Theresa and his 10-year-old brother Curtiss. On meeting Wilson for the first time, everyone believes he is either on his way to a hospital or has just come out of one. His mother, Mrs. Claudia Diver, claims the boy eats as much as his brothers and sisters and has the energy of his brothers and sisters, but that he just looks sickly most of the time. It does not help young Wilson's condition that he and his family are among the poorest families in Massachusetts.

It was very clear to Claudia Diver that her eighth baby, even at birth, was not as strong as the others. Wilson had a fine disposition and seemed to walk and talk at the normal time, but he was, somehow, an unwell child. The first sign of illness came when he was two, when for weeks at a time he would lie in his crib whimpering, unable to breathe, and running high temperatures. As he grew up, these bouts of asthmatic bronchitis—as they later were diagnosed—came more frequently, eight, nine times a year. Wilson would show the beginning signs of a cold. He would cough and sneeze and find his nose running. Then, usually at night, the coughing became unbearable. He would cough without respite until his chest would sag and deep rings lined his eyes. He could not talk, and by flaring his nostrils and opening his mouth, he barely got sufficient air into his lungs. The cold weather made his life miserable, particularly at night when there was no heat in the Diver apartment. There was no way to keep him warm or provide him with any relief. His mother would prop him up in bed and hold him while she and his sleepy brothers and sisters would stare at him, expecting him, surely, to die at any moment. No one could believe how sick Wilson could become in such a short time. One day he was fine, the next morning he would show symptoms of a cold, and by that night he would look to be on the brink of death.

Wilson was examined once by a medical student in the large hospital six miles from the Diver house. The doctor said that he heard nothing in Wilson's chest to indicate a chronic problem. "Some kids," he told Mrs. Diver, "are just susceptible to pulmonary and bronchial complications when they get sick." He prescribed medicine to use the next time Wilson became ill. The medicine seemed to help; at least it gave Wilson relief in breathing. Strangely though, it also seemed to stimulate him so that he was unable to sleep. Mrs. Diver had to decide which was more important, relief in breathing or sleep.

By his 12th year, Wilson was more than used to his periodic illnesses. He did his best to avoid catching colds, but he simply was more susceptible to them than anyone he knew. No matter how warmly he dressed or wisely he ate, the infections got to him. Claudia Diver kept promising she would move the family to a warmer climate, for she had relatives in Birmingham, Alabama, but her shortage of money never allowed for this. There was no way she could find a job as good as the one she held in the small wool factory near her home. "Wilson has survived this long," she said, "and he's getting bigger and stronger. He'll survive the rest of the way. Has to."

In February, two months before Wilson's 13th birthday, he became sick again. All the usual signs appeared; the unstoppable coughing at night, the runny nose and eyes, the pains in the sinus areas behind his cheeks and forehead, chest aching from strain and fatigue. This time, however, the infection seemed to hang on longer than ever before, and a new symptom was present. Early one morning, Wilson grew nauseated and began to vomit violently. Even when he had rid his stomach of its contents, a muscular reflex continued, and he gagged until he felt he would expel his lungs. Blood appeared in the vomit.

Awakened by the sounds of Wilson retching and crying, McCay, his older brother, found him in the bathroom and promptly woke his mother. At six o'clock in the morning the family decided that, as difficult as it would be, they had to take Wilson to the hospital. A portion of the hospital trip was described by Wilson himself several months later:

"First we called the police, you know, and they said they couldn't send nobody 'round to our house 'less we could prove it was an emergency. McCay said I should get on the phone and cough for 'em. He wasn't joking neither. But they wouldn't come out, so we went down to the corner and waited for the bus. It was so cold out there we might as well froze together. Everybody was standing around me, trying to keep me warm, you know. Must have had ten coats and jackets on me. And I kept up this gagging and choking I was doing. So after half an hour, the bus comes, and we get on.

"Then we had to transfer to another bus, and finally we got there. We were real early too, but this waiting room they got there was crowded with people, it was like we were going to a bus station or something. Every chair was filled up. Some old man, you know, gave his seat to my mother, but McCay and me, we sat on the floor. Place was cold too, man, and there wasn't nothing to eat. They had a real nice water fountain, I remember.

"Now here's the truth: we must have got there by eight o'clock, and we didn't talk to no one, no one, man, 'til eleven, or maybe later. And that was this woman who took our names and stuff like that, you know. She wasn't even a nurse! She was just taking our names. And the place was getting more crowded every minute. You should have seen the people coming in there too, man. Broken legs, and bleeding. They brought this one guy in on a table and they said he died. Man died there after the doctors saw him.

"So then, like at twelve, maybe, the woman calls our name and we go up to this desk, and she tells my mother we don't have the right kind of insurance. She needed to prove where she worked or something, but anyway, McCay has to go all the way home and get this card, like, that proves she can come to the hospital, that we live in the neighborhood. And 'cause we don't have no telephone we can't call up at home, and anyway no one was home 'cause they was all at school.

"So McCay goes and he comes back, this time with the police. He just went there and told him his problem and this cop gave him a ride all the way. Now it's like one thirty and I ain't seen no doctor yet. Finally they get all the stuff straightened out on the papers. Oh, here's what it was. They thought it would be better for my mother to say she was on welfare than to say she had a job. It worked out better for me and them if they did it like that. So they did. She didn't care none, she just wanted me to see the doctor 'cause I wasn't getting no better. Finally, they call my name and I see this doctor. He tells me to take off my shirt and lie on a table, one of those tables like that guy died on, only this one had a clean sheet. So I get on the table and I'm thinking to myself, this doctor looks too young. And it's cold in this hall they got me in too, 'cause it's not a room, it's just a hall with a sheet hanging down from the ceiling to kind of hide me, you know what I mean. Then the doctor goes out and he don't come back. I'm lying there with my shirt off freezing. So finally I get up and walk out and ask somebody, can I put my shirt on and this man there he say, 'you can put your hat on for all I care. If you can walk and ask questions you ain't sick enough to be in no emergency room.' So I get disgusted and go back to my little sheet room in the hall, you know, and get dressed.

"While all this is going on, McCay goes home 'cause he's so hungry he can't stand it no more. But he asked someone before he left, how come no one's helping *me*, and the woman tells him it's her job to choose which people coming into the room look sickest. I guess since I didn't look that sick to her she kept me waiting. So then I go out again and tell someone I'm really hungry, man. This time it's a doctor, and he looks at this little piece of paper they had me carrying with me and he say, 'You've been vomiting, so you better not eat.' When I went back again to my sheet room I saw the clock said five thirty. Still nobody had come to see me.

"You ain't going to believe that nobody came until six thirty. Then this other doctor comes, not the first one, but a different one, and he's looking so tired, and he's talking to so many people he looks sick himself. So he say, 'Take your shirt off Mr. Wilson.' I say, 'My *first* name's Wilson.'

He don't hear me. He's got that thing in his ears already and he's starting to listen on my chest and on my back. Then he lays me down and pushes his hands so hard on my stomach I thought he was going to kill me 'stead of cure me. Then he asks if I'm hungry. I say I ought to be, haven't eaten since last night. So he gives me this hard candy he's got in his pocket, and he tells me where he buys it and pats my face. Nice guy.

" 'How you feel?' he say. I tell him I want to go home. 'You're going to be fine, Wilson my boy,' he say. 'You're going to be good as new. You just got to eat my special candy.' Man, did I feel good after that. I ask him, 'Can I go, doc?' 'Hold still a bit longer,' he say. All this time he's writing on a sheet of paper. 'You got a phone number?' he say. 'No.' 'What's your address?' I tell him. 'Now can I go?' 'Hold still,' he say. Tough too. So now I have to wait some more. But when he leaves he promises me he'll come right back. 'Don't worry.' Then he leaves and I hear him tell this nurse there's a boy in there who's very sick. We got to find him a bed. I didn't know what he meant. Then I figured maybe they want me to go to the hospital 'cause I wasn't fine, and I started to cry. Real soft 'cause I didn't want no one to find me. When nobody came back I put my shirt on for like the tenth time and went out to get my mother, but she was gone. The room wasn't crowded no more, neither. Then I really got scared. But there was this new woman there and she had a note saying my mother would come back and I shouldn't worry. Shouldn't worry, why not? They wanted to put me in the hospital, which meant I was real sick. I'd been there all day and only one person saw me and he only was there a couple minutes. 'Course he gave me that candy which was my breakfast, lunch and dinner. They did give me *that*! So then I waited some more.

"Then, like about ten o'clock in the night, a nurse comes in the room where they got the television to say a policeman's outside waiting to take me home. She says I should be in the hospital and they've been waiting for a bed to open up, but since they had no room they was sending me home. Before I left she had to take some blood from me which hurt, man, like out-of-sight pain! 'You going to drink it?' I say. 'I been here all day, lady,' I told her. 'Me, too,' she say. Angry old bitch. Anyway, the cop took me home! I fell asleep and the cop had to carry me into the house. Everybody was asleep 'cept my mother and McCay. They tried to get back to the hospital, but the buses wasn't running no more. That was the longest day of my life, man. Started out with me vomiting up my lungs, ended with a policeman carrying me home. I knew I had to go back to the hospital. I told my mother, couldn't she find a better hospital? She say they were all the same, and anyway, this one had my records. I was doomed, man. I told McCay: 'If I go back there I'm going to die,

man. Hospital's going to kill me off just by all that waiting.' My mother
told me not to talk that way, but McCay, he say 'Wilson's right. What
about that man we saw who died on the table like the one they put Wilson on!' My mother told him to shut up, but he was right. Only I didn't
want nobody to talk about it like he did. He didn't have to go back there
like I did."

Ten days after Wilson Diver's examination, the hospital sent a letter to
Mrs. Diver saying that the results of his blood tests indicated that Wilson
should enter the hospital for further tests. The hospital would notify the
Divers when a bed was free, but it would be helpful if they could return
to the hospital before that time for a chest X ray. It was three weeks before the X ray was taken.

"This time," Wilson said, "I only waited three hours, only I was by
myself. But it was all right 'cause I didn't have to go to school all that
day. People were nice to me too. The woman remembered me from before. 'Bout a week later they wrote to my mother saying they had a record of me coming in for X rays but no record of the X rays. So I had to
go back all over again. And you got to remember that each trip to the
hospital, man, takes about two hours, if you don't have to wait too long
for the buses. Each time you got to wait outside in the cold, you know
what I mean, and you're getting so cold you don't know whether to go
on or go back. One time I went back and told my mother I went. Then I
had to cut school another day so I could go for real. So they did the same
X ray all over. I was feeling how my chest seemed to be getting smaller.
For a while I was thinking so much about going to the hospital and worrying about if I was sick, I didn't even think about *being* sick. But I never
vomited again like I did that one night. I just couldn't shake my cold, you
know. It was stuck to me, like I was going to have it forever. I don't
know. Maybe I will."

Four months after his first examination and the decision to hospitalize
him, Wilson Diver was admitted to the hospital. He was placed in a
room with five other boys. New doctors examined him this time; he
rarely saw the same doctor twice. A third chest X ray was taken and a
variety of medical tests performed. On the third afternoon of his hospitalization, Mrs. Diver was called into the doctor's office on the second
floor for consultation. Her son was suffering with pulmonary problems,
she was told. But there was more. The X rays had revealed a spot on his
right lung which indicated tuberculosis. Furthermore, while the doctors
were not certain, several tests suggested the possibility of his also having
leukemia, although it was, hopefully, a treatable form. He also was malnourished. As Claudia Diver reports it, the doctor was stern but helpful
He was about to remonstrate with her for the way she had failed to pro-

vide her son proper medical attention. But after looking at her, he had stopped himself. She did not have to explain Wilson's circumstances, or her own.

No one could rightly argue that Doreen Grainger is a dreamy child, a child who fantasizes more than she approaches life realistically. To be sure, Doreen, 11 years old, one of six children living in a three-and-a-half-room flat in Clapham, spends a great deal of time by herself, just sitting and thinking. Her family reports that she does; she admits she does. But when I ask her if she is willing to share some of her feelings and thoughts of these private moments with me, we both can see there is nothing dreamy or fantasy-like about them. One could say that much of what she contemplates is fantastic. I have told her this on numerous occasions, but she doubts my words.

No, she tells me again and again, her interest lies in the study of history. She is fascinated with the events of long ago and the people who preceded her in time. She reads history books for children, mainly ones on the history of England, and one of her most common expressions is "in the olden days." In the olden days, she will begin a sentence, sounding very much like a school teacher, the people carried their goods to the market place on animals. Then, misinterpreting the expression of fascination and delight on my face as doubt, she will invariably add, "It's true. Really. It's true. They used animals, like donkeys." All of this is said in the calm, placid, but hardly emotionless manner that is so characteristic of her.

Her brothers and sisters as well as her parents are well aware of her placid way and the sense of inner peace that emanates from her. Everybody notices it. She is a placid child, not passive, retiring, without feeling, merely calm. One relaxes in her presence and feels one's own irritabilities and anxieties receding. There is always time with Doreen Grainger, always enough hours in the day to do what has to be done. The single day seems to be long enough for one to fulfill one's projects and dreams, not that Doreen is wholly optimistic about all the outcomes. No one living in the poor circumstances she has always known could be wholly optimistic. It is simply that at this point in her life, she rarely reveals impatience or despair, or even intense personal frustration. If she does not reveal enormous displays of energy, it just may be that she is storing up her strength for use sometime in the future. And, while it may seem ironic that a child fascinated with history should be storing up her reserves for future use, Doreen herself would not think so. She would say: I am certain, that no one can plan for the future, much less attempt to catch glimpses of it, without concentrating long and hard on the past. So her involvement with time, and history in particular, seems perfectly right for her, and perfectly natural.

As is always the case when one offers only samples, snippets really, of what a person has said in many conversations, much of the richness of thought and language is lost. Not only that, but even by presenting extended passages of speech, a person still may come across in a somewhat thin or unfinished way. Speaking with some people causes me to feel this reservation intensely; one of these people is Doreen. In recalling what she has said, I often fear I have omitted too much or not caught precisely enough the delicacies of her associations and combinations of thoughts. Perhaps this is because she has a peculiarly acute sense of time, which means a special alertness to the sequence of events and possible causation. It is not bending the truth to say that the large majority of our conversations focus on matters of time, however implicitly they may be drawn. But her awareness of and concern with the predicaments of England's black communities is never far from the surface of these conversations. We share many interests in common, Doreen and I, and while she describes feelings and attitudes for me which she believes are what *I* am looking for—as if I always knew what I was looking for—she is also eager to tell me what matters most to *her*. Here then is a sample of what this child, my friend of two years, has told me.

The words that follow are taken from a recent conversation in which Doreen's normal calmness seemed more brittle than ever before. It seemed to me that anger was trying to break through her usually peaceful nature.

"I was thinking," she said that afternoon, "about what it must be like when people die. I keep thinking—probably they put you in a grave and you don't feel anything. At least that's what people say, you don't feel anything. But what if you do? What if dying means feeling everything, but you can't get anything to move, like your eyes and your mouth, so you can't say, stop putting me in the grave. I can hear you, just don't bury me. What if too, when people die with their eyes open, they can see? Only nobody knows they can because their eyes never move and they can't tell anybody what they're seeing. If people can't talk when they're dead, how do we know what dying is? Maybe people are lying in their graves still thinking about things. It could be, nobody knows for sure. Even my mother said it *could* be true. I was thinking, maybe I like to read history so when I die, if I can still think, I can think about all the things that went on before I was born and after I was born, too.

"Some children are afraid to die, but I'm not afraid. They think it's awful to die, so they never think about people long ago dying, or think of themselves getting older and older and pretty soon dying. I don't think about it all that much but sometimes I'm afraid of getting older and not just because when you get old you get sick, and your body gets stiff. And you cough a lot. What I worry about is that, like, I have many things I want to do with my life, many people I would like to be, you know. Then I get worried, maybe there won't be enough time. Maybe I'll start too many things too late, then I'll run out of time. My mother laughs at me when I talk this way. She says, there's enough time; children should never worry about things like that. But all I ever hear *her* talking about is how there's never enough time and she'll be dead before she knows it. So she tells me one thing and herself something different. And she isn't *that* old. She thinks she is, but she isn't. People, I hear, they always tell each other, oh, you aren't that old. Then the other person says, I don't care how old I am, I *feel* old and that's all that matters. Well, I feel old lots of the time. People think children only think about getting old but never that they're old. But everybody is only as old as they are, so they feel *that* old. Children can die too. Adults forget this.

"You know what I think? I think families that don't have lots of money always feel older than they really are. Maybe it's like no one gives them a chance to be children. They pretend they're children, and everybody pretends to treat them like children, but everybody knows they aren't regular children. In the old days they made children work. Then they had laws that said they couldn't work that way any more. But the children who live around here, they do all the same things other children do, except the rich children who have their own houses and things like that; but I don't think they're really children, like children are supposed to be. You remember before when I told you I think sometimes there isn't going to be enough time for me to do all the things I want to do? Well, children like us, we're afraid too many things are going to happen that are going to make it bad for us. So that's what we worry about some of the time. Most children, though they don't think like that. They do whatever they want or whatever they have to do, and don't care about what happens to them all that much. But we can't do that. We have to worry about it or pretend there's nothing to worry about.

"So we act like we're children, which *is* what we are, but we don't always feel like children because we're worrying about those other things. I think maybe I like history because I'm afraid to find out what's going to happen to me. Or maybe something even worse; maybe I already know what's going to happen to me.

"See what's important about history is that you can sort of be alive when you weren't really alive. That's why teachers should tell you about the people who were alive then, and not just the *things* that happened. Because then you can pretend that you were alive too, when they were alive, or you'll pretend that you will be alive when you know you won't be alive any more. You can pretend that what's going to happen when you're not here is what happened to people a long time ago when you weren't here either. That way, learning about history is like making believe you could live three different lives instead of just one life: The life you have, the life people had before you were born, and the life people are going to have after you die. So you can know about things and pretend about things too. Maybe things have always been the same; I don't think so, but maybe for some people they are. But people don't look like they did millions of years ago, so how could other things be the same?

"I was just thinking, maybe what I want to know about history is whether everything will be for my family like it is now. I mean, it's fun to know about other people, but I want to know whether it will always be like this for me and my family. And then how will it be when I get older, and then very old. Nobody can see the future, but they can see what history was like, only not the kings. The kings don't tell me anything about me, or anybody I know. They only tell what it's like for the important people, like in government. Maybe that's why we study them, because the rich people in government like the kings, they tell the rest of us how we have to be. One thing that isn't fair is just reading about the rich people who lived long, long ago. They, for sure, don't tell me anything about me or people like us. All you have to do is figure out a little what happened to your own family long, long ago, and you know *that's* never going to happen. I guess history makes me sad sometimes.

"My mother says, you never know what tomorrow will bring. That's the wonderful thing about going to sleep every night. But why does she say that when we all know what tomorrow's going to bring? Tomorrow's going to bring another day like today, and yesterday. So who she trying to kid? She gets me wound up when she talks like that. She must know she is too, and there she is always telling us, no matter what we do or say, we must never lie to anybody and especially to people in our family. But she's doing it. She's lying, and it's not because she wants us to go to bed on time. She could tell us a million other things to get us into bed. My father does. He tells my brother Frederick every night: If you don't get into that bed in one minute I'm going to pull down your pajamas and whack your backside. It gets him in bed all right.

"So why does my mother lie? I'll tell you why. Because no matter what she tells us, she knows nothing is ever going to get better for us. She pretends by saying you never know what tomorrow will bring that maybe she won't know, but she knows. She tells us how nothing will ever be better for her, which would be all right if she knew it was going to be better for us. But she thinks she's going to die with the world being just as bad for us as it is for her now and when she was a child. All she's doing is telling us a fairy story so she can get us into bed, but the rest of the time she'll tell her friends, how is it ever going to be better.

"So maybe that's why I worry a lot of the time. If she says it's going to be tomorrow and tomorrow and tomorrow like it is today, then why should I grow up at all? Or if it's going to be the same when I'm an adult like it is now, then it's like I'm already an adult, and that means I'm an adult and a child—a little adult, that's all. Now that kind of thinking is much more scary than wondering what it's like to die. I can't even figure out what it's like to be alive. You could tell me all children think like I do, but I wouldn't believe it. I know they don't, especially rich children. You ask them if they think tomorrow, or when they grow up, they're going to be living just like they're living now? They'll say, oh no, I'm not. I'm going to be living here, or I'm going to be going there and doing this. Maybe I'll keep changing where I live and what I do. That's the kind of thing they'll tell you. But the kids that live near me, they might tell you those same things, but they know they're only making up those words because that's the way children *like* to think. That's how we're different from them. When I'm pretending, I *know* I'm pretending. I could tell you when I grow up I'll have lots of houses and travel all over the world like the Queen, but I know I'm telling you a big lie. And I can't really be all that happy when I know I'm telling you a lie, even if you asked me to tell you what I'm going to do when I get older. Or, I could say, well, I don't know, come back and see me in twenty years, and you and I will both know what I did, or what I'm doing then. But you don't need to come and see me in twenty years. Because if I'm alive I'll know where I'll be and what I'm doing. I won't be able to leave England. Where could I go? Maybe they'll make us go somewhere, but I hope not, because this is where I come from and this is where I should be. I bet if you come to see me in twenty years you won't have any trouble finding me because I bet I'll be living where I live right now. Nobody I know moves away. Some new people come in and live near us, but nobody moves away. My father always says, if people like us are moving away, it means either they're giving up for good, or they're foolish enough to think there's a better chance for them somewhere else. They pretend maybe there's a good thing waiting for them somewhere, but all they're doing is pretending so they can feel better about themselves. I say if they're pretending, then they're acting more like children than we are.

"I know everything about the future because I find out about history. I don't think the world changes so much. That's another thing people want to pretend about, that everything is changing, getting worse, or getting better. It stays the same, that's why I know for sure what's going to be. When you live around here, the most exciting thing sometimes is to wonder whether this might be the day when you're going to die. I know that sounds like a horrible thing to say, but it isn't. It's true.

"We see the same people everyday, and the same places, and most of us keep thinking the same things and saying the same things. I know people who read, and all they do is read the same thing over and over again. The newspapers are always the same, and the telly is always the same. People get so cross when they change shows on the telly. They want to know that every Monday is the same as every other Monday. They change shows and people get upset. But you know when they get excited? When someone dies, like in a fire, or a little baby, or some old person. That's the only thing that gets people even a little interested. They come running into the streets, and they talk louder and make a lot of noise which is different from the way they usually are. Maybe they don't *want* people to die, although it sure looks like they do when you see how they act when someone's been killed, like in an accident. That's all everybody talks about. And that's because their lives are so boring.

"Sometimes I hope something horrible will happen, too. I mean, I don't wish it, but I say to myself, it's about time for something exciting to happen. I mean, I don't *want* anybody to get hurt, but I know if they do we can all get excited about it. You see all these people sitting in front of the windows, you know. They have their tellys on, but they rather look out the window, just in case something happens they wouldn't want to miss it. It might be the most exciting thing that ever happened to them. I wouldn't want to miss it either. When I get to be my mother's age, I'll probably *really* feel this way. I don't want you to think the people 'round here are mean. It's just they don't have anything else to be interested in. They never go anywhere, they never do much of anything except be at home and go to work. I don't blame them. Maybe I wish they were different, but I don't see how they could be. No one lets them do what they want to do, so what else *can* they do? They don't *want* to be the way they are; they just are. They know they're never going to be any different, even if there was excitement in the streets every day of their lives. All it is is a little excitement; it doesn't make anyone change."

References

Cottle, T. J. *Busing*. Boston: Beacon Press, 1976.
Cottle, T. J. *Barred from school*. Washington, D.C.: The New Republic Book Co., 1976.
Cottle, T. J. *Children in jail*. Boston: Beacon Press, 1977.
Cottle, T. J. *Black testimony*. London: Wildwood House, 1978.
Roszak, T. *Person/planet*. New York: Anchor Press, Doubleday, 1978.

The Case of Sophie

Burton Blatt

❖
...While there may not be a law or regulation allowing a given practice, there does not seem to be very much precedent forbidding it. Or conversely, while there may not be something on the books forbidding a practice, it does not seem to be in good taste. Some examples of quasi-legal practices in the field of mental retardation must certainly include the continued approval of sterilization, inmate employment without compensation, and assignment of the recently deceased as medical school cadavers.

For many years, I have written about all of this and more. Indeed, I have spent the last 20 years cataloging virtually every type of legal, illegal, and quasi-legal abuse perpetrated on the mentally retarded. I have described the work of the cadaver committee in a New England city, sterilization practices at various state schools; the pulling of teeth of inmates who bite themselves or others; the pulling of plugs at distinguished medical centers; other premature or strange deaths, even stranger autopsy investigations; peonage in its almost infinite forms; a severe spastic choking to death on a whole hard boiled egg; a severely retarded bed patient nearly bleeding to death after his groin was ripped open by an assailant in the night and he was not seen by a doctor until morning infirmary call; inmates involuntarily volunteered for dangerous experiments at Ivy League medical schools; children raped by older inmates; and older inmates brutalized by marauding adolescents. And of course, although many of these atrocities could have been classified as illegal and the perpetraters could have been prosecuted, they hardly ever were; there is hardly a disruption of institutional routine when such situations occur.

I rummaged through my files, but there seemed nothing new to say about quasi-legal practices. Yet, I knew that I must say something. The very idea of "least restrictive environment" was born out of a history of quasi-legal practices applied to people. I then went to my diary, which is used, if anything, as a last resort. I knew exactly what I was looking for,

From Burton Blatt, "Bureaucratizing Values," in Justin M. Joffe and George W. Albee (eds.) *Prevention Through Political Action and Social Change.* Copyright © 1981 by the Vermont Conference on the Primary Prevention of Psychopathology. Reprinted by permission.

the raw notes and description that provided the background for a book I started alone in late 1975 and, luckily for me, finished in 1978 with Andrejs Ozolins and Joe McNally.

Now I have read all of those pages and I want to tell you about Sophie, who was a resident of the state school for the retarded and died at a local hospital, and may have died of neglect. To this day, the only consequence of Sophie's quasi-legal demise was the withdrawal of medical services to the state school by the group of physicians in the community who had then been serving that place. There have been other inadequately explained deaths since Sophie's, and there have been other medical groups attending residents of the state school.

I am sure that somebody somewhere in America today has just seen an inmate die needlessly, or has just learned that a medical group is withdrawing its favors from the state's bughouse, or has just attended a meeting where promises were made to finally fix up the state school, or is right now reading in the evening paper that the state has finally found a way to serve the residential needs of the mentally retarded. But the deaths continue, nearly unnoticed and sufficiently legal. I am not surprised. If everything about Sophie's life was legal, why should not everything about her death be legal?

What follows was written at the time it happened in late 1975.

This has been a strange week, very strange indeed. My mind wanders to thoughts about last evening's meeting of our Advocacy Board. I could kick myself for getting so angry, for showing my anger. Why can't these good people realize, as I realize, that case-by-case advocacy will consume us, will play into the hands of those who want to maintain the status quo or regress further toward a segregated and bureaucraticized society? We "win" victory after victory on behalf of this family or that one—no mean achievements—and I am not knocking those accomplishments. However, while we win those skirmishes, the city breaks ground for a new segregated facility, this one to contain the so-called "trainables." Case by case, we advocate for children and their families. Some we win, some we lose; the record is fairly impressive. But, we are losing too many; too many children are still denied educations; too many people sit in back rooms receiving little or nothing of society's interest or services; too many are in locked institutions, not because they must be locked up but, rather, because there is no other "place" to be, because the (only) "place" was created for them. The debate wore me out, driving me eventually to leave the meeting, not because of my anger—though I was angry—but because I was weary, and wanted to go home, and remove those stale clothes and drive out of my head the morbid thoughts of practical people.

Indeed, it has been a strange week. I forced myself to think about Sophie, but not to cheer myself up. Last Monday was scheduled to be a low-keyed, routine day. Nobody knew very much earlier than Monday—therefore nobody told me— that Sophie was to be buried on Monday. And, even had they known it would happen that she needed to be buried on Monday, nobody would have suspected earlier that I would have been asked to attend the funeral, or that I would have accepted the invitation had the offer come. You see, the very first time I ever laid eyes on Sophie was this past Monday at the Garfield Funeral Home. I saw her, but she didn't see me.

Sophie was a resident at the State Developmental Center, near the State School, near the Asylum for Idiots. She had been there for many, many years, leading what I was told was an uneventful and unhappy life. She became ill, very ill, so ill that she was removed to the Community General Hospital. There she died, approximately one week later.

What was interesting about all this, quite inflammatory in this community, concerned the allegation that Sophie did not die of natural causes. There were charges, confused and contradictory but strong charges, that—as we have lately learned to say—the plugs were pulled. Sophie was euthanized; she was rewarded with a dignified death. A big cheer for Death With Dignity, and the Happy Angel that supervises it all. Rejoice, some told us. Sophie has left this vale of misery to an eternal peace and happiness that she did not find on earth. So we gathered together at the funeral home, the priest gave his blessings and read from the Scriptures, some said their Hail Mary's or Hail whatevers, we signed the guest book—guests!—and went on our own ways.

The Death With Dignity Society, and there is one here, should be pleased. The crazy thing about it all is that, in the Cosmos, there may be some explanation for all of this; and, it would not surprise me if such an explanation agreed with the death wishers. Yet, there is also something evil here, something that would tell a human being that it is time for her to die; but if we were in your shoes, sister, we would live! It's best that you die now, first because you're sick. If you were not sick, we would not kill you. Yet, not only are you sick, you are old (is 63 really that old) and, not only are you sick and old, you are defective. Sickness, we sometimes tolerate if it's not too much sickness. And, even the defectives need not be marked early or, especially, with the Terrible Decree. But, Sophie, even you must agree that you gave us no choice. Being sick, old, and defective necessarily must strip you of the rights other people have guaranteed to them. Don't blame us, Sophie, this is all your fault. Besides, you'll be happier up there than down here. It's all over for you, and we have yet to face the terror that is now behind you. What we have done for you is the stuff that causes ordinary people to become true humanitarians.

It is the day after Sophie's funeral. It is 8:00 P.M., then 9, then the hour approaches midnight. We are in Room 407 of the County Courthouse. The County Legislative Commission to Investigate Mental Health and Mental Retardation is holding its last formal hearing prior to its report to the citizens. I am a member of the Commission and, just before termination of the long evening's discussions, I ask the superintendent of the State Developmental Center to reflect upon the future: "In the best of all possible worlds, what do you envision for the Developmental Center in ten years?"

He responded: "In ten years things will not be very much different than they are today. Can I speculate about the world in 50 years?"

"Will the people wait 50 years? There are people who desperately need help, not even in 10 years, tomorrow," I said.

"Don't misunderstand me. If I had my way," he replied, "we would evacuate the Developmental Center in 10 years, five years, or sooner if we could. We would give it to the State, or to your university to use as a dormitory, or for some other educational purpose."

I do not misunderstand. I am embarrassed for him. I think about those times six years ago when it might not have been too late to stop the construction of this $25,000,000 monstrosity. I attempt to avoid remembering the pleadings and arguments, even the threats we made, anything to block construction of the new State School. I remember too much.

Quite early the next morning, I am back in my office . . . The phone rings. It's the Executive Director of the President's Committee on Mental Retardation. Not any president's committee, *The President's*! Would I do a study for them! Would I visit the institutions that continue to defy extinction? Would I expose the rottenness, the abuse, the mismanagement, the inhuman treatment?

"Sure" I reply, "what else do I have to do? As a matter of fact, I was just thinking about those problems today. I'll study these state schools for you. I hope you don't think I've been sitting by this phone all morning waiting for you to call, though. You just happened to catch me in, between assignments, so to speak. Between life and death. You caught me just as I was beginning to believe that Sophie was the lucky one."

I have been arguing that, as Robert Frost might have said if he had been a poet of the human service industry. Something there is that doesn't love a definition. No sooner do we build a row of definitions—definitions of restrictiveness or abuse, freedom or dignity—than it begins to crumble into loopholes, exceptions, and quasi-legal rubble. I have been trying to show that this is not so much because we do not build good definitions, but because life simply will not be captured in definitions.

Yet even as I describe our failure to define things better, even as I read my notes on Sophie whose life slipped away over the edge of a definition of human rights, I too have to agree that we need better definitions. Perhaps, to burden Robert Frost a little more: Good definitions make good neighbors. And though they fall down in the winter of our inattentiveness, each spring we must build them anew, as though they would stay.

Mental Retardation in the Slums

F. Rick Heber

❖ Our research, which has come to be known as the Milwaukee Project, was designed to add to our factual knowledge of the etiology of cultural-familial mental retardation and its susceptibility to preventive measures. Those adhering to either the hereditary or the social deprivation hypothesis have cited virtually the same data in support of their respective positions: principally epidemiological data on population and family group incidence frequencies of mental retardation.

It should be obvious, however, that simple awareness of the high frequency of mental retardation in areas where the economically or otherwise disadvantaged are concentrated is sufficient neither to validate the prepotence of genetic determinants nor to conclude that social deprivation in the slum environment causes the retardation encountered there. Such a generalization ignores the fact that most children reared by economically disadvantaged families are by no means mentally retarded. In actual fact, a majority of children reared in city slums grow and develop and learn relatively normally in the intellectual sense.

Before we could begin any prospective research it was necessary to learn more about the distribution of cultural-familial mental retardation. We conducted a series of surveys in a residential section of Milwaukee, a city of 800,000, characterized by census data as having the lowest median family income, the greatest population density per living unit, and the greatest rate of dilapidated housing in the city. For the United States it was a typical urban slum of the 1960's and it yielded by far the highest prevalence of identified mental retardation among school children in the city. In our first survey, all of the families who had a newborn

From F. Rick Heber, "Sociocultural Mental Retardation: A Longitudinal Study," in Donald G. Forgays (ed.) *Environmental Influences and Strategies in Primary Prevention.* Copyright © 1978 by the Vermont Conference on the Primary Prevention of Psychopathology. Reprinted by permission.

infant and at least one other child of up to the age of six were
selected for study.

The major finding relevant to this discussion is that the variable
of maternal intelligence proved to be by far the best single predictor of the level and character of intellectual development in the
offspring. Mothers with IQ's of less than 80, although comprising
less than half the total group of mothers, accounted for almost
four-fifths of the children with IQ's below 80 (see Table 1).

It has been generally acknowledged that slum-dwelling children
score lower on intelligence tests as they grow older;

Table 1
Distribution of Child IQ's as a Function of Maternal Intelligence

Mother's IQ	Percent of Mothers	Children's IQ		
		%>90	%80-90	%<80
>80	54.6	65.8	47.3	21.9
<80	45.4	34.1	52.7	78.2

> = greater than   < = less than

Table 2
Probability of Child IQ Following Within IQ Ranges
As a Function of Maternal IQ

		Mother IQ		
Child IQ	>100	84-99	68-83	52-67
>100	1	.98	.67	.25
84-99	1	1.02	.95	.93
68-83	1	1.57	1.24	2.20
52-67	1	2.36	3.70	14.20

...however, the mean measured intelligence of offspring of
mothers with IQ's above 80 is relatively constant. And it is only
the children of mothers with IQ's below 80 who show a progressive decline in mean intelligence as age increases.

Further, the survey data showed that the lower the maternal IQ, the greater the probability of offspring scoring low on intelligence tests. For example, as Table 2 shows, the mother with an IQ below 67 had roughly a fourteen-fold increase in the probability of having a child test below 67 as compared with the mother whose IQ fell at or above 100.

These surveys convinced us that the prevalence of mental retardation associated with the slums of American cities is not randomly distributed but, rather, is strikingly concentrated within individual families who can be identified on the basis of maternal intelligence. In other words, the source of the excess prevalence of mental retardation appeared to be the retarded parent residing in the slum environment, rather than the slum itself.

These population survey data have been taken by some as support for the prepotence of hereditary determinants of cultural-familial mental retardation. Our simple casual observation, however, suggested that the mentally retarded mother residing in the slum creates a social environment for her offspring which is distinctly different from that created by her next-door neighbor of normal intelligence.

Most importantly, these survey data suggested that it would be feasible to conduct the longitudinal, prospective research essential to achieving a more adequate understanding of what determines the kind of retardation that perpetuates itself from parent to child in the economically deprived family. That is, the survey data suggested that parental intelligence could be utilized as a tool to select a sample which would be small enough for practical experimental manipulation but would still yield a sufficient number of cases who would later become identifiable as mentally retarded.

An Alabama Prison Experience

Stanley L. Brodsky and Kent S. Miller

❖ An elderly Black inmate named Worley James wrote a penciled letter to federal district judge Frank M. Johnson, explaining that in many years in Alabama prisons he, James, had simply become worse and worse in many ways. This letter became transformed into the class action suit of *James* v. *Wallace* against the State of Alabama, and subsequently was combined with two other suits—one for adequate medical treatment and the other for the right to be free from physical harm in the Alabama prisons (*Newman* v. *Alabama* and *Pugh* v. *Locke*).

In January, 1976, Judge Johnson ruled in favor of the plaintiffs in this suit. The rulings severely denounced the conditions in the prisons, criticizing the unacceptable sanitary conditions, the food, the pervasive overcrowding of men into less than 24 square feet of living space, and the untreated and undiagnosed physical and mental illnesses. The court ordered that no more prisoners be admitted to the prison system until the population was reduced to the design capacity of the buildings. Immediate changes in sanitation, food, and living conditions were ordered. Eleven constitutional rights of inmates were identified. And a major effort was begun to change the barbaric, violent, and oppressive circumstances in which Alabama inmates found themselves.

Psychologist participation in this legal action began early. Attorneys for the plaintiffs consulted with many mental health professionals about issues to pursue and minimum standards for maintaining human adjustment. One psychologist, Carl Clements, inspected the prisons repeatedly and testified in court about the effects of these prison living conditions. Following the court order, the Psychology Department of the University of Alabama conducted a prisoner classification project, under the direction of the department chairman, Raymond Fowler. Over a period of four months, 3,191 prisoners were assessed, and approximately 1,000 judged as appropriate for "community custody." The court order had required evaluation to determine which prisoners were fit for noninstitutional living, and most of the 1,000 men and women were

From Stanley L. Brodsky and Kent S. Miller, "Coercing Changes in Prisons and Mental Hospitals: The Social Scientist and the Class Action Suit," in Justin M. Joffe and George W. Albee (eds.) *Prevention Through Political Action and Social Change.* Copyright © 1981 by the Vermont Conference on the Primary Prevention of Psychopathology. Reprinted by permission.

transferred to work release centers or other community placements, or released.

The prison classification project was not an unqualified success, and many problems arose in implementation of the court standards and order (Brodsky, 1977; Schuster and Widmer, 1978). Nevertheless, the class action suit and court order present some important lessons in understanding the social change–primary prevention process.

First, no amount of direct service would have been able to ameliorate the emotional harm wrought by the day-to-day living environment. In some prisons, over half of the men were victims of physical or sexual assaults, and carrying a weapon for self-protection was normative behavior. For the men there, as well as for future inmates, the system change allowed the potential for maintaining an emotional status quo. And while the Alabama prison system is worth describing because of the seriousness of the problems, the same process exists in other prisons. In our experience, only a minority, and perhaps a small minority, are not vulnerable to the stresses of prison confinement, and the sweeping change by class action suit and court order is a preventive strategy of much value. The right to avoid cruel and unusual punishment is often abrogated, and the symptoms from such punishment may be severe.

Second, a familiar pattern emerged in the wake of the order. The prison system budget rose, the inmate census and overcrowding dropped dramatically, and attention of citizens at large, newspapers, and legislators became forcibly directed toward prison problems.

Third, much of the evidence in court and the post-order action was based on assessments by social science and mental health professionals. This evidence and these assessments were utilized by the attorneys for the plaintiffs who were suing the system. Thus the social scientists' role could be defined as a system challenger.

Lastly, the resistances to system change persisted even in the presence of the court order. The state is far from being in full compliance. Many of the originally identified constitutional violations continue, although the overcrowding and other violations have been corrected or alleviated.

SOLITARY CONFINEMENT ON DEATH ROW

Long confinement under circumstances of isolation has been studied both in sensory deprivation research and in investigations of solitary confinement in prisons. Several books in the last two decades have considered effects of sensory deprivation (for example, Schutz, 1965; Zubek, 1969). A great range of disturbance has been reported, including cognitive and perceptual disorganization, anxiety, and inappropriate emotional reactions. Within prison settings, so-called isolation sickness occurs with great frequency. The process of developing cabin fever, if one is a solitary explorer wintering over in the Arctic, or going stir crazy in solitary confinement, appears well validated (Lugg, 1977; Taylor, 1961), although a few behavioral scientists have attempted to develop the argument that solitary confinement can be beneficial (for example, Suedfeld, 1975).

The present concern is with *Jacobs* v. *Britton*, C.A., No. 78–309–H, filed in the U.S. District Court for the Southern District of Alabama. This class action suit alleged that the "treatment of death row inmates constitutes cruel and unusual punishment and a denial of equal protection." The alleged violations of state law, and of the Eighth and Fourteenth Amendments to the Constitution, included unsanitary food, improper toilets, physical brutality by the guards, limited visiting, minimal exercise and recreation, and indefinite confinement in these conditions. The plaintiffs' attorneys asked one of us to assess the psychological impact of living on death row. In particular, the issue was raised of whether the conditions themselves had adverse effects on the mental well-being of the inmates. If a substantial hazard to the health of the inmates *was* discovered, this finding would indicate a violation of the inmates' constitutional protection against cruel punishment.

Our investigation centered around the nature of existing psychopathology in the death row inmates—its extent, and whether it was peculiar to these death row conditions. If the disorder existed prior to death row confinement, then no causal inferences could be drawn. A final necessary complication was whether anticipation of execution—that is, having an assigned death penalty—was pathology-producing by itself. If it was, then the effects of the living conditions would be less clear.

Thirty-three prisoners were confined on death row at the time of our study. Initially, the full prison records of each were examined. It was found that these records were generally skimpy and useless for our purposes. Because the prisoners were under the death sentence, and because they were officially under the administrative control of the county jail authorities, no classification testing or assessment process was undertaken.

Interviews were conducted with the two psychologists, the classification officer, and the medical-technical assistant who had some contact with the prisoners. Further discussions were held with the warden and with the correctional officers in charge of the unit.

The medical records were studied, and all doctors' contacts, medical examinations, chart entries, and prescribed medication were abstracted. Two instruments were used in extensive interviewing of a selective sample of the prisoners. The prisoners were seen in interviews lasting from 30 minutes to one hour, and the Omnibus Stress Index and a checklist of solitary confinement related symptoms were administered. The index used is a 12-item schedule for which prisoner norms were available in David Jones's book *The Health Risks of Imprisonment* (1976). The latter checklist was especially constructed from a content analysis of the litera-ture on solitary confinement. While a portion of the results was derived from brief interviews with inmates through their cell doors, the major substance including the present information came from ten detailed interviews.

The Psychological Consequences

Two of the ten men were assessed as seriously disturbed, five as moder-ately disturbed, and three as mildly disturbed or no maladjustment seen. The medical records of the two most disturbed inmates included items such as "laughs all the time . . . a psychotic depressive . . . hebephrenic schizophrenic diagnosis" and "tears paper up in piles . . . wild-eyed and does not answer." The inmates themselves offered self-reports about the serious emotional consequences of death row confinement. Their state-ments included:

"If I ever were to get out. I would not be the same person. I just want them to leave me alone."

"They are all out to get you."

"If I am sitting up, I get to shaking, my hands go back and forth."

"I'm confused now. I'm so confused I don't understand. I'm not a killer."

"You just can't sleep . . . you are wide awake."

The reactions reported as characteristic were crying, dejectedness, an-ger, hostility toward specific persons, confusion, inappropriate giggling, and obsessive ruminations. Headaches were reported as well as anxiety: "The anxiety goes right through you." The milieu was described in negative terms:

"They treat you like an animal here."

"They try to degrade you and break your spirits."

"Respect of the inmate is abused."

"[there are] 23½ hours of [cell] confinement every day."

The physical milieu was described as having bad smells, unsanitary conditions, cold food, limited exercise and visiting, and clothing restric-tions beyond those of other prisoners. The general sentiment was that "living conditions here ain't worth a shit." When the inmates were asked if they were aware of sensory deprivation, they agreed and reported that they experienced losses in ability to think clearly, and in recognition ca-pacity, as well as perceptual alterations and hallucinations.

Omnibus Stress Index

In response to the query "Do you experience these symptoms?" eight of the ten intensively interviewed men endorsed the following four items: nervousness, inertia, insomnia, and trembling hands. Seven men reported perspiring hands; six reported a nervous breakdown or feelings of an impending nervous breakdown; and six reported headaches. Five men reported nightmares and dizziness; four reported heart palpitations; and one reported fainting spells. Overall, these patterns were higher than the 50 percent rate reported in the Jones study of the Omnibus Stress Index with Tennessee prisoners.

In the Ferracuti, et al. (1978) study of mental deterioration in prisoners in Ohio and Italy, 21 percent of the older prisoners were found to be susceptible to deterioration, as well as nineteen percent and sixteen percent of two younger prisoner groups. Again, the present prisoners appeared to be suffering more symptoms, more severely. The checklist of solitary confinement symptoms revealed parallel findings. The prisoners tended to report quiet withdrawal, talking to themselves, feeling stir crazy, hostility, confusion, lessened concern about physical appearance, apathy, and memory losses.

The Exceptions

Three of our sample seemed to have adapted reasonably well. They were unhappy about the living conditions, and complained at length, but there were few or no signs of psychopathology. These men generally experienced little current or past anxiety about their lives, and were often flip, and occasionally quite humorous. The interviews were conducted in the one available room, the observation room that adjoined the electric chair chamber. One of these inmates looked through the observation window and quipped, "So that's what old sparky looks like." Another, when offered a Life-saver candy while walking down the corridor replied, "If they really work, I'll take two or three."

Implications of the Death Row Suit

The three interrelated factors—preexisting pathology, effects of being under death sentence, and actual living conditions—could not be fully differentiated. Nevertheless, from the best information available to us, there were many men who had not shown significant earlier disorder and men who reported at least some strongly noxious effects of the living conditions. Our conclusion was that emotionally vulnerable men were very likely to deteriorate, and that the cell confinement, combined with little to do and virtually no positive social contact, represented a substantial stress.

The primary prevention implications concern dealing with such problems. It would be possible to mobilize a team of expert mental health professionals who would treat these men as needed. If prison officers spotted a man acting in bizarre ways or showing signs of psychotic processes, then a prompt referral could be made, and if necessary, the inmate transferred to a hospital or prison treatment unit.

However, the class action suit in this case suggested that a variety of contextual and environmental circumstances caused the emotional problems. If indeed the death sentence was believed to be a causal factor, one preventive strategy might have been to use that factor as a vehicle for changing the law through the legislature or courts. Our own observations of men on death row for years at a time have documented patterns of emotional trouble. Before the death penalty was frozen in the 1960s, we observed men slipping in and out of psychotic episodes as they waited with some uncertainty about their futures. These men, however, were also isolated from other people, prisoners, and staff—and thus precise cause and effect events were not available to us.

The case of *Jacobs* v. *Britton* has been subjected to a series of delays and a trial is pending. If a decision is ordered affirming the positions of the plaintiffs, the long-term effects will extend to future prisoners. As they go through the long wait before a clemency decision (the likely outcome for most death row prisoners in most states) typically commuting the death penalty to life imprisonment without parole, they will be given the opportunity to maintain some sense of personal integrity and worth. The role of the mental health professional in this suit is similar to many other such cases. Clinical knowledge is applied, but not in the interests of direct client service. Rather, the clinical knowledge is directed toward evaluation of an entire living complex and looks at the full range of factors that influence personal equilibrium. These evaluations are in the service of the court, rather than in the service of the immediate individual clients or agencies. It is arguably the court that has the most power to command an immediate change in these environmental factors, and if this is so, then the clinicians' work has a very broad impact.

Hospitals, Prisons, and Primary Prevention

In the face of the considerable attention that has been given to distinctions between primary, secondary, and tertiary prevention, the relationships between institutions and primary prevention may not be readily apparent. By the time the individual is in prison or a mental hospital, the perceived need is not for prevention, but for helping and treatment services. Yet there are a number of ways in which these institutions can be related to concepts of prevention and a number of reasons they should continue to be a focus of reform efforts.

1. The proportion of the population in institutions of one kind or another has not dropped as dramatically as is generally assumed.
2. The institutions consume a disproportionate amount of the resources available for services.
3. The emphasis upon the development of community programming frequently involves institutional populations.
4. The people in institutions represent ultimate powerlessness and these places are the clearest point where the state exercises its coercive powers (frequently in the name of good).
5. Continued support for total institutions as they are now constituted hinders the development of alternative and more effective means of dealing with troublesome behavior.
6. It is in these settings that many mental health professionals have knowingly or unknowingly played a conservative and system-supportive role.

There are a number of basic concepts or practices that could be judged to reflect primary prevention efforts in general. Among these would be included the following: the minimization of dependency; the fostering of a sense of community; maximizing the client's role in decision making; minimizing coercion; and, the reduction of stress. Our prisons and mental hospitals tend to work in directions opposite to each of these concepts. These negative aspects are harmful not only to the clients but also to the staff who work in the institution, and thus in this sense are antithetical to primary prevention. For all of these reasons, a continued effort at reform is important and of consequence to a large number of people.

❖ The point is that we may not as yet have made a significant commitment to serving those at the bottom of the ladder, and more specifically, to those in our institutions. There is substance to the argument of some that no amount of money could overcome the inherent abuses in institutions. We tend to endorse this view, but highlight here the fact that such an attempt has not yet been made.

There is a need for system change and system advocacy in the broadest sense, and an approach through the courts by means of class action or public interest suits continues to hold considerable promise. There can be no doubt about the changing role of the judiciary in this country.

Roles that were unacceptable to the courts two or three decades ago are now assumed to be a reasonable responsibility for them (Horowitz, 1977, p. 4–21). We noted above the expansion of judicial responsibility into the administration of public programs, because of the failure of other branches of government to handle problems satisfactorily. The courts now determine entire courses of governmental agency conduct over a period of time, involving changing identities of the named defendants and plaintiffs. There has been a subordination of the significance of individual cases, although these frequently provide a departure point, and the assumption is that the public has an interest in the judicial resolution of important issues.

We are now hearing expressions of concern about the courts having overstepped their bounds, and we can expect the criticism to continue to mount. In the not too distant future, the courts may be a less significant force for change. If or when that occurs, those seeking reform will shift to other avenues. For example, when the American Civil Liberties Union found that under the Nixon courts the percentage of cases it was winning was cut in half, an increased emphasis was placed upon legislative change.

References

Aaron, H. J. *Politics and the professors*. Washington, D.C.: The Brookings Institution, 1978.

Abramson, M. F. The criminalization of mentally disordered behavior: Possible side-effects of a new mental health law. *Hospital & Community Psychiatry*, 1972, *20*, 13–16.

Barton, W. E., and Sanborn, C. J. *Law and the mental health profession*. New York: International Universities Press, 1978.

Bazelon, D. L. Psychiatrist and the adversary process. *Scientific American*, 1974, *230*, 18–23.

Bradley, V., and Clarke, G. (Eds.). *Paper victories and hard realities: The implementation of the legal and constitutional rights of the mentally disabled*. Washington, D.C.: The Health Policy Center, Georgetown University, 1976.

Brodsky, S. L. *Psychologists in the criminal justice system*. Urbana: University of Illinois Press, 1973.

Brooks, A. D. Foreword to J. Rubin, *Economics, mental health and the law*. Lexington, Mass.: D. C. Heath, 1978.

Chayes, A. The role of the judge in public law litigation. *Harvard Law Review*, 1976, *89*, 1281–1316.

Crouse & McGinnis v. Murray, No. 575–191 (N.D. Ind., filed Nov. 17, 1975).

Davis v. Balson, No. C73–205 (N.D. Ohio, Jan. 21, 1977).

Doe v. Hudspeth, No. J75–36(c) (S.D. Miss., Feb. 17, 1977).

Ferracuti, F., Dinitz, S., and Piperno, A. *Mental deterioration in prison*. Columbus: Program for the Study of Crimes and Delinquency, School of Public Administration, Ohio State University, 1978.

Forst, M. L. *Civil commitment and social control*. Lexington, Mass.: Lexington Books, 1978.

Gaylin, W., Glasser, I., Marcus, S., and Rothman, D. *Doing good: The limits of benevolence*. New York: Pantheon, 1978.

Glazer, N. Should judges administer social services? *Public Interest*, 1978, *50*, 64–80.

Halderman & United States v. Pennhurst, C. A., No. 74–1345 (E.D. Pa., Nov. 30, 1976).

Halleck, S. L. A troubled view of current trends in forensic psychiatry. *Journal of Law and Psychiatry*, 1974, *2*, 135–157.

Halleck, S. L., and Witte, A. D. Is rehabilitation dead? *Crime & Delinquency*, 1977, *23*, 372–382.

Herbert, W. The politics of prevention. *APA Monitor*, May, 1979, *10*, #5, 8.

Himmelsbach, J. T. Consequences of cooperation between police and mental health services: Issues and some solutions. In R. Cohen, R. P. Sprafkin, S. Oglesby, and W. Claiborn (Eds.), *Working with police agencies: The interrelations between law enforcement and the behavioral scientist*. New York: Human Sciences Press, 1976.

Horack v. Exxon, No. 72-L-299 (D. Neb., 1973).

Horowitz, D. L. *The courts and social policy*. Washington, D.C.: Brookings Institution, 1977.

Jacobs v. Britton, C. A., No. 78-309-H (S.D. Ala.).

Jones, D. *The health risks of imprisonment*. Lexington, Mass.: Lexington Books, 1976.

Krantz, S., Smith, C., Rossman, D., Froyd, P., and Hoffman, J. *Right to counsel in criminal cases: The mandate of Argersinger vs. Hamlin*. Cambridge, Mass.: Ballinger, 1976.

Lipton, D., Martinson, R., and Wilkes, J. *The effectiveness of correctional treatment: A survey of treatment evaluation*. New York: Praeger, 1975.

Lottman, M. S. Enforcement of judicial decrees: Now comes the hard part. *Mental Disability Law Reporter*, 1976, *1*, 69–76.

Lugg, D. J. Physiological adaptation and health of an expedition in Antarctica, with comment on behavioral adaptation. Canberra, Australia: Australian National Antarctic Research Expeditions, ANARE Scientific Report, Series B (4) Medical Science, publication No. 126, 1977.

Miller, K. S., Fein, S. B., and Schmidt, W. C. The therapeutic state and current court cases. In K. S. Miller (Ed.), *Conflict and collusion: The criminal justice and mental health systems*. Final Report, LEAA Grant No. 77NI-99-0061, 1979.

Morse, S. J. Law and mental health professionals: The limits of expertise. *Professional Psychology*, 1978, *9*, 389–399.

Navarro v. Hernandez, No. 74-1301 (D.P.R., Apr. 20, 1977).

NYSARC & Parisi v. Carey, 393 F. Supp. 715 (E.D. N.Y., 1973).

NYSARC & Parisi v. Carey, 393 F. Supp. 717 (E.D. N.Y., 1975).

Ohio Assn. for Retarded Citizens v. Moritz, No. C2-76-398 (S.D. Ohio, Apr. 19, 1977).

Patients v. Camden Co. Bd. of Chosen Freeholders, No. L-33417-74-P.W. (N.J. Sup. Ct. Camden Co., filed Oct. 17, 1975).

Patients v. Camden Co. Bd. of Chosen Freeholders, No. L-33417-74-P.W. (N.J. Sup. Ct. Camden, Co., filed April 29, 1977).

President's Commission on Mental Health. Vol. II, Washington, D.C.: U.S. Government Printing Office, 1978.

Robitscher, J. Isaac Ray Award Lectures, George Washington University, Schools of Medicine and Law, in conjunction with the American Psychiatric Association, Washington, D.C., November 6, 7, and 8, 1977.

Rosenberg, N. S. Symposium presented at the annual meeting of the American Society for Public Administration, Baltimore, Md., 1979.

Rubin, J. *Economics, mental health, and the law.* Lexington, Mass.: D. C. Heath, 1978.

Sanford, N., Comstock, C. and associates. *Sanctions for evil: Sources of social destructiveness.* San Francisco: Jossey-Bass, 1971.

Scallet, L. The realities of mental health advocacy: State ex rel. Memmel v. Muncy. In L. E. Kopolow and H. Bloom (Eds.), *Mental health advocacy: An emergency force in consumer rights.* DHEW Publication No. (ADM) 77–455, NIMH, Rockville, Md., 1977.

Schindenwolf v. Klein, No. A-2695-76 (N.J. Sup. Ct. App. Div., filed July 27, 1977).

Schuster, R. L., and Widmer, S. A. Judicial intervention in corrections: A case study. *Federal Probation,* 1978, *42,* 10–17.

Schutz, D. P. *Sensory restriction.* New York: Academic Press, 1965.

Sosowsky, L. Crime and violence among mental health patients: Reconsidered in view of the now legal relationship between the state and the mentally ill. *American Journal of Psychiatry,* 1978, *135,* 33–42.

State v. Alton, 362 A.2d, 545 (N.J., 1976).

Stone, A. A. *Mental health and law: A system in transition.* Washington, D.C.: National Institute of Mental Health, Center for Studies of Crime and Delinquency, DHEW Publication No. (ADM) 75–176, 1975.

Stone, A. A. Recent mental health litigation: A critical perspective. *American Journal of Psychiatry,* 1977, *63,* 273–279.

Suedfeld, P. The benefits of boredom: Sensory deprivation reconsidered. *American Scientist,* 1975, *63,* 60–69.

Taylor, A. J. W. Social isolation and imprisonment. *Psychiatry,* 1961, *27,* 323–326.

Wuori v. Bruns, No. 75–80 (D. Me., filed Oct. 1, 1975).

Wyatt v. Stickney, 344 F. Supp. 373, 387 (M.D. Ala., 1972), aff'd. 503 F2d 1305 (5th Cir. 1974).

Zubek, J. P. *Sensory deprivation: Fifteen years of research.* New York: Meredith, 1969.

A Welfare Funeral

Stephen E. Goldston

❖ ...I
call to the reader's attention a circumstance reported in April 1979 on the front page of the *Washington Post*. The news story detailed the travails of a welfare mother as she made funeral arrangements for her five-year-old daughter who had been killed in a fire. Specifically, this mother was entrapped in the obscure world of "welfare funerals" in Washington, an arena of private grief and public, tax-paid "contract" burials involving several hundred of the city's poor and costing about a quarter of a million dollars each year. The burial practices to be described are associated with social, racial, and financial conflicts having decided mental health components.

Basically, the contract burials provided for the essentials of a funeral, but not the "extras," such as flowers, a newspaper notice, an extra death certificate, and a guest book for the wake and funeral. The contractor used the occasion of the first meeting with the bereaved to obtain payment for these "extras." After the cash was exchanged, this welfare mother was told that because of the tight schedule of funerals, the service would have to be limited to one-half hour, that the coffin could not be open for viewing since this would cause further delays, and that due to a backlog the funeral could not be held for a week! What stark oppression and extreme insensitivity directed at the helpless at a point of crisis. The article brought to public knowledge the practices of the white-owned funeral business that had a contract from the municipal government of what is a predominately black populated city. At the time, black undertakers asserted that the contract business was insensitive to black funeral tradition, especially open caskets and prolonged emotional grieving. As a result of complaints to the appropriate city agency, as well as of the news story, new legislation was promulgated to permit welfare recipients to choose among a number of funeral homes for city-financed services, thereby closing out the monopoly previously enjoyed by a single firm.

Preventionists reading about this incident would probably observe

From Stephen E. Goldston, "Messages for Preventionists," in Justin M. Joffe and George W. Albee (eds.) *Prevention Through Political Action and Social Change.* Copyright © 1981 by the Vermont Conference on the Primary Prevention of Psychopathology. Reprinted by permission.

three factors: (a) the gross insensitivity on the part of the undertaking business having the welfare contract; (b) the mother's grief compounded by this difficult situation; and (c) the fact that at no point, before, during or after, did mental health workers appear to have any involvement whatsoever in either exposing existing procedures or advocating more appropriate practices consistent with the psychological, racial, social, and cultural needs of the bereaved.

This incident deals with a stressful and damaging environmental condition, which certainly seems to be linked with excessive imbalances in power. Moreover, this incident typifies the public health dictum to seek out "foci of infection." But yet, mental health workers played no role in either exposing or changing the oppressive contract burial practices.

Even when we clearly are on the side of the angels, everyone is not always going to agree. Perhaps I have stacked the deck with my choice of words, "clearly" and "always," but the message is that what may well appear to make good sense, can be perceived otherwise by some folk. My illustration of this message harks back to an experience I had during the Nixon years. I had proposed, with considerable written justification, and had secured the necessary funding for a series of short educational films on the theme of helping children to understand death. After reviewing the professional literature on the imperatives of promoting parent-child communications about death in order to sensitize, educate, and detraumatize children, I concluded that some graphically beautiful films on this subject were needed. As are the ways of a bureaucracy, final clearance on films rested well up in the departmental hierarchy. Consequently, late one afternoon I received a copy of the following memorandum from the Assistant Secretary for Public Affairs:

I have reviewed the initial proposal and summary memorandum to produce several films on "Death and the Child" and concluded that we cannot approve this proposed project in any form.

Films of this nature would be more appropriately developed by theologians and philosophers than HEW.

I drew a black crayoned border around that memo, and to this very day it appears on the bulletin board over my desk, a constant reminder of the message with which I began this segment.

Sexual Exploitation

George W. Albee

❖ The problem we face in attempting to prevent rape and the sexual abuse of children becomes an instructive paradigm that helps us clarify our thinking about the more general problem of the prevention of psychopathology. Rape is a specific form of exploitation of women and children by the more powerful male for his own gratification. It often occurs in the context of a family situation where there is no escape. A wife without the skills to be economically independent and unable to support herself and her children may acquiesce hopelessly to her fate and fail to protest the sexual abuse of her children. She may have no support system and no hope of rescue. This pathological form of culturally sanctioned exploitation and oppression is characteristic of a social system that supports patriarchy. The victims suffer a variety of damaging consequences to their personhood and their self-esteem. Too frequently the society, supporting patriarchal myths, blames the victims. Sometimes the victims, not the perpetrators, are stigmatized. Certainly they learn to regard themselves as persons of low worth.

But so it is with many other forms of emotional disorder. I suggest to you that most forms of emotional disturbance are interpersonal in origin, and that the process begins with the exploitation of persons when they are defenseless and powerless (often during infancy and childhood). As in the instance of rape, we often blame the victim—he or she was flawed by bad genes or bad chemistry.

Less overt, more symbolic, rapes occur with great frequency in our patriarchy. Our society provides a subtle but nurturant climate for the exploitation of the weak by the powerful. Unequal pay for equal work; sexual harassment in the workplace, the kitchen, and the bedroom; the endless media depiction of women as mindless sex objects adorning automobiles, or chortling with glee over whiter washes or shinier floors; the constant media modeling of males as warriors, as powerful manipulators of machines

From George W. Albee, "Introduction," in George W. Albee, Sol Gordon, and Harold Leitenberg (eds.) *Promoting Sexual Responsibility and Preventing Sexual Problems*. Copyright © 1983 by the Vermont Conference on the Primary Prevention of Psychopathology. Reprinted by permission.

and people (often women); the portrayal of males on the TV screen as law-givers, priests, overpaid sports gladiators, diplomats and judges, outlaws and sheriffs—all of these images put social pressure on marginal men, susceptible men, psychopathic men, to buttress their shaky self-esteem by brutalizing a woman or a child. Only a small proportion of men who are potential rapists actually carry out the overt act with a stranger. A larger number act out in their families and help produce the next generation of hysterics, obsessives, and schizophrenics. But an even larger number of men carry out "little rapes" in their daily lives—exploiting women as objects, as nonpersons—and the cumulative effects on the victims may be as destructive as overt assault.

Sexual Abuse of Children

Gertrude J. Rubin Williams

There is a Jewish legend about the fools of Chelm, a community of smug simpletons who lacked insight into their incredible stupidity. They lived at the top of a steep mountain from which they had to traverse a narrow, winding path to reach the market at the foot of the mountain. In the course of their frequent journeys, droves of Chelmsians were killed or maimed as they dropped from the narrow path into the valley below. After decades of ignoring the carnage, the surviving fools of Chelm took action to control the problem. They built a hospital at the bottom of the valley to treat those unfortunates who dropped off the mountain.

Descendants of the fools of Chelm are now attempting to bring child abuse under control.

In his call for the prevention of sexism, Albee (1981) observes that "no mass disorder . . . afflicting humankind has ever been brought under control by attempts to treat afflicted individuals." This observation is applicable to the mass disorder of child abuse, which treatment is failing to control. Child abuse will be eradicated only by the prevention of sexism, pronatalism, the sexual exploitation of children, and other irresponsible sexual ideologies and practices, to which professionals themselves have often contributed.

Futility of a Treatment Approach

The Child Abuse Prevention and Treatment Act of 1974 refers to prevention as a major goal, yet it has received insignificant attention in child abuse programs. The overriding emphasis on the treatment of child abuse to the virtual exclusion of prevention mirrors the American health care

From Gertrude J. Rubin Williams, "Responsible Sexuality and the Primary Prevention of Child Abuse," in George W. Albee, Sol Gordon, and Harold Leitenberg (eds.) *Promoting Sexual Responsibility and Preventing Sexual Problems.* Copyright © 1983 by the Vermont Conference on the Primary Prevention of Psychopathology. Reprinted by permission.

model which deals almost exclusively with the treatment of illness, rather than with the maintenance and enhancement of health. Social agencies struggling vainly to meet the unremitting demands for emergency and long-term treatment of abuse families are too depleted to develop the imaginative programs and well-coordinated service delivery systems required for the primary prevention of child abuse (Fraser, 1979).

There are less obvious reasons for the overemphasis on treatment and the avoidance of primary prevention. The prevention of child abuse lacks concreteness, drama, and sensationalism, whereas treatment evokes the graphic images, righteousness, and rescue fantasies that inspire public support. Of paramount importance is the reality that if child abuse is ever to be prevented, radical transformations must occur in social ideologies, practices, and programs. Few professionals or politicians have been willing to sacrifice the good press, public approval, or government grants they receive for touting treatment and to risk the controversy related to exposing and working to annihilate the roots of child abuse.

Many critics contend that primary prevention is an overly idealistic, unaffordable fantasy and that we are entitled to rest on the laurels of the manifold programs across the nation treating child abuse. But is the treatment of child abuse effective? The answer, tragically, is a resounding no. The limited focus on treatment has opened a Pandora's box of travail devoid of the hope assured in the myth.

Helfer (1978) states that "every year 1½-2 percent of our children are reported as suspected victims of child abuse. While social agencies are working to help this year's 2 percent, they are still trying to figure out what to do with last year's 2 percent and are pleading with legislators for more money to deal with next year's 2 percent. The problems of abuse and neglect accumulate at the rate of 1½-2 percent each year." Nevertheless, child protection agencies continue on the treatment treadmill despite the impossibility of meeting these ever-increasing demands. Kempe (1979) describes child protection workers as "the only public servants willing to constantly stretch their case loads to meet demands . . . because they are not a militant profession with defined duties" (p.x). These workers are expected to help abuse families with their manifold problems, despite inadequate training in carrying out tasks that would tax even expertly trained professionals; many workers have only an undergraduate degree. Despite recommendations by national child welfare groups of no more than 20 child abuse families per worker, case loads are often twice that amount.

In light of these dismal realities, it is not surprising that the field is characterized by low job satisfaction, burnout, and large turnover. Few abuse families see the same worker throughout the treatment process. Compounding these crushing problems, the treatment focus of child protection agencies does not necessarily assure that abuse families will even receive treatment. According to the U.S. Department of Health, Education and Welfare (1975), "Of the three components of the community-team program—identification and diagnosis, treatment, and education—treatment tends to be most notably lacking. It is not uncommon for a community to develop extensive identification and diagnostic resources and then find itself ill-equipped to help identified families" (p. 65). In many agencies that do provide treatment, treatment is often equated with medical care, casework, or psychotherapy, rather than with the wide range of services required for such multiproblem families (Cohn and Miller, 1977).

In line with the dubious philosophy of keeping abused children with their parents except as a last resort, treatment programs are directed to the abusive parents, not to the children they abused. Indeed, only adult members are receiving treatment services in 85 percent of the nationwide federally funded child abuse programs (Cohn and Miller, 1977). The treatment focus on abusive parents has been based on the 'trickle down' theory . . . the credo of protective services for one hundred years" (Kempe, 1979, p. xi). Help for the parents is unquestioningly assumed to trickle down to the abused child, who receives little or no treatment. The only study found on the effects of treating parents on child variables is that of Taitz (1980), in England, who reported that, of 38 abused infants whose families had received casework during a 5-year period, only 12 were classified as satisfactory in mental development, speech attainment, and growth outcome.

Recidivism in Treated Abusive Parents

Recidivism of abuse is a crucial measure of the effects of treatment on parents and, indirectly, on children. Early investigators (Friedman, 1972; Skinner and Castle, 1969) of recidivism reported ranges from 20 to 60 percent. Even higher recidivism rates are found in recent, more methodologically sophisticated research. In a follow-up study of 328 abuse families who had received services, Herrenkohl, Herrenkohl, Egolf, and Seech (1979) found 66.8 percent of verified incidents of parental reabuse compared to 25.4 percent officially reported incidents. Depending on the number of types, targets, and perpetrators of abuse in a family, recidivism ranged from 45 to 85 percent. Even after cases had been closed, presumably because abuse was no longer believed to be present, recidivism was found in 18.5 percent of the cases, 25 percent of which had received over 3 years of treatment. These grim findings were corroborated in England by Butterfield, Jackson, and Nangle (1979) in a 2½-year follow-up of extensive services to abusive parents. They reported that 46 of 69 children remained at risk, were reabused, or had a sibling who was abused.

Perhaps the most significant study of the effects of treatment is Cohn's (1979) evaluation of 11 federally funded demonstration projects on the treatment of child abuse. She found that a combination of highly skilled professional counseling and lay services was more effective than professional individual or group treatment alone in alleviating problems that trigger abuse. Recidivism remained high in all treatment groups, however, ranging from 47 to 62 percent of treated abusive parents. Regardless of treatment modality, recidivism of severe abuse occurred in 56 percent of cases considered serious at intake. Thirty percent of the entire sample of parents reabused the child during the course of treatment. Inasmuch as these measures of recidivism excluded mild physical abuse and neglect and emotional abuse and neglect, the findings are an underestimation of the recidivism likely to have been found had a broader definition of child abuse been used. It can also be assumed that recidivism rates are even higher in abuse families in treatment programs that do not have the benefits of services, consultation, funding, and other resources offered in the demonstration projects.

Irresponsible Sexuality and Child Abuse

Research evidence is demonstrating that current treatment programs cannot stem the ever burgeoning tide of child abuse, which will continue indefinitely unless the focus is changed to primary prevention. It is true that the causes of child abuse are complex, multiple, and interrelated, but there is little doubt about the major contributors to the problem. These include poverty, the oppression of children or reverse ageism, manifested in socially sanctioned corporal punishment, and irresponsible sexuality, manifested in inadequate provision for and utilization of contraception, abortion, and sex education, and in sexism and pronatalism (Gil, 1970; Light,

1973; Williams, 1976, 1980). This paper focuses on three kinds of irresponsible sexuality that are related to child abuse: unwanted pregnancy, irrationally wanted pregnancy, and father-daughter incest in childhood.

Unwanted Pregnancy and Child Abuse

The paucity of attention paid to contraceptive and abortion services, and sex education and counseling in the prevention of child abuse is especially remarkable because the circumstances of the conception and the attitudes toward pregnancy have been linked to child abuse in numerous investigations. Steele and Pollack (1968) state that "an infant born as the result of a premaritally conceived pregnancy or who comes as an accident too soon after the birth of a previous child, may be quite unwelcome to the parents and start life under a cloud of being unwanted and unsatisfying to the parents. Such infants may be perceived as public reminders of sexual transgression or as extra, unwanted burdens rather than need-satisfying objects" (pp. 128-129). Wasserman (1967) notes that a child conceived out of wedlock often becomes a "hostility sponge" for an unwanted marriage, reminds the mother of the man who deserted her during pregnancy, or is beaten by the mother and step-father who perceive the unwanted child as a public reminder of sexual transgression.

Numerous investigators (Bishop, 1971; Gaddis, Monaghan, Muir, and Jones, 1979; Gil, 1970; Green, 1976; MacCarthy, 1977; Prescott, 1976; Scott, 1980; Spinetta and Rigler, 1972) report significant relationships between child abuse and unwanted pregnancy, pregnancy occurring shortly after the birth of a previous child, and/or being a member of a large family with four or more children. Oates, Davis, Ryan, and Stewart (1979) in England, and West and West (1979) in Australia, found a significantly higher frequency of unplanned, unwanted, and illegitimate pregnancies among abusive parents compared to control samples. Ferguson, Fleming, and O'Neil (1972) report higher rates of child abuse and neglect among illegitimate children and in larger families in New Zealand.

Adolescent childbearing, two-thirds of which is unplanned (Green and Pottzeiger, 1977), is associated with a multitude of variables related to child abuse (Friedrich and Boriskin, 1976; Lynch and Roberts, 1977). These variables include a high risk of complications during the adolescent's pregnancy, labor, and delivery, and of prematurity, low birth weight, mental retardation, cerebral palsy, and epilepsy among infants of adolescent mothers.

Resnick (1970) reviewed the world literature since 1751 on the murder of the newborn and found that the vast majority of parents attributed the murder simply to not wanting the infant. Passivity was a prominent characteristic of these young women who planned neither the pregnancy nor the murder. However, "When reality is thrust upon them by the infant's first cry, they respond by permanently silencing the intruder" (p. 1416). Resnick contrasts the passivity of neonaticidal women with those who seek abortions; the latter recognize the reality of the unwanted pregnancy early and cope actively with the problem. So if abortion is murder, when shall the murder take place? *In utero* or at birth?

In these times of right-wing fanaticism, a statement made in 1969 by Dr. Lester Breslow, then the president of the American Public Health Association, is especially relevant:

Can anyone estimate how much physical harm is a byproduct of rigid abortion laws? The unwanted child, resulting from contraceptive failure or failure to abort, may be born only to be victimized by hostile parents . . . . Not only are battered children sometimes killed and often disabled but they are usually psychologically distorted. An enlightened policy on abortion would prevent much of this waste and callous infliction of pain.

Irrationally Wanted Pregnancy and Child Abuse

Although unwanted pregnancy is linked to child abuse, contraceptive and sex education and counseling, which should be mandatory components of all child abuse programs, are absent from most of them. Many abusive parents whose children have been removed from them keep bearing more children whom they abuse. Some abusive parents are ignorant of or indifferent to contraception and abortion. Others purposely bear more children to prove to themselves and society that they are good parents. For example, one pair of abusive parents, from whom four children had been removed, planned their current pregnancy because, as they put it, "We just love children to death." This sentiment is almost literally true. Two of the children they battered are brain damaged and one is nearly blind. All five have psychological problems. The agency permitted them to keep their fifth child, an infant who is already showing developmental delays. These abusive parents are eagerly awaiting the birth of their sixth "wanted" child.

Thus, though not wanting the pregnancy is a parental attitude related to child abuse, wanting the pregnancy is insufficient to prevent abuse.

Indeed, extreme yearning for a child may increase the probability of abuse. Lenoski (1974) describes a group of mothers who intensely wanted the child they subsequently abused. They were more likely than a nonabusive control group to name the child after a parent or to have worn maternity clothes earlier.

Martin and Beezley (1974) explain the seemingly contradictory findings of abusive parents who wanted the pregnancy, or adoptive parents who abuse their wanted adoptive children, as an extension of the findings of Steele and Pollack (1968), namely, that abusive parents typically expect the child to meet their own intense emotional needs. The parents lash out at the child, who is irrationally viewed as withholding love. Steele and Pollack also refer to a "splitting" in abusive parents between love for the child and a sense of righteousness about beating a disobedient, unrewarding child. These two contradictory systems, walled off from each other yet coexisting, are manifested in the abuse of children who were also wanted by their parents.

Walsh (1977) describes a group of abusive adolescent mothers who viewed pregnancy and motherhood as ways of defining their identity and social role and of providing the security absent during their own childhoods. When the baby they wanted so intensely failed to meet their irrational expectations, the adolescent mother expressed her frustration and rage by abusing the child.

The relationship between child abuse and wanting a child intensely is reported by Helfer (1975). He describes a group of abusive young women who refused contraception and abortion because of their strong desire to become pregnant, and with whom "family planning and birth control measures must be pursued even though frequently resisted" (p. 29). He recommends special counseling for such women, because referral to a family planning agency is ineffective.

These women had experienced the "world of abnormal rearing" (WAR), a pattern of abusive, rejecting, emotionally damaging relationships with their own parents. Their motivations for the pregnancy were "to free themselves from their unhappy home, prove to their parents and themselves they could indeed be good parents, provide them with someone to keep them company, or [they expect] the baby to role reverse and begin to parent the parents" (p. 34). The infants, incapable of granting these irrational wishes, became the target of their mothers' frustration.

The relationship between child abuse and wanting a child highlights the crucial importance of competent counseling for women with unplanned pregnancies. These distraught women are often exposed to a brand of "counseling" by antichoice proponents that can only be described as incompetent and unethical. Are these women helped to make informed, reflective, personally valid decisions at these significant points in their lives? This is the general goal of quality counseling services, including reputable abortion centers which do not try to dictate the pregnant client's choice. Yet fanatical antichoice advocates, under the guise of counseling, use brainwashing techniques on conflict-ridden clients such as dogmatically preaching that abortion is "killing the preborn child," displaying fetuses in bottles, reinforcing unfounded fears of sterility and death as outcomes of abortions, and other scare tactics.

If such propagandizing occurred with other clients, professional associations and the public would raise vociferous objections. Indeed, action, in the form of charges of violation of ethical standards, expulsion from professional associations, and malpractice suits, needs to be taken against counselors who use such tactics. The fact that abortion is a sensitive social issue does not alter the essential guideline of client-counselor relationships: *the counseling relationship should not be exploited for propagandistic purposes by the counselor, who is committed to fostering an emotional atmosphere conducive to the free choice of the client.*

Inasmuch as few women with problem pregnancies place their children for adoption, agencies which exhort distraught clients to carry the child to term are inadvertently contributing to child abuse. The irresponsible naiveté of antichoice proponents is manifested in their insistence on the ease with which their clients "discover" through "counseling" that they really want the child. They overlook the reality that wanting a child in no way rules out abuse of wanted children after they are born, especially if wanting the child is based on irrational motivation.

The children of these mothers are at especially high risk for abuse. Not only was the pregnancy unwanted, but the circumstances of the birth were likely to have been tumultuous. The mothers are often young, poor, uneducated, under stress, and unlikely to have received adequate prenatal care, variables that significantly increase the risk of child abuse, especially in combination. Their children are in further jeopardy because they are likely to possess medical problems that also predispose them to abuse, such as prematurity, low birth weight, and a variety of other vulnerabilities.

Valid questions regarding follow-through by agencies demand clear answers, for the postpartum period is an opportunity to put reverence-for-life preachings into practice. Do these agencies support the lives of the mother and fetus they rescue from abortion? Do they educate her for responsible sexuality by contraceptive education? Do they educate her for responsible parenthood so that the born child will, in fact, be able "to laugh and love," as their bumper stickers righteously proclaim? On the contrary, once the preborn becomes the *newborn*, their interest in the new mother and her child disappears and is redirected to further fetus rescuing. By obstructing abortion rights on clinical and public policy levels, counselors and agencies are perpetuating child abuse.

Findings that some women abuse the child they wanted also highlight the influence of sexism and pronatalism in the perpetuation of child abuse. If child abuse is ever to be eradicated, attitudes toward women's roles, childbearing, and the definition of the family must be transformed. The abysmal failure of these women in a role they had sought with joyful expectations poignantly depicts the destructiveness of sexist and pronatalist upbringing. No doubt, these women learned to accept unquestioningly the major tenets of these destructive ideologies: sex role stereotyping and the views that anatomy is destiny, that the only fulfilling life-style for women is motherhood, and that a woman becomes validated as a person only when she bears a child. Despite their harsh backgrounds, these women need not have become child abusers. Had the culture offered these abusive mothers a range of choices in addition to motherhood, they might have become contributors to the community rather than a drain on its resources.

Clear social sanctions for the tenets of the women's movement and the National Alliance for Optional Parenthood would significantly contribute to the primary prevention of child abuse. These tenets include the view that anatomy is not destiny for either women or men, that the family should be redefined as families, a pluralistic institution with a wide variety of life-styles, and that child-free marriage and singlehood merit social sanctions equal to marriage and parenthood. Sexist and pronatalist ideologies continue to be promoted, not only in textbooks and advertising, but in some sex education courses. For example, few family life education courses give equal time to nonparenting life-styles. Some are preparing youth for the 1940s by perpetuating the myth that children define a family. Indeed, the substitution of courses on life-styles for courses on traditional family life would contribute to the primary prevention of child abuse. By being presented with a varied range of equally sanctioned, fulfilling life-styles, youths who learn that they lack generative motivation for childbearing or that they possess the negative attitudes toward childrearing associated with abuse could opt for a child-free life-style. Other youths who opt for parenthood on the basis of informed choice, rather than social pressure, are more likely to raise children nonviolently.

Father-Daughter Incest in Childhood

Sexism is also a major contributor to father-daughter incest, a form of child abuse which will be eliminated only by radical changes in power relations between females and males and between children and adults. Over 90 percent of child victims of sexual abuse by adult relatives are female, and the vast majority of abusers are male even when the child victim is male (Herman, 1981). The pattern of intergenerational incest parallels that of other sex crimes in that most assailants are males and most victims are females. The transcendence of parents' rights over those of their children also contributes to victimization. For example, "Fathers confronted with detection . . . often express surprise that incest is punishable by law and frequently insist that they have done nothing wrong. Some fathers believe sexual access to be one of their parental rights" (Hennepin County Attorney's Office, no date). Their dual status as females and as children intensifies the powerlessness of female victims of father-daughter incest. Therefore, it is understandable that the women's movement and child advocacy lobbies have promoted public recognition of this form of incest as a social problem.

The average age when incest is initiated is between 6 and 11 years (Browning and Boatman, 1977; Maisch, 1972), but infants and younger children are also sexually abused by their fathers. The abuse usually consists of fondling the genitals, masturbation, exhibition, and oral-genital contact. Some mental health professionals and judges erroneously minimize the harmful impact of incest on children because sexual intercourse is not ordinarily involved. The sexual abuse is likely to occur over many years beginning with the oldest daughter and to continue serially with the younger daughters (Cavallin, 1966).

In many cases, incest is not only a family affair but a sociocultural manifestation, in caricature form, of traditional sex role stereotypes played out in a patriarchal family scenario (Cormier, Kennedy, and Sangowicz, 1962; de Young, in press; Herman, 1981; Herman and Hirschman, 1977; Sgroi,

1979; Weinberg, 1955). The father, a "good family man," is also a tyrant; one arch-chauvinistic father even constructed a throne for himself (Summit and Kryso, 1978). The mother is passive, compliant, and extremely dependent on her husband for emotional and financial security. She is sometimes further trapped in the traditional female role by chronic illness or repeated childbearing. The oldest daughter, who is especially vulnerable to sexual abuse by her father, has strong, unmet affectional needs and models the submissiveness of her mother. She is expected to play the role of "little mother" and assume responsibility for housework and child care. This role reversal is an adaptive response to a dysfunctional family environment and is also present in many battered children. This precocity combined with the little girl's affect-hunger and poignancy may be viewed by the authoritarian father as sexual seductiveness.

The old saw that the male offers love to get sex and that the female gives sex to get love is applicable in these cases, for the father's power and the daughter's submissiveness, needfulness, and admiration of him constitute a major dynamic in the relationship. As Geiser (1979) explains: "The best summary of what went on in a father's mind when he turned to his daughter for sex was given by one father in response to his daughter's question, 'Why did you do it to me?' The father's answer: 'You were available and you were vulnerable'" (p. 52). The relationship is sustained by the father's intimidation of his daughter by threats that exposure of the incestuous secret will break up the family, punishment of both of them, and loss of financial security. Fear of loss of familial, emotional, and financial security may also contribute to the mother's denial of the incestuous relationship.

Sexism characterizes not only father-daughter incest per se but also the way in which incest is viewed. As in rape, wife battering, and other crimes against females, the response to incest has been to exonerate the criminal and blame the victim, a response that dates back to the Bible. In Chapter 19 of the Book of Genesis, Lot's wife was turned into a pillar of salt, a symbol of her emotional unavailability. Lot's daughters got him drunk and seduced him, thus justifying his participation in the incest. Some professionals are perpetuating this timeworn bias in incriminating the incest victim in the same way they incriminated the rape victim, namely, by depicting her as seductive and thus provocative or compliant. The wife, too, is viewed as blameworthy. Her coldness and rejection are presumed to explain her husband's incest with their daughter, but the basis of the wife's emotional unavailability because of his tyranny or her entrapment in a psychologically numbing sex role is rarely addressed. The injured party in the family is not the daughter but the father, an innocent victim of his wife's, his daughter's—and sometimes, his mother's—personality flaws. He is thus exempted from responsibility for the sexual abuse of his daughter who, like the rape victim, is viewed as "asking for it."

What are these children actually asking for? According to several investigators, they are asking for affection, attention, and caring. Peters (1976) concluded that the fathers were in a state of reduced ego control when they mistakenly interpreted their daughters' emotional needfulness as seductiveness. He urges professionals not to indict these children for their affection-seeking behavior, for it was the adult who initiated the specifically sexual behavior. Meiselman (1978) refers to adultomorphic misperception, the ascription of adult sexual motives to the child. After psychologically evaluating children at the National Center for the Prevention and Treatment of Child Abuse, Johnston (1979) contended, "It is difficult to understand the characterization of the child as the initiator or seductress since the child is frequently involved in sexual activity which she does not understand, to which she has not given informed consent and which is characteristic of a psychosexual stage beyond her developmental level" (p. 943).

❖   Cormier, Kennedy and Sangowicz (1962) state that incestuous fathers claimed that their daughters had provoked the sexual contacts, whereas the daughters claimed to have been coerced by their fathers. Gebhard, Gagnon, Pomeroy, and Christenson (1965) report that the matter of coercion was sidestepped in their interviews with convicted incest offenders because "the authoritarian position of the father makes the differentiation between threat, duress, acquiescence, and willingness almost impossible" (p. 207). Studies of court records by Gligor (1966) and Maisch (1972) indicate that daughters had shown seductive behavior in a small minority of cases, 12 percent and 6 percent respectively. McGaghy (1968) refers to incest offenders' projection of responsibility onto the child victims as one of the techniques of deviance disavowal used to preserve a normal, healthy self-image.

But what if the little girl was seductive or failed to resist the sexual advances of her father? Does this render incest harmless? The seductiveness and failure to resist of rape victims have often been used to discount the effects of rape, which, nevertheless, have been found to be serious and long term. The same is true of incest. Recent research is demonstrating an array of psychologically damaging effects of father-daughter incest which include interpersonal, marital, sexual, and identity problems, revulsion at being touched, school problems, antisocial behavior, and suicidal attempts (Anderson, 1979; Densen-Gerber, 1979; Finklehor, 1979; Geiser, 1979; Herjanic and Bryan, 1980; Johnston, 1979; Jorné, 1979; Kempe, 1978; Peters, 1976; Rush, 1980).

Seventy-five percent of a sample of adolescent female prostitutes in Minnesota had been victims of incest (Weber, 1977). Meiselman (1978) found that psychotherapy patients with a history of incest had more social, psychological, and sexual problems than those without a history of incest. The majority of women who volunteered to discuss their childhood incest experiences reported marked to severe effects on a number of indices of psychological and social functioning (Courtois and Watts, 1980). Herman and Hirschman (1977) described a syndrome in women who experienced incest in childhood. This included difficulty in forming intimate relationships, low self-esteem, and a predisposition to becoming repeatedly victimized. In many cases, symptoms may not be present during childhood but may occur in adulthood when the victims become overwhelmed by greater emotional and sexual demands (Peters, 1976).

An early study of adult-child sex relations by Bender and Blau (1937) is often cited as evidence for the negligible effects of incest. Their sample of a total of 16 cases included only 4 cases of incest, 2 of them involving father-daughter incest, hardly a basis for scientific generalization. Furthermore, their conclusions were based on the remaining sample of 12 children who had been sexually molested by *strangers*. Other investigators took these conclusions out of context and erroneously applied them to child victims of incest. Even on the basis of their four incest cases, Bender and Blau concluded that incest was harmful. They state:

Anxiety states with bewilderment concerning social relations occur especially in children who are seduced by parents. Such incest experiences undoubtedly distort the proper development of their attitudes toward members of the family, and subsequently, of society in general. (p. 516)

Apparently sexist and child-oppressive attitudes clouded the objectivity of some professionals to such an extent that they distorted evidence actually supportive of the harmful effects of father-daughter incest on the child into support of its negligible effects.

Despite the findings of psychological damage to victims of intergenerational incest, a few liberal professionals and parents are promoting the practice as beneficial to children (Yudkin, 1981). This irresponsible view further perpetuates the sexual victimization of children. In the past and in some current households, wife battering has also been viewed as beneficial to family harmony or even to the wife, as this old adage illustrates: "A wife, a spaniel, and a walnut tree/ The more they're beaten, the better they be." Some abusive parents and extremist educators even tout severe corporal punishment as beneficial to children, in the face of the evidence of serious damage to them. In the opinion of author C. S. Lewis, the most oppressive tyranny is that exercised for the benefit of its victims.

Some women have survived the effects of intergenerational incest, just as some have survived the effects of other forms of child abuse. Indeed, some victims may learn to transform these and a variety of childhood traumas into exceptional personality invulnerabilities during adulthood. Nevertheless, no rational individual would use these outcomes as a basis for recommending childhood trauma as a means of strengthening personality in adulthood.

The consequences of sexual initiation of children by parents and other adults in our society differ from those in primitive cultures. The direct motor expression of sexual initiation is supported by the entire ethos and rituals in primitive cultures, whereas it is dysfunctional in ours. In modern technological societies, the intergenerational incest taboo is essential to protect children from sexual exploitation by adults. There can be no informed consent in sexual relationships between adults and children in our society. Here, children are victims of reverse ageism. Our laws and mores offer them minuscule protection against violent coercion and no protection against emotional coercion. The passivity of incest victims is not surprising. In our society, when a child is sexually exploited by an adult, "The entire world of adult authority bears down to confuse and confound the hapless victim" (Brownmiller, 1976, p. 300). Female children are the most vulnerable of all groups, for they are the victims of double oppression: sexism as well as reverse ageism.

The indirect transmission of sexual knowledge to youths by their elders through the mediation of language and conceptualization is the appropriate mode in our society. The modern equivalent of sexual initiation is sex education, not sexual exploitation.

Throughout history and into the present, crimes against the female have been rationalized by incriminating her and absolving the criminal. Father-daughter incest adds a new dimension of oppression in that the female child is blamed and the male adult exonerated. The extent to which child protection was sacrificed in the interests of father protection is incisively illustrated in Freud's intensely conflicted attempts to grapple with the problem of father-daughter incest.

❖ Courtois and Watts (1980) found that women in their sample who had sought psychotherapy reported having gone to several therapists before they found one who believed them. Although the finding requires further exploration, it is noteworthy that those who received psychotherapy for the incest suffered significantly more severe psychological effects than those who did not. Peters (1976) states:

> It is my thesis . . . that both cultural and personal factors combined to cause every-one, including Freud himself at times, to welcome the idea that reports of child-hood sexual victimization could be regarded as fantasies. This position relieved the guilt of adults....
>
> Psychiatrists have in the past erred in the direction of ascribing to childhood fantasy real cases of sexual assault upon children. Experience in the rape victim clinics . . . and with patients in private psychoanalytic practice seem to indicate that reports of sexual assaults upon children are ignored or discounted at the expense of the psychologic well-being of the child victim. (pp. 401, 420)

The prejudices of many psychotherapists have contributed to the perpetuation of sexual abuse of the child by their denial of the victimization, by blaming the victim, and by overidentification with the adult male aggressor. They have added insult and more injury to the injury of father-daughter incest by probing the victim's role in allegedly eliciting the abuse, rather than helping her cope with it, protecting her from reabuse, and empathizing with her confusion, terror, rage, powerlessness, degradation, and despair. Like the rape victim, she is accused of lying, fantasizing the sexual victimization, or bringing it on herself because of her seductiveness, passivity, or failure to struggle. In *Sanctions for Evil* (Sanford and Comstock, 1971), Opton describes the psychosocial processes that permit individuals to tolerate the most inhumane acts. One such psychological mechanism, "It never happened and besides they deserved it," applies to the inhumane act of father-daughter incest.

Toward Responsible Sexuality and the Primary Prevention of Child Abuse

How can child abuse be prevented? By changing entrenched, worn-out solutions to the problem. Child abuse is but the tip of the iceberg. The glacier from which that iceberg formed consists of manifold expressions of irresponsible sexuality and the sanctioning of sexist, pronatalist, child-oppressive ideologies. The child abuse industry, with its overemphasis on treatment, creates the illusion that the glacier of social pathology undergirding child abuse does not exist and that treatment is all that is required to control the problem. This illusory optimism does not change the forecast that child abuse will continue indefinitely unless professionals and the public actively support sexually enlightened, egalitarian, child-advocating ideologies and programs directed toward primary prevention.

References

Abraham, K. The experiencing of sexual trauma as a form of sexual activity. In K. Abraham (Ed.), *Selected papers on psychoanalysis*. New York: Basic Books, 1954.

Albee, G. W. The prevention of sexism. *Professional Psychology*, 1981, *12*, 20-27.

Anderson, D. Touching: When is it caring and nurturing or when is it exploitative and damaging? *Child Abuse and Neglect*, 1979, *3*, 793-794.

Bender, L., and Blau, A. The reactions of children to sexual relations with adults. *American Journal of Orthopsychiatry*, 1937, *7*, 500-518.

Bishop, F. I. Children at risk. *Medical Journal of Australia*, 1971, *1*, 623.

Breslow, L. Unpublished paper presented at the first national Conference on Abortion Laws. Chicago, Illinois, 1969.

Breuer, J., and Freud, S. [Studies on hysteria.] In J. Strachey (Ed. and trans.), *The complete works of Sigmund Freud* (Vol. 2). London: Hogarth Press, 1955. (Originally published, 1895.)

Browning, D., and Boatman, B. Incest: Children at risk. *American Journal of Psychiatry*, 1977, *134*, 69-72.

Brownmiller, S. *Against our will: Men, women and rape*. New York: Bantam Books, 1976.

Butterfield, A. M., Jackson, A. D. M., and Nangle, D. Child abuse: A two year follow-up. *Child Abuse and Neglect*, 1979, *3*, 985-989.

Cavallin, H. Incestuous fathers: A clinical report. *American Journal of Psychiatry*, 1966, *122*, 1132-1138.

Cohn, A. H. Essential elements of successful child abuse and neglect treatment. *Child Abuse and Neglect*, 1979, *3*, 491-496.

Cohn, A. H., and Miller, M. K. Evaluating new modes of treatment for child abusers and neglectors: The experience of federally funded demonstration projects in the USA. *Child Abuse and Neglect*, 1977, *1*, 453-458.

Cormier, B., Kennedy, M., and Sangowicz, J. Psychodynamics of father-daughter incest. *Canadian Psychiatric Association Journal*, 1962, *7*, 203-215.

Courtois, C. A., and Watts, D. *Women who experienced childhood incest: Research findings and therapeutic strategies.* Paper presented at the annual meeting of the American Psychological Association, Montreal, Canada, 1980.

Densen-Gerber, J. Sexual and commercial exploitation of children: Legislative responses and treatment challenges. *Child Abuse and Neglect*, 1979, *3*, 61-66.

De Young, M. Promises, threats and lies: Keeping incest secret. *Journal of Humanics*, in press.

Dostoyevsky, F. *Crime and punishment.* New York: Laurel Press, 1962. (Originally published, 1886.)

Ferguson, D. M., Fleming, J., and O'Neil, D. P. *Child abuse in New Zealand.* Wellington, New Zealand: Department of Social Welfare, 1972.

Finkelhor, D. *Sexually victimized children.* New York: Macmillan, 1979.

Fraser, B. Child abuse in America: A de facto legislative system. *Child Abuse and Neglect*, 1979, *3*, 35-43.

Freud, S. [*The origins of psycho-analysis, letters to Wilhelm Fliess, drafts and notes: 1887-1902.*] (M. Bonaparte, A. Freud, and E. Kris, eds., and E. Mosbacher and J. Strachey, trans.). New York: Basic Books, 1954.

Freud, S. The aetiology of hysteria. In J. Strachey (Ed. and trans.), *Standard edition of the complete psychological works of Sigmund Freud* (Vol. 3). London: Hogarth Press and the Institute of Psychoanalysis, 1955. (Originally published, 1896.)

Freud, S. *The standard edition of the complete psychological works of Sigmund Freud.* (J. Strachey, Ed. and trans.) (Vols. 1, 2, and 3). London: The Hogarth Press and the Institute of Psychoanalysis, 1924/1955.

Freud, S. [*The complete introductory lectures on psychoanalysis.*] (J. Strachey, Ed. and trans.). New York: W. W. Norton, 1966. (Originally published, 1933.)

Friedman, S. B. The need for intensive follow-up of abused children. In C. H. Kempe and R. E. Helfer (Eds.), *Helping the battered child and his family.* Philadelphia: J. B. Lippincott, 1972.

Friedrich, W. N. and Boriskin, J. A. The role of the child in abuse: A review of the literature. *American Journal of Orthopsychiatry*, 1976, *46*, 580-590.

Gaddis, D. C., Monaghan, S., Muir, R. C., and Jones, C. J. Early prediction in the maternity hospital. *Child Abuse and Neglect*, 1979, *3*, 757-766.

Gebhard, P. H., Gagnon, J. H., Pomeroy, W. B., and Christenson, C. *Sex offenders: An analysis of types.* New York: Harper and Row, 1965.

Geiser, R. L. *Hidden victims: The sexual abuse of children.* Boston: Beacon Press, 1979.

Gil, D. G. *Violence against children.* Cambridge, Mass.: Harvard University Press, 1970.

Gil, D. G. *Testimony.* Hearing before the Subcommittee on Children and Youth of the Committee on Labor and Public Welfare, 93rd Cong., 1st session. Child Abuse Prevention Act, 1973. Washington, D.C.: U.S. Government Printing Office, 1973.

Gligor, A. M. Incest and sexual delinquency: A comparative analysis of two forms of sexual behavior in minor females (Doctoral dissertation, Western Reserve University, 1967). Dissertation Abstracts International, 1966, 27B. (University Microfilms No. 67-04588, 3671)

Green, A. A psychodynamic approach to the study and treatment of child abusing parents. *Journal of Child Psychiatry,* 1976, *15,* 213-224.

Green, C. P., and Pottzeiger, K. *Teenage pregnancy: A major problem for minors.* Washington, D.C.: Zero Population Growth, 1977.

Helfer, R. E. *Child abuse and neglect: The diagnostic process and treatment programs.* Washington, D.C.: U.S. Department of Health, Education and Welfare, Publ. No. OHD75-69, 1975.

Helfer, R. E. *Prevention of serious breakdowns in parent child interaction.* Unpublished paper presented at the National Committee for Prevention of Child Abuse, Denver, Colorado, 1978.

Hennepin County Attorney's Office. *Sexual assault: The target is you.* Brochure prepared by the Hennepin County Attorney's Office, Minneapolis, Minnesota, no date.

Herjanic, B., and Bryan, B. Sexual abuse of children. *Medical Aspects of Human Sexuality,* 1980, April, 92-99.

Herman, J. Father-daughter incest. *Professional Psychology,* 1981, *12,* 76-80.

Herman, J., and Hirschman, L. Father-daughter incest. *Signs: Journal of Women in Culture and Society,* 1977, *2,* 735-756.

Herrenkohl, R. C., Herrenkohl, E. C., Egolf, B., and Seech, M. The repetition of child abuse: How frequently does it occur? *Child Abuse and Neglect,* 1979, *3,* 67-72.

Johnston, M. S. K. The sexually mistreated child: Diagnostic evaluation. *Child Abuse and Neglect,* 1979, *3,* 943-951.

Jones, E. *The life and work of Sigmund Freud.* New York: Basic Books, 1961.

Jorné, P. S. Treating sexually abused children. *Child Abuse and Neglect,* 1979, *3,* 285-290.

Kempe, C. H. Sexual abuse: Another hidden pediatric problem. *Pediatrics,* 1978, *62,* 382-389.

Kempe, C. H. Recent developments in the field of child abuse. *Child Abuse and Neglect,* 1979, *3,* ix-xv.

Lenoski, E. F. Unpublished paper presented at the Seminar on Child Abuse, Denver, Colorado, September 1974.

Light, R. J. Abused and neglected children in America: A study of alternative policies. *Harvard Educational Review,* 1973, *43,* 556-598.

Lynch, M. A., and Roberts, J. Predicting child abuse: Signs of bonding failure in the maternity hospital. *British Medical Journal,* 1977, *1,* 624.

MacCarthy, D. Deprivation dwarfism viewed as a form of child abuse. In A. W. Franklin (Ed.), *The challenge of child abuse.* London: Academic Press, 1977.

Maisch, H. *Incest*. New York: Stein and Day, 1972.

Martin, H. P., and Beezley, P. Prevention and the consequences of child abuse. *Journal of Operational Psychology*, 1974, *6*, 68-77.

McGaghy, C. H. Drinking and deviance disavowal: The case of child molesters. *Social Problems*, 1968, *16*, 43-49.

Meiselman, K. C. *Incest: A psychological study of causes and effects with treatment recommendations*. San Francisco: Jossey-Bass, 1978.

Oates, R. K., Davis, A. A., Ryan, M. G., and Stewart, L. F. Risk factors associated with child abuse. *Child Abuse and Neglect*, 1979, *3*, 547-553.

Opton, E. M. It never happened and besides they deserved it. In N. Sanford and C. Comstock (Eds.), *Sanctions for evil*. San Francisco: Jossey-Bass, 1971.

Peters, J. J. Children who were victims of sexual assault and the psychology of the offenders. *American Journal of Psychotherapy*, 1976, *30*, 398-417.

Prescott, J. Abortion of the unwanted child: A choice for a humanistic society. *Journal of Pediatric Psychology*, 1976, *1*, 62-67.

Resnick, P. J. Murder of the newborn: A psychiatric review of neonaticide. *American Journal of Psychiatry*, 1970, *126*, 1414-1420.

Rush, F. *The best kept secret: Sexual abuse of children*. Englewood Cliffs, N.J.: Prentice-Hall, 1980.

Sanford, N., and Comstock, C. (Eds.), *Sanctions for evil*. San Francisco: Jossey-Bass, 1971.

Scott, W. J. Attachment and child abuse: A study of social history indicators among mothers of abused children. In G. J. Williams and J. Money (Eds.), *Traumatic abuse and neglect of children at home*. Baltimore: Johns Hopkins University Press, 1980.

Sgroi, S. M. The sexual assault of children: Dynamics of the problem and issues of program development. In Community Council of Greater New York (Ed.), *Sexual abuse of children*. New York: Community Council of Greater New York, 1979.

Skinner, A. E., and Castle, R. L. *78 battered children: A retrospective study*. London: National Society for the Prevention of Cruelty to Children, 1969.

Spinetta, J. J., and Rigler, D. The child-abusing parent: A psychological review. *Psychological Bulletin*, 1972, 77, 296-304.

Steele, B. F., and Pollack, C. B. A psychiatric study of parents who abuse infants and small children. In R. E. Helfer and C. H. Kempe (Eds.), *The battered child*. University of Chicago Press, 1968.

Summit, R., and Kryso, J. Sexual abuse of children: A clinical spectrum. *American Journal of Orthopsychiatry*, 1978, *48*, 237-251.

Taitz, L. S. Effects on growth and develoment of social, psychological, and environmental factors. *Child Abuse and Neglect*, 1980, *4*, 55-65.

United States Department of Health, Education, and Welfare. *Child abuse and neglect: An overview of the problem*, (Vol. 1). Washington, D.C.: DHEW Publication (OHD) 75-30073, 1975.

Walsh, T. *Premature parenting and child abuse*. Unpublished paper presented at the Workshop on Teen Parenthood, Onondaga Community College, New York, March 8, 1977.

Wasserman, S. The abused parent of the abused child. *Children*, 1967, *14*, 175-179.

Weber, E. Sexual abuse begins at home. *Ms.*, April 1977, p. 64.

Weinberg, S. K. *Incest behavior*. New York: Citadel, 1955.

West, J. E., and West, E. D. Child abuse treated in a psychiatric hospital.*Child Abuse and Neglect*, 1979, *3*, 699-707.

Williams, G. J. Origins of filicidal impulses in the American way of life. *Journal of Clinical Child Psychology*, 1976, *5*, 2-11.

Williams, G. J. Toward the eradication of child abuse and neglect at home. In G. J. Williams and J. Money (Eds.), *Traumatic abuse and neglect of children at home*. Baltimore: Johns Hopkins University Press, 1980.

Yudkin, M. Breaking the incest taboo: Those who crusade for family "love" forget the balance of family power. *Progressive*, May 1981, pp. 27-28.

Symptoms in Women

Marcia Guttentag

❖ *SEX DIFFERENCES IN MENTAL HEALTH SYMPTOMATOLOGY*

Women—especially young women—are more depressed than men. In adolescence, female mental hospital admission rates exceed those of males. In the age group 25 to 44, women's frequency of admission peaks over men's: the figures for 1969, for example, were 766,744 females compared with 666,389 males.[1]

The percentage of men and women suffering from personality disorders, neurosis, and schizophrenia are roughly equivalent, but twice as many women as men are diagnosed as suffering from depressive disorders.[2] These disorders peak in women between the ages of 25 and 44, accounting for 49 percent of total disorders.[3]

In all types of facilities except state and county mental hospitals, depressive disorders are the leading diagnoses for women. This includes community mental health centers, private mental hospitals, general hospital in-patient services, and out-patient services. Only in state and county mental hospitals is schizophrenia the leading diagnosis for women admitted, with depressive dis-

---

1. *Socio-economic characteristics of admissions and out-patient psychiatric services, 1969*. National Institute of Mental Health, Department of Health, Education, and Welfare Publication No. (HSM)-72-9045 (U.S. Government Printing Office, Washington, D.C., 1971), Table 7, p. 26.

2. As a percentage of total episodes, 9.8 percent males—as against 21.1 percent females—have depressive disorders. *Utilization of Psychiatric Facilities by Persons Diagnosed with Depressive Disorders*. National Institute of Mental Health, Department of Health, Education, and Welfare Publication No. ADM 74-5 (1974), Table 2, p. 7.

3. Ibid., Table 6, p. 16.

From Marcia Guttentag, "The Prevention of Sexism," in George W. Albee and Justin M. Joffe (eds.) *The Issues: An Overview of Primary Prevention*. Copyright © 1977 by the Vermont Conference on the Primary Prevention of Psychopathology. Reprinted by permission.

orders second. For men, in contrast, alcoholic disorders, schizo-phrenia, and personality disorders—in that order—are the leading diagnoses for state and county mental hospital admissions, while in community mental health centers, schizophrenia and per-sonality disorders lead (Cannon and Redick, 1973). For hospital admissions overall, females always outnumber males for depressive disorders, while males always outnumber females for alcoholic and drug disorders.

Throughout the countries of the developed world, mental health utilization figures show a significantly greater number of depressed females than males (Weissman, 1975). Only in a few underdeveloped countries does the rate of depression in women appear to be slightly lower than for men (see Table 2).

Nearly all studies of treated cases of depression in the United States show a marked increase in young females diagnosed as depressed during the past two decades (see Table 2). I recently returned from Hungary—a country that has undergone rapid in-dustrialization during the past two decades—where I was permitted to examine the diagnostic data of the National Institute of Mental Health. These revealed that in Hungary, too, there was a startling increase in the number of treated cases of depression in young females since World War II.

EPIDEMIOLOGICAL STUDIES

Rates of treated illnesses must be viewed cautiously. Women are much more likely than men to go to doctors and are therefore more likely to turn up in statistics on treated mental illness. It is therefore important to ask whether there are significant differ-ences in rates of depression for untreated cases. Weissman (1975) has compiled figures from community mental health surveys conducted in the United States and Western Europe during the past twenty years showing that untreated women were indeed significantly more depressed than men in all the developed countries. (See Table 3.)

One must be initially skeptical about such findings, since a number of plausible alternative hypotheses may account for them. Could it not be, for example, that women are more willing to admit distress? Perhaps their response biases make them look more depressed. Perhaps women are freer to express all feelings, or it

Table 1

The Three Leading Diagnoses among Male and Female Admissions
to State and County Mental Hospitals and to Community Mental Health Centers in 1970

(From Cannon and Redick, 1973)

	MALES	FEMALES
State and County Mental Hospitals	1. Alcohol Disorders 32.1%	1. Schizophrenia 37.7%
	2. Schizophrenia 24.0%	2. Depressive Disorders 16.9%
	3. Personality Disorders 16.3%	3. Organic Brain Syndromes 10.6%
Community Mental Health Centers	1. Schizophrenia 14.6%	1. Depressive Disorders 20.7%
	2. Transient Situational Personality Disorders 13.5%	2. Schizophrenia 15.6%
	3. Personality Disorders 13.3%	3. Transient Situational Personality Disorders 13.5%

Table 2*
Sex Ratios in Depression: Treated Cases
(From Weissman and Klerman, 1977. Reproduced by permission).

TREATED CASES:UNITED STATES

Place and Time	Sex Ratios Female/Male	References
Baltimore, Maryland 1936	2/1 (Psychoneurosis, including depression and manic-depressive)	Lemkau
Boston, Massachusetts 1945, 1955, 1965	Marked increase in young females with diagnosis of depressive reaction.	Rosenthal
Pittsfield, Massachusetts 1946-68	2.4/1 (Patients treated with ECT)	Tarnower and Humphries
New York State 1949	1.7/1	Lehmann
Massachusetts 1957-58	2.5/1 (All depressives)	Wechsler
Ohio 1958-61	First admissions 1.9/1 (White) 2.7/1 (Nonwhite)	Duvall et al.
Madison, Wisconsin 1958-69	Increase in depression for women over decade (patients referred for psychological testing)	Rice and Kepecs
Monroe County, New York	2.1/1 (Affective psychosis)	Gardner et al.
United States	Outpatient Admissions 1.4/1 (Psychotic depression) 1.2/1 (Manic-depression) 1.8/1 (Involutional psychosis) 1.6/1 (Depressive reactions)	Rosen, Bohn, and Kramer
Monroe County, New York 1961-62	1.6/1 (Prevalence) 1.3/1 (Incidence)	Pederson
Northern Florida 1963	26% female and 16% male medical patients were depressed. In the lower class, more men than women were depressed.	Schwab
New Haven, Connecticut 1966	3/1 (All depressions)	Paykel et al.
United States 1970	Admissions to All Psychiatric Facilities 2.1/1 (All depressive disorders)	Cannon and Redick
St. Louis, Missouri 1971	2.1/1 (Excluded bipolar depressives)	Baker

TREATED CASES: OUTSIDE UNITED STATES

Amsterdam 1916-40	2.3/1 Ashkenázim Jews 2.4/1 Gentiles	Gewel
Gaustad, Norway 1926-55	Life Time Risk of First Admission 1.37/1 (1926-35) 1.36/1 (1946-50) 1.33/1 (1951-55)	Odegaard

*References can be found in Guttentag and Salasin, 1976.

Table 2 (continued)

Place and Time	*Sex Ratios* *Female/Male*	*References*
Buckinghamshire, England 1931–47	1.8/1 (1931–33) 1.9/1 (1945–47	Lehmann
Basle, Switzerland 1945–57	1.5/1 (approximately)	Kielholz
London, England 1947–49	2/1	Lehmann
Scania, Sweden 1947, 1957	1.8/1 (Life time prevalence of severe depression)	Essen-Moller and Hagnell
Hertfordshire, England 1949–54	Neurotic Depression 3.5/1 (Admissions) 2.2/1 (Consultations)	Martin
England and Wales 1952, 1960	1.6/1 (1952) 1.7/1 (1960)	Lehmann
Tanganyika 1954	.5/1	Smartt
Aarhus County, Denmark 1958	2/1 (Endogenous Depression) 4/1 (Psychogenic Depression) 3/1 (Depressive Neurosis)	Juel-Nielson
Salford, England 1959–63	1.9/1 (Depressive Psychosis)	Adelstein et al.
Dakar, Guinea 1960–61	.5/1	Collomb and Zwingelstein
Madras and Madurai, India 1961–63	0.2/1	Venkoba Rao
Tokyo, Japan and Taiwan, China 1963–64	Women have more depressive symp- toms.	Rin
Madurai, India 1964–66	0.56/1 (Endogenous Depression)	Venkoba Rao
Bulawayo, Rhodesia 1965–67	1.1/1 (N=76)	Buchan
Baghdad, Iraq 1966–67	1.1/1	Bazzoui
Honduras 1967	1.6/1 (Admissions) 6.7/1 (Outpatients)	Hudgens et al.
New Delhi, India 1968	0.55/1	Teja et al.
Jerusalem, Israel 1969–72	2.1/1 (Affective disorders)	Gershon and Liebowitz
Papua, New Guinea 1970–73	.4/1 (Based on a few cases)	Torrey et al.
Denmark 1973	1.9/1 (First admissions for manic- depression)	Dupont et al.
Bangkok, Thailand	1.3/1 (Far East Orientals) .8/1 (Occidentals)	Tongyonk

may be that the same stress has different effects on men and women. After carefully analyzing a number of studies that have investigated these questions, Weissman (1975) concurred with Clancy and Gove (1974) that sex differences "in the degree of symptoms found in community studies appear to reflect actual differences and are not an artifact of response bias" (p. 6).

Interestingly, although the older psychiatric literature has emphasized involutional melancholia as the most prevalent form of depression in women, all of the recent data show that the highest rates of depression occur among young women in the 21- to 44-year age category.

Another source of data on the increase in depression among young women comes from epidemiological studies of suicide attempts. Weissman (1974) reviewed all studies conducted from 1960 to 1971. Throughout the developed world, suicide attempters were overwhelmingly young females, predominantly 20 to 30 years old. The average age has decreased in the past decade, and there has been an increase in suicide attempts among married and separated or divorced women. Several studies of the personality of suicide attempters have found most of them to be clinically depressed at the time of the attempt.

Other studies report an excess of attempters in the lower social classes. Still others have found that such attempts usually take place "in the context of a recent and serious inter-personal conflict—typically including marital or family discord" (p. 742).

Studies of the suicide attempters indicate which women are the most depressed. Very recent epidemiological work confirms this indication.

One such study, conducted by NIMH (Radloff, 1975; see Table 4) in Kansas City and in Washington County, Maryland, found that the married women and divorced or separated women in the community were significantly more depressed than men of similar status. Both working wives and housewives were more depressed than comparable working married men. The most depressed women were those who were poorly educated, were working at low-status jobs, and were married, with children at home. (As Bernard, 1973, has pointed out, mothers whose children no longer lived with them were significantly *less* depressed than women whose children were living with them or women who had no children). It is the young married working blue-collar mother

Table 3
Sex Differences in Depression: Community Surveys
(From Weissman, 1975)

COMMUNITY SURVEYS: UNITED STATES

Place and Time	Sex Ratios Female/Male	References
Brooklyn and Queens, New York 1960	Women were more depressed.	Benfare et al.
Baltimore, Maryland 1968	1.6/1 (Includes wives of blue-collar workers only)	Siassi et al.
Northern Florida 1968	1.8/1	Schwab
Carroll County, Maryland 1968	Women were more nervous, helpless, anxious	Hogarty and Katz
New Haven, Connecticut 1969	2/1 (Suicidal feelings)	Paykel et al.
St. Louis, Missouri 1968–69	No significant sex difference in depression in bereaved spouse	Clayton et al.
New York, New York 20-year period	More referrals for minor depression in female employees in one company	Hinkle et al.

COMMUNITY SURVEYS: OUTSIDE UNITED STATES

Iceland 1910–57	1.6/1 (All depressions)	Helgason
Samsø, Denmark 1960	3.5/1 (All depressions)	Sørenen
Ghiraz, Iran 1964	3.6/1 (N=23)	Bash and Bash-Liechti
Lucknow, India 1969–71	2/1	Sethi
Hertfordshire, England 1949–54	2.4/1	Martin
Agra, India	1.6/1 (Manic-depression)	Dube and Kuman

who is most likely to be depressed; and the risk has apparently increased dramatically during the past two decades.

Why? A recent study (Warren, 1975) done in urban communities provides some insight into this question. Warren observed where people turned for help when they had problems. She found considerable differences between blue- and white-collar women. Blue-collar men, for example, turned to their wives for help 58.2

Table 4
Mean Depression Score (CES-D):
Sex by Age, Education, Income for Currently Married
(Combined sites, Whites Only)
(From Radloff, 1975)

SEX vs. AGE

		Less than 25	*25–64*	*65+*
Male	x̄	9.47	7.38	5.78
	n	62	611	106
Female	x̄	12.41	9.26	8.14
	n	109	747	74

F-test: Sex $p < .01$
Age $p < .01$
Interaction Sex x Age $p > .69$

SEX vs. EDUCATION

		Less than HS	*HS*	*Some College*	*BA+*
Male	x̄	7.75	7.79	6.39	6.12
	n	301	254	111	113
Female	x̄	10.92	9.61	7.42	7.54
	n	335	360	151	84

F-test: Sex $p < .01$
Education $p < .01$
Interaction Sex x Education $p > .19$

SEX vs. INCOME

		Less than $4,000	*$4,000– $11,000*	*$12,000+*
Male	x̄	9.33	7.98	6.47
	n	68	327	342
Female	x̄	11.05	9.81	8.85
	n	84	413	362

F-test: Sex $p < .01$
Income $p < .01$
Interaction Sex x Income $p > .77$

percent of the time, whereas blue-collar women turned to their husbands only 40.5 percent of the time. This difference was significantly greater than among white-collar spouses. Again, although blue-collar men could turn to their co-workers for help 34.6 percent of the time, blue-collar women could do so only 18.9 percent of the time. Blue-collar women, in contrast with white-collar women, were also much less able to turn for help to informal neighborhood organizations or professionals.

If depression is indeed related to powerlessness and a sense of helplessness (Seligman, 1974), then it would appear that the blue-collar married young mother has both the greatest number of stresses to cope with and the fewest possible sources of help.

In their review of adult sex roles and mental illness, Gove and Tudor (1972) concluded that role conflicts and demands are probably at the root of these symptoms. During the past two decades, women's entry into the labor force—both blue-collar and white-collar women—has increased markedly (Levine, 1974). However, although the family role demands for white-collar women have changed in a slightly less sexist direction (they can turn to their husbands for help as well as vice versa), the same has not been true for the blue-collar married mother. She is caught within the traditional sexist family role requirements. Her entry into the labor force, in a low-level job, has meant that she must fulfill all of the traditional family role requirements in addition to working at a poorly paid and unsatisfying job. She has few sources of aid (though her husband can turn to her for aid with his problems). No wonder she feels trapped and powerless. The situation of the divorced or separated blue-collar mother is even worse.

If these mental health findings are viewed in relation to sex role stereotypes, the conclusion is inescapable that it is the sex-stereotyped familial and socioemotional roles that women now carry in addition to occupational burdens which are causing the greatly intensified stresses they experience.

REFERENCES

Bem, S. L. Psychology looks at sex roles: where have all the adrogynous people gone? Paper presented at the UCLA Symposium on Women, May 1972.

Bernard, J. *The future of marriage*. New York: Bantam Books, 1973.

Cannon, M. S., and Redick, R. W. *Differential utilization of psychiatric facilities by men and women, U.S. 1970*. (NIMH Biometry Branch, Statistical Note 81), Washington, D.C., 1973.

Clancy, K., and Gove, W. Sex differences in mental illness: an analysis of response bias in self report. *American Journal of Sociology*, 1974, *80*, 205–216.

Gove, W., and Tudor, J. Adult sex roles and mental illness. *American Journal of Sociology*, 1972, *78*, 812–835.

Guttentag, M., Bray, H., Amsler, J., Donovan, V., Legge, G., Legge, W. W., Littenberg, R., and Stotsky, S. *Undoing sex stereotypes: A How-to-do-it guide with tested non-sexist curricula and teaching methods.* New York: McGraw-Hill, 1976.

Guttentag, M., and Salasin, S. Women, men, and mental health. In L. Cater, W. Martyna, and A. Scott (Eds.), *Changing roles of men and women.* Aspen, Colo.: Aspen Press, 1976.

Levine, A. Women at work in America: History, status, and prospects. Unpublished paper, 1974.

Radloff, L. Sex differences in mental health: the effects of marital and occupational status. *Sex Roles*, 1975, *3*, 249–265.

Spence, J., Helmreich, R., and Stapp, L. The Personal Attributes Questionnaire: A measure of sex role stereotypes and masculinity and femininity. *Catalog of Selected Documents in Psychology*, 1974, *4*, 29–39.

Warren, R. B. The work role and problem coping: sex differentials in the use of helping systems in urban communities. Unpublished paper.

Weissman, M. M. The epidemiology of suicide attempts, 1960–1971. *Archives of General Psychiatry*, 1974, *30*, 737–746.

Weissman, M. M. Sex differences and the epidemiology of depression. Unpublished paper, 1975.

Weissman, M. M., and Klerman, G. Sex differences in the epidemiology of depression. *Archives of General Psychiatry*, 1977, *34*, 98–111.

Women: Dependence and Independence

Grace K. Baruch and Rosalind C. Barnett

The major theme of this paper is that in our society the psychological well-being of women is facilitated: (a) by the development of occupational competence and of the capacity for economic independence; and (b) by involvement in a variety of roles. With respect to the first point, we shall argue that neither psychological well-being nor full social competence in adulthood is compatible with occupational incompetence and economic dependence. Unfortunately, women still fail to grasp this social reality and thus do not prepare for it. Many women, therefore, find themselves unable to cope successfully with the circumstances in which they find themselves. They are at high risk for psychiatric symptomatology, poverty, and diminished well-being, especially as they grow older. As for the second point, we shall argue that when one considers the whole life span, the gratifications provided by multiple role involvement usually outweigh any conflict and stress such involvement may entail.

We begin by discussing the social changes that have made occupational competence and economic independence critical for women's successful adaptation. We then review evidence about the effects of multiple role involvement on psychological well-being in a group of married women with young children who differ in employment status. Women who occupy the traditional pattern of wife and mother are compared with those who combine these roles with that of paid worker, a pattern shared by increasing numbers of women.

The issues to be discussed must be viewed in the context of at least two sets of social changes. The first set includes the ability to control fertility, the problems of overpopulation, and the lengthening life span. An increasing proportion of women need no longer face frequent or unpredictable childbearing (Hoffman, 1977), and the social value of children has decreased. Furthermore, female life expectancy now exceeds 75 years, of which perhaps 10, or no more than about 1/7 of a lifetime, may be spent in intensive child-rearing, and that not for all women. A view of women that focuses on the wife and mother role and socializes girls mainly for such a role reflects serious lags in our perceptions, beliefs, and, perhaps most important, our emotions.

The second set of social changes revolves around what is really not a change at all, but a return to the way things have usually been in human history. We refer to the increasing participation of women, including mothers of young children, in the paid labor force. What is old about this is the restoring to women of their historic role as economic providers. In hunter-gatherer and agricultural societies, which together have constituted the human life style for over 90 percent of our history, women have always provided a substantial proportion of the economic basis for survival and for support of their families through food-gathering, farming, and other economically productive activities.

The East African women studied by the anthropologist Beatrice Whiting (1977), for example, grow crops on small plots, earn cash, and provide food and clothing required by their children. Doing their work in the company of other adults, they spend four or five hours a day away from their children, yet their lives provide what Whiting sees as the critical components of human well-being: a sense of competence—that is, having a valued impact on one's environment; sufficient variation in stimulation; and the assurance of support and comfort. But as their husbands move into stable paid employment in urban settings, the women follow, leaving their family farms. Landless and jobless, they become economically dependent for the first time and must take sole, full-time responsibility for the care of their children in isolated homes. Boredom and irritability increase; self-esteem decreases; well-being suffers. But to take on eight hours a day of poorly paid work in the labor force is not an answer to their demoralization. Such work creates overwhelming difficulties with child care, fatigue, and other problems so familiar to many women in our society. What should strike us is that these new social changes in Kenya that trouble Beatrice Whiting so much are frighteningly similar to our norm, indeed our social ideal, for the American family: the man as sole economic provider, the woman, jobless and in sole charge of children, economically dependent and isolated in her own home.

But for women not to be involved in economically productive work is in fact a new-fangled pattern in human society. With a cross-cultural perspective, we can see that our pattern, which otherwise might appear to reflect some kind of natural law about the division of labor between men and women, may actually be very unstable as well as painful and dysfunctional.

Of course, which patterns are adaptive and which are not depends obviously upon the social context, but given the context we have described, we believe that all adults must be able to function as economic providers. This simple idea is a cliché if one is thinking about men, but it remains controversial when applied to women. When men cannot support themselves or their families, we read about it in the newspapers. And as such cases multiply, they command the attention of social workers and economists, psychiatrists and senators. When a woman is unable to provide for herself and any dependents, that is as expected, unless and until she enters particular social categories of persons who threaten to impinge upon public monies: separated mothers, pregnant teenagers, elderly widows. Like magic, her economic dependence suddenly becomes all too visible and regrettable, attaining the status of a social problem, a label that is a passport to social concern. But this concern should have been present in the minds of parents and educators, mental health workers and public officials from her cradle days on. Yet the situations of the divorced mother, the unmarried pregnant teenager, the poor elderly widow, the battered wife unable to leave home—all are simply visible crises that punctuate the course of an otherwise undetected disease. The twin components of this disease are occupational incompetence and economic dependence; among the various milder manifestations are low self-esteem and depression.

Much current literature on mental health and well-being documents these and other negative impacts of what we might call our recent "traditional" patterns, and conversely, the positive consequences of "nontraditional" lifestyles. For example, when the famous group of gifted children first studied by Terman was followed up recently—they are now in their 60's—the women in the group were asked to describe their life pattern and their satisfaction with it (Sears and Barbee, 1977). The women who reported the highest level of satisfaction were income-producers, that is, they were working for pay, and were heads of households, that is, not currently married. These findings were contrary to expectations, perhaps because our psychological theories (and national mythologies) say that marriage and children are the route to a sense of well-being. These women, of course, were very able and in many cases were relatively successful occupationally. But in a study of working-class women all of whom were married and had children, Myra Ferree (1976) found that despite the routine nature of their jobs, those who worked felt happier and had higher self-esteem than did the unemployed housewives.

A second illustration is the work of George Brown and his colleagues (Brown, Bhrolchain, and Harris, 1975). Their study of the development of psychiatric symptomatology in women living in London showed that among women most at risk—that is, those with small children, who did not have a confidante—employment was a powerful antidote to stress; psychiatric symptoms developed in 79 percent of those women who were not employed, compared with only 14 percent of those employed.

Finally, in a large-scale study of households in the Chicago area, Frederic Ilfeld (1977) found that women have higher rates of symptomatology than do men. However, the only group of women with symptomatology rates as low as those of men were those who worked in high-prestige occupations. The mental health implication, Ilfeld concluded, is to get more women into high-status jobs.

Intellectual well-being, we believe, is also a component of mental health. Consider a very disturbing longitudinal study of children given IQ tests in the 1930's (Kangas and Bradway, 1972). Results of a follow-up when the subjects were in their middle years showed that the brighter a man was as a youngster (in terms of IQ scores), the more he had gained in IQ with age; the brighter a woman, the less she had gained. Since the patterns of "average" women resembled those of men, biological differences are an unlikely explanation for the results found for the bright women. Therefore it may be that their lives had not provided the elements necessary for cognitive growth. On this point, Melvin Kohn and his associates (Kohn and Schooler, 1977) have recently demonstrated that the structure of work affects aspects of personality previously thought to be relatively stable and fixed early in life. The cognitive complexity of the work their subjects did was found to be related both to their intellectual flexibility and to their self-esteem. For those engaged in repetitive work, as are some housewives, the implications for well-being are ominous.

Furthermore, while the family is often viewed as a valuable refuge from the occupational world, we often forget that the workplace can be a valuable refuge from family life, from strong emotions, conflicting demands, petty annoyances. Work can provide variety, challenge, clear-cut responsibilities, even respectful underlings. Certainly if unemployment can contribute to mental illness, employment, for women as well as men, can contribute to mental health. Yet we rarely conceptualize unemployment as a social problem for women. Their unemployment is often hidden; analyses of the National Longitudinal Survey data (Blau, 1978) suggest that the effect of recessions, at least among white women, is to discourage them from entering the labor force. Furthermore, among black women, those who want to work form a larger group than those who actually hold jobs (Sullivan, 1977). When employed women lose their jobs, moreover, the social supports available are minimal (Warren, 1975) compared to those available to men.

It is almost a cliché now for people who work long hours at demanding jobs, aware of what they are missing in terms of time with family, long talks with friends, concerts, all kinds of opportunities for leisure, to express the sentiment that "there is more to life than work." The problem is that life *without* productive work is terrible. We assume this for men in thinking about their unemployment and their retirement, but we do not think about the situation of women in this way. We want to stress here that as Linda Fidell (1978) has shown, for some women the activities associated with child-care and home-making are truly productive and satisfying in terms of engaging their interests and talents, at least for part of their lives, as are volunteer activities. However, for others, the lack of economically productive work is associated with the absence of one or more of the previously mentioned requirements postulated by Beatrice Whiting (1977): a sense of competence; support and comfort; and variations in stimulation.

Many women settle for support and comfort at the expense of their other needs.

Unfortunately, our norm of married women economically dependent upon their husbands is not viable in many circumstances. Husbands lose their jobs or die without leaving an adequate estate; inflation makes two incomes increasingly necessary; and perhaps most important, marriages dissolve. It is projected that 40 percent of current marriages will end in divorce. Divorce too often brings poverty to many middle-class women who thought it could never happen to them. About half of the women now on welfare are separated or divorced, and the situation of divorced and separated women *not* on welfare is precarious. Dorothy Burlage (1978) in a new study of such women asks the question, How do these women manage to avoid welfare? The answer is, barely and painfully, and by being breadwinners. Their major source of support is their own earnings, not alimony or child support. Their economic situation after divorce is much worse than before, and considering income in relation to need, is much worse than that of their ex-husbands. Because of the limitations of their training and experience and the absence of social supports, many are living out Beatrice Whiting's nightmare alternative for mothers: eight hours of paid drudgery. The low pay of women's occupations, the need to work full time to receive not only income but desperately needed health benefits, and barriers to further education constrain both their current and future income. In their book *Time of Transition*, Heather Ross and Isabel Sawhill (1975) report finding that of separated women who are on welfare, only about one quarter could earn even $1000 more a year than welfare provides.

So we return to the question of occupational competence, and to its roots in socialization, because in mentioning such phenomena as divorce and widowhood, one is reciting the list of disasters that young girls are warned may force them to work. Thus they are encouraged to prepare themselves for some sort of fall-back occupation. In this way economic independence is associated not with pride and pleasure but with misfortune, stigma, and failure. For girls to develop maximum occupational competence has been a goal neither for them nor for their parents. The images of girls as future wives and mothers and boys as

economic providers are powerful influences on the values, attitudes, practices, and feelings of parents, who have been very
concerned not to jeopardize the wife-and-mother part of a girl's
future role. We are only now beginning to think about what may
jeopardize optimal development of a girl's occupational life.
The problem may be seen in a study by Barnett (1975), who
found that when one ranks occupations in terms of how prestigious they are, the more prestige an occupation has, the more
boys, but not girls, desired to enter it. For girls the more prestigious an occupation, the more they expressed an aversion to
entering it. Traditional parental values and attitudes can therefore be hazardous for daughters' future occupational options.
Having a challenging and satisfying occupation can be a central
source of self-esteem, identity, and satisfaction and it is increasingly important that women derive these from sources beyond
the roles of wife and mother.

Theoretical and empirical literature relevant to these topics
is unfortunately inadequate. Depending upon whose book one
is reading, one is told that marriage and children are a health
hazard for women, that career-oriented women are unhappy,
neurotic, conflicted about femininity, and so forth. Available
data are limited in various ways, but at least researchers are
asking important questions, such as whether marrying and having children are necessary for well-being.

On the question of marriage, studies of depression indicate
that among married people, women are more depressed than
men; among the unmarried, men are more depressed than women.
In reviewing these data, Lenore Radloff (1975) concluded that
marriage is a mental health advantage to men, but not to women.
However, a large-scale survey by Angus Campbell and his associates (1976) found no evidence that women were less satisfied
than men, and married women were more satisfied and happier
than unmarried women. So far, then, the data on marriage are
mixed.

Data on the relationship between rearing children and well-
being are somewhat clearer. Depression and a lower sense of
well-being are associated with caring for young children; indeed,
women in the so-called empty nest years are in fact lower in risk
for depression and higher in sense of well-being (Radloff, 1975).

Thus intensive involvement in child care is no sure route to happiness for women.

Work, in contrast, has until recently been seen as peripheral to women's well-being. Moreover, even studies that do focus on women's employment status tend to ignore variations among employed women which are due to differences in occupational status and in commitment to work (Campbell, Converse, and Rodgers, 1976; Kanter, 1977). Similarly, Linda Fidell (1978) has recently pointed out that women at home are not all alike; some are committed to the role of housewife, some want to work, and these variations affect well-being.

REFERENCES

Bailyn, L. Personal communication, 1978.

Barnett, R. C. Sex differences and age trends in occupational preference and occupational prestige. *Journal of Counseling Psychology*, 1975, *22*, 35–38.

Bart, P. Depression in middle-aged women. In J. M. Bardwick (Ed.), *Readings on the psychology of women*. New York: Harper and Row, 1972.

Baruch, G. K. Feminine self-esteem, self-ratings of competence, and maternal career-commitment. *Journal of Counseling Psychology*, 1973, *20*, 487–488.

Baruch, G. K. Girls who perceive themselves as competent: Some antecedents and correlates. *Psychology of Women Quarterly*, 1976, *1*, 38–49.

Birnbaum, J. A. Live patterns and self-esteem in gifted family-oriented and career-committed women. In M. Mednick, S. Tangri, and L. W. Hoffman (Eds.), *Women and achievement: Social and motivational analysis*. New York: Hemisphere-Halstead, 1975.

Blau, F. D. *The impact of the unemployment rate on labor force entries and exits*. Paper presented to Secretary of Labor's Invitational Conference on the National Longitudinal Surveys of Mature Women, Washington, D.C., 1978.

Brown, G. W., Bhrolchain, M. N., and Harris, T. Social class and psychiatric disturbance among women in an urban population. *Sociology*, 1975, *9*, 225–254.

Burlage, D. *Divorced and separated mothers: Combining the responsibilities of breadwinning and childrearing*. Unpublished doctoral dissertation, Harvard University, 1978.

Campbell, A., Converse, P. E., and Rodgers, W. L. *The quality of American life*. New York: Russell Sage, 1976.

Coopersmith, S. *The antecedents of self-esteem*. San Francisco: Freeman, 1968.

Ferree, M. M. The confused American housewife. *Psychology Today*, 1976, *10*, 76–80.

Fidell, L. *Employment status, role dissatisfaction and the housewife syndrome.* Unpublished manuscript, California State University, 1978.

Gove, W. R., and Tudor, J. F. Adult sex roles and mental illness. *American Journal of Sociology*, 1973, *78*, 812–835.

Hoffman, L. W. Changes in family roles, socialization, and sex differences. *American Psychologist*, 1977, *32*, 644–657.

Ilfeld, F., Jr. *Sex differences in psychiatric symptomatology.* Paper presented at American Psychological Association meeting, San Francisco, 1977.

Kangas, J., and Bradway, K. Intelligence at middle age: A thirty-eight-year-follow-up. *Developmental Psychology*, 1972, *5*, 333–337.

Kanter, R. M. *Work and family in the United States: A critical review and agenda for research and policy.* New York: Russell Sage Foundation, 1977.

Kohn, M. L., and Schooler, C. *The complexity of work and intellectual functioning.* Paper presented to American Sociological Association meeting, Chicago, 1977.

Lipman-Blumen, J. *The vicarious achievement ethic and non-traditional roles for women.* Paper presented to Eastern Sociological Association, New York, 1973.

Macke, A. S., and Hudis, P. M. *Sex-role attitudes and employment among women: A dynamic model of change and continuity.* Paper presented to Secretary of Labor's invitational conference on the National Longitudinal Surveys of Mature Women, Washington, D.C., 1978.

Radloff, L. Sex differences in depression: The effects of occupation and marital status. *Sex Roles*, 1975, *1*, 249–265.

Rosenkrantz, P., Vogel, S., Bee, H., Broverman, I., and Broverman, D. Sex-role stereotypes and self-concepts in college students. *Journal of Consulting Psychology*, 1968, *32*, 287–295.

Ross, H. L., and Sawhill, I. V. *Time of transition: The growth of families headed by women.* Washington: The Urban Institute, 1975.

Sears, P. S., and Barbee, A. H. Career and life satisfaction among Terman's gifted women. In J. Stanley, W. George, and C. Solano (Eds.), *The gifted and the creative: Fifty year perspective.* Balitmore: Johns Hopkins University Press, 1977.

Spence, J., and Helmreich, R. The attitudes towards women scale: An objective instrument to measure attitudes towards the rights and roles of women in contemporary society. JSAS *Catalog of Selected Documents in Psychology*, 1972, *2*, 66.

Sullivan, T. A., *Black female breadwinners: Some intersections of dual market and secondary worker theory.* Paper presented to American Sociological Association, Chicago, 1977.

Treiman, D. J. Problems of concept and measurement in the comparative study of occupational mobility. *Social Science Research*, 1975, *4*, 183–230.

Warren, R. B. *The work role and problem coping: Sex differentials in the use of helping systems in urban communities.* Paper presented at meeting of American Sociological Association, San Francisco, 1975.

Whiting, B. B. Changing life styles in Kenya. *Daedalus*, 1977, *106*, 211–225.

Family Stress and Children's Response

Michael Rutter

There is a regrettable tendency to focus gloomily on the ills of mankind and on all that can and does go wrong. It is quite exceptional for anyone to study the development of those important individuals who overcome adversity, who survive stress, and who rise above disadvantage. It is equally unusual to consider the factors or circumstances that provide support, protection, or amelioration for the children reared in deprivation. This neglect of positive influences on development means that we lack guides on how to help deprived or disadvantaged children. It is all very well to wish for the children to have a stable, loving family which provides emotional support, social stability, and cognitive stimulation. But we are almost never in a position to provide that. All we can do is alleviate a little here, modify a little there, and talk to the child about coming to terms with his problems. On the whole, the benefits that follow our therapeutic endeavors are pretty modest in the case of severely deprived children. Would our results be better if we could determine the sources of social competence and identify the nature of protective influences? I do not know, but I think they would. The potential for prevention surely lies in increasing our knowledge and understanding of the reasons why some children are *not* damaged by deprivation. My purpose in this paper is to consider some of the very limited evidence so far available on the topic.

Among children in Britain today about one in six live in conditions of extreme social disadvantage characterized by poverty *and* poor housing *and* family adversity (Wedge and Prosser, 1973). Nearly half of these children are well adjusted, one in seven has

From Michael Rutter, "Protective Factors in Children's Responses to Stress and Disadvantage," in Martha Whalen Kent and Jon E. Rolf (eds.) *Social Competence in Children.* Copyright © 1979 by the Vermont Conference on the Primary Prevention of Psychopathology. Reprinted by permission.

some kind of outstanding ability, and one in eleven shows above average attainment in mathematics. Thus, in spite of profound social deprivation, some of these children not only develop adequately but are well above average in their educational attainments.

Even in a deprived neighborhood, it is unusual for a child to suffer the constellation of disadvantages of parental criminality, bad child-rearing, poverty, low intelligence, and large family size (West and Farrington, 1973, 1977). Yet, of the children who do experience all these sources of risk, over a quarter show no evidence of any kind of delinquent or antisocial behavior as assessed in multiple ways on several occasions during a longitudinal study.

It is difficult to imagine the dreadful stresses experienced by youngsters who are brought up by mentally disturbed parents with a lifelong personality disorder whose marriages show extreme discord, hostility, and disruption. Everything appears against them, but a proportion of such children developed normally without any evidence of disorder at any time during the course of an intensive four-year longitudinal study (Rutter, Quinton, and Yule, 1977).

The three studies I have quoted all placed great emphasis on the severe risks for later psychosocial development which attend being brought up in grossly deprived or disadvantaged family circumstances. Their research findings provide ample evidence of the extent of the risks. Children who suffer in this way are much more likely than other children to develop psychiatric disorder, become delinquent, or remain educationally retarded. Nevertheless, as the figures I have quoted illustrate, some children do come through unscathed. This is a phenomenon shown by all investigations, but it has been systematically studied only rarely. In particular, although various writers have drawn attention to the importance of coping skills in children at risk and their resistance to stress (e.g. Hersov, 1974; Murphy, 1962; Garmezy, 1974; Anthony, 1974; Rutter, 1974, 1977a), there have been very few attempts to determine why and how some children appear relatively invulnerable.

❖   *INTERACTIVE EFFECTS BETWEEN STRESSES*

The first point to make is the very great importance of interactive effects. We tend to overlook their importance because several stresses so often come together, and most research data are not analyzed in such a way as to reveal the cumulative and interactive effects of single stresses. The usual approach is to take account of intercorrelations between variables by some form of statistical regression or standardization procedure. The resulting comparison shows whether or not a particular stress still has an effect after taking into account its associations with other forms of stress or disadvantage. However, it is necessary to appreciate that while the result shows whether the stressor has an effect over and above that of other factors, it does not show whether the stressor has an effect when it occurs entirely on its own.

We looked at this point in relation to the data collected in the Isle of Wight and inner London epidemiological studies (Rutter et al., 1975a, 1975b) of 10-year-old children. First, we identified six family variables all of which were strongly and significantly associated with child psychiatric disorder: (1) severe marital discord; (2) low social status; (3) overcrowding or large family size; (4) paternal criminality; (5) maternal psychiatric disorder; and (6) admission into the care of the local authority (Rutter and Quinton, 1977). Next we separated out families which had none of these risk factors, those with only one risk factor, those with two, and so on. We then compared these groups in terms of the rates of psychiatric disorder in the children.

The results, summarized in Figure 1, were interesting and surprising. The children with just one risk factor—that is, those with a truly isolated stress—were no more likely to have psychiatric disorder than children with no risk factors at all. It appeared that even with chronic family stresses the children were not particularly at psychiatric risk so long as it was really a single stress on its own. On the other hand, when any two of the stresses occurred together, the risk went up no less than fourfold. With yet more concurrent stresses, the risk climbed several times further still. In other words, the stresses *potentiated* each other so that the combination of chronic stresses provided very much more than a summation of the effects of the separate stresses considered singly.

These findings refer to interactions between chronic stresses. It appears that much the same thing may also apply to acute stresses. In the same set of studies we examined the long-term effects of hospital admission. We found, as had Douglas (1975) previously, that there were no detectable long-term sequelae of

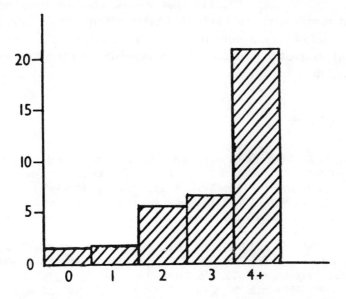

Figure 1. Multiplicity of Risk Factors and Child Psychiatric Disorder

single admissions to hospital regardless of the age at which they occurred (Quinton and Rutter, 1976). On the other hand, we found, as had Douglas, that *multiple* hospital admissions were associated with a substantially (and significantly) increased risk of psychiatric disorder in later childhood.

This finding is of interest from several points of view. First, it demonstrates the greatly increased effects of a cumulation of stresses. One hospital admission did no long-term harm, but two admissions were damaging. An interaction effect again. Secondly, there were two quite different types of associations between chronic stresses and hospital admission. On the one hand, children from deprived and disadvantaged families were more likely to *have* multiple admissions to hospital. In other words, the presence of chronic family stress meant that the children were more likely to experience a series of multiple acute stresses during development. Sameroff (1975) has called this a transactional effect.

On the other hand, there was also a potentiating or interaction effect. Not only were children from disadvantaged homes more likely to have multiple admissions, they were also more likely to suffer from the long-term adverse effects.

184   MICHAEL RUTTER

❖   ...In other words, children from more
favored homes were less likely to develop psychiatric disorder following multiple admissions. It seemed that a favorable home environment exerted a protective effect in relation to the stresses of
recurrent hospitalization.

REFERENCES

Anthony, E. J. The syndrome of the psychologically invulnerable child. In E.
    Anthony and C. Koupernick (Eds.), *The child in his family*. Vol. 3, *Chil-
    dren at psychiatric risk* (New York: Wiley, 1974), pp. 529–544.
Aronson, E., and Mettee, D. R. Dishonest behavior as a function of differen-
    tial levels of induced self-esteem. *Journal of Personality and Social Psy-
    chology*, 1968, *9*, 121–127.
Berger, M., Yule, W., and Rutter, M. Attainment and adjustment in two geo-
    graphical areas. II. The prevalence of specific reading retardation. *British
    Journal of Psychiatry*, 1975, *126*, 510–519.
Brown, G. W., Bhrolchain, M. N., and Harris, T. Social class and psychiatric
    disturbance among women in an urban population. *Sociology*, 1975, *9*,
    225–254.
Chavez, A., Martinez, C., and Yaschine, T. The importance of nutrition and
    stimuli on child mental and social development. In J. Cravioto, L. Ham-
    bracus, and B. Vahlquist (Eds.), *Early malnutrition and mental develop-
    ment*. Symposia of the Swedish Nutrition Foundation. Stockholm: Alm-
    quist and Wilksell, 1974.
Conway, E. S. *The institutional care of children: A case history*. Unpublished
    Ph.D. thesis, University of London, 1957.
Coopersmith, S. *The antecedents of self-esteem*. San Francisco: W. H. Freeman
    and Co., 1967.
Crowe, R. R. An adoption study of antisocial personality. *Archives of General
    Psychiatry*, 1974, *31*, 785–791.
Dixon, P. Unpublished data. 1977.
Douglas, J. W. B. Early hospital admissions and later disturbances of behaviour
    and learning. *Developmental Medicine and Child Neurology*, 1975, *17*,
    456–480.
Garmezy, N. The study of competence in children at risk for severe psycho-
    pathology. In E. Anthony and C. Koupernick (Eds.), *The child in his
    family*. Vol. 3, *Children at psychiatric risk* (New York: Wiley, 1974), pp.
    77–98.
Gath, D., Cooper, B., Gattoni, F., and Rockett, D. *Child guidance and delin-
    quency in a London Borough*. Institute of Psychiatry. Maudsley Mono-
    graph No. 24. London: Oxford University Press, 1977.
Glueck, S., and Glueck, E. *Predicting Delinquency and Crime*. Cambridge:
    Harvard University Press, 1959.

Graham, P., Rutter, M., and George, S. Temperamental characteristics as predictors of behavior disorders in children. *American Journal of Orthopsychiatry*, 1973, *43*, 328–339.

Hersov, L. Introduction: Risk and mastery in children from the point of view of genetic and constitutional factors and early life experience. In E. J. Anthony and C. Koupernick (Eds.), *The child in his family*. Vol. 3, *Children at psychiatric risk* (New York: Wiley, 1974), pp. 67–76.

Hutchings, B., and Mednick, S. A. Registered criminality in the adoptive and biological parents of registered male adoptees. In S. A. Mednick et al. (Eds.), *Genetics, environment, and psychopathology*. Amsterdam: North-Holland, 1974.

Jahoda, M. *Current concepts of positive mental health*. New York: Basic Books, 1959.

Moerk, E. Changes in verbal child-mother interactions with increasing language skills of the child. *Journal of Psycholinguistic Research*, 1974, *3*, 101–116.

Murphy, L. B., and associates. *The widening world of childhood: Paths toward mastery*. New York: Basic Books, 1962.

Offer, D., and Sabshin, M. *Normality: Theoretical and clinical concepts of mental health*. New York: Basic Books, 1966.

Osofsky, J. D., and O'Connell, E. J. Parent-child interaction: Daughters' effects upon mothers' and fathers' behaviors. *Developmental Psychology*, 1972, *7*, 157–168.

Power, M. J., Alderson, M. R., Phillipson, C. M., Schoenberg, E., and Morris, J. N. Delinquent schools? *New Society*, 1967, *10*, 542–543.

Power, M. J., Benn, R. T., and Morris, J. N. Neighbourhood, school and juveniles before the courts. *British Journal of Criminology*, 1972, *12*, 111–132.

Pringle, M. L. K., and Bossio, V. Early prolonged separations and emotional adjustment. *Journal of Child Psychology and Psychiatry*, 1960, *1*, 37–48.

Pringle, M. L. K., and Clifford, L. Conditions associated with emotional maladjustment among children in care. *Educational Review*, 1962, *14*, 112–123.

Quinton, D., and Rutter, M. Early hospital admissions and later disturbances of behavior: An attempted replication of Douglas' findings. *Developmental Medicine and Child Neurology*, 1976, *18*, 447–459.

Reynolds, D., Jones, D., and St. Leger, S. Schools do make a difference. *New Society*, 1976, *37*, 223–225.

Reynolds, D., and Murgatroyd, S. Being absent from school. *British Journal of Law and Society*, 1974, *1*, 78–81.

Rutter, M. Sex differences in children's responses to family stress. In E. J. Anthony and C. Koupernick (Eds.), *The child in his family*. Vol. 1, (New York: Wiley, 1970), pp. 165–196.

Rutter, M. Parent-child separation: Psychological effects on the children. *Journal of Child Psychology and Psychiatry*, 1971, *12*, 233–260.

Rutter, M. *Maternal deprivation reassessed*. Harmondsworth, England: Penguin, 1972.

Rutter, M. Epidemiological strategies and psychiatric concepts in research on the vulnerable child. In E. J. Anthony and C. Koupernick (Eds.), *The child in his family*. Vol. 3, *Children at psychiatric risk* (New York: Wiley, 1974), pp. 167–180.

Rutter, M. Early sources of security and competence. In J. S. Bruner and A. Garton (Eds.), *Human growth and development*. London: Oxford University Press, 1977. (a)

Rutter, M. Individual differences. In M. Rutter and L. Hersov (Eds.), *Child psychiatry: Modern approaches* (Oxford: Blackwell Scientific, 1977), pp. 3–21 (b)

Rutter, M. Maternal deprivation 1972–1977: New findings, new concepts, new approaches. Paper read at the Biennial meeting, Society for Research in Child Development, New Orleans, 16–20 March 1977. (c)

Rutter, M., Birch, H. G., Thomas, A., and Chess, S. Temperamental characteristics in infancy and the later development of behavioural disorders. *British Journal of Psychiatry*, 1964, *110*, 651–661.

Rutter, M., Cox, A., Tupling, C., Berger, M., and Yule, W. Attainment and adjustment in two geographical areas. I. The prevalence of psychiatric disorder. *British Journal of Psychiatry*, 1975, *126*, 493–509. (a)

Rutter, M., Graham, P., and Yule, W. *A neuropsychiatric study in childhood*. Clinics in Developmental Medicine 35/36. London: Heinemann/SIMP, 1970.

Rutter, M., and Madge, N. *Cycles of disadvantage*. London: Heinemann Educational, 1976.

Rutter, M., and Quinton, D. Psychiatric disorder: Ecological factors and concepts of causation. In H. McGurk (Ed.), *Ecological factors in human development*. Amsterdam: North-Holland, 1977.

Rutter, M., Quinton, D., and Yule, B. *Family pathology and disorder in children*. London: Wiley, 1977.

Rutter, M., Tizard, J., and Whitmore, K. (Eds.). *Education, health and behaviour*. London: Longmans, 1970.

Rutter, M., Yule, B., Quinton, D., Rowlands, O., Yule, W., and Berger, M. Attainment and adjustment in two geographical areas. III. Some factors accounting for area differences. *British Journal of Psychiatry*, 1975, *126*, 520–533. (b)

Sameroff, A. J. Early influences on development: Fact or fantasy? *Merrill-Palmer Quarterly of Behavior and Development*, 1975, *21*, 267–294.

Sameroff, A. J. Concepts of humanity in primary prevention. In G. W. Albee and J. M. Joffe (Eds.), *Primary prevention of psychopathology*. Vol. I, *The issues* (Hanover, N.H.: University Press of New England, 1977), pp. 42–63.

Shaffer, D., Chadwick, O., and Rutter, M. Psychiatric outcome of localized head injury in children. In R. Porter and D. FitzSimons (Eds.), *Outcome of severe damage to the central nervous system*. Ciba Foundation Symposium 34 (new series). Amsterdam: Elsevier-Excerpta Medica-North Holland, 1975.

Shields, J. Heredity and psychological abnormality. In H. J. Eysenck (Ed.), *Handbook of abnormal psychology*, 2nd ed. London: Pitman Medical, 1973.

Shields, J. Polygenic influences. In M. Rutter and L. Hersov (Eds.), *Child psychiatry: Modern approaches*. Oxford: Blackwell Scientific, 1977, pp. 22–46.

Stacey, M., Dearden, R., Pill, R., and Robinson, D. *Hospitals, children, and their families: The report of a pilot study*. London: Routledge and Kegan Paul, 1970.

Tizard, B., and Hodges, J. The effect of early institutional rearing on the behaviour problems and affectional relationships of eight year old children. *Journal of Child Psychology and Psychiatry*, 1978, *19(2)*, 99–118.

Tizard, B., and Rees, J. The effect of early institutional rearing on the behaviour problems and affectional relationships of four year old children. *Journal of Child Psychology and Psychiatry*, 1975, *16*, 61–74.

Varlaam, A. Educational attainment and behaviour at school. *Greater London Intelligence Quarterly*, 1974, No. 29, December, pp. 29–37.

Wedge, P., and Prosser, H. *Born to fail?* London: Arrow Books, 1973.

West, D. J., and Farrington, D. P. *Who becomes delinquent?* London: Heinemann Educational, 1973.

West, D. J., and Farrington, D. P. *The delinquent way of life*. London: Heinemann Educational, 1977.

White, R. W. Competence and the growth of personality. *Science and Psychoanalysis*, 1967, *11*, 42–49.

Wilson, H. Parenting in poverty. *British Journal of Social Work*, 1974, *4*, 241–254.

Wolkind, S. N. Sex differences in the aetiology of antisocial disorders in children in long-term residential care. *British Journal of Psychiatry*, 1974, *125*, 125–130.

Wolkind, S. N., Kruk, S., and Chaves, L. P. Childhood separation experiences and psychosocial status in primiparous women: Preliminary findings. *British Journal of Psychiatry*, 1976, *128*, 391–396.

Wolkind, S. N., and Rutter, M. Children who have been "in care": An epidemiological study. *Journal of Child Psychology and Psychiatry*, 1973, *14*, 97–105.

Unmet Needs of Children

Edward Zigler and Matia Finn

Infant Mortality

❖ Among 42 nations keeping comparable statistics, in 1975 the United States, the richest and technologically most advanced country in the world, ranked 16th in the incidence of infant mortality and death of mothers in child birth (U.S. Department of Health, Education and Welfare, 1976). While significant, these statistics for the nation as a whole mask the disparity in infant mortality and maternal death rates between whites and minority groups as well as between regions of the country. In 1974 the infant mortality rate for nonwhites was 1.5 times greater than for whites and the maternal death rate was 3.5 times greater. There were 14.9 deaths per 1,000 births in the Pacific states in 1973, as compared with 21.6 deaths per 1,000 births in the southeastern United States (Advisory Committee on Child Development, 1976).

Poverty, poor sanitation, malnutrition in pregnant women, and lack of prenatal care are leading contributors to the high infant mortality rate in this country. It is now generally accepted that prenatal care should begin during the first three months of pregnancy in order to have the greatest success in preventing infant mortality and handicapping conditions in children. However, many pregnant women receive no prenatal care during the first trimester. In 1977, 47 percent of black women and 24 percent of white women did not have the minimal level of care suggested by the American College of Obstetrics and Gynecology. This neglect condemns many infants still in the uterus to death at birth or to a variety of physical and psychological handicaps which no amount of intervention can fully remediate.

Teenage Pregnancy

The number of pregnant teenage girls reached epidemic proportions during the last decade. The phenomenon of children having children is associated with complications during pregnancy and delivery. The risk of having infants in poor health and of low birthweight is greater for women

From Edward Zigler and Matia Finn, "A Vision of Child Care in the 1980s," in Lynne A. Bond and Justin M. Joffe (eds.) *Facilitating Infant and Early Childhood Development.* Copyright © 1982 by the Vermont Conference on the Primary Prevention of Psychopathology. Reprinted by permission.

below the age of 20. Low birthweight is associated with developmental delays and disabilities later in life. Although some experts believe that this is due to the physical immaturity of the teenage mother, a recent study in Copenhagen suggests that teenage mothers given proper care had the least complications in childbirth (Mednick, Baker, and Sutton-Smith, 1979). The study indicates that the high risk associated with teenage pregnancy may be due to lack of prenatal care rather than young age. No matter what the risks are attributed to, the fact remains that over 550,000 girls age 19 and under are giving birth each year. Of these girls, 10,000 are 10 to 14 years old (U.S. Department of Health and Human Services, 1980). Over 93 percent of girls choose to keep their babies (Zelnick and Kantner, 1978). The effects on the children are devastating. Infants born to teenage mothers often face a life of poverty and neglect because their mothers lack the emotional and financial capability to raise a child.

Health

Good health care for infants and young children is crucial to their chances for healthy and productive lives. Yet over 30 percent of children in the United States receive inadequate medical care and about 25 percent of the children do not receive physical examinations over the course of a year (Advisory Committee on Child Development, 1976). Half the children in this country under age 15 and 90 percent of those under age 5 have never made a single visit to the dentist over their entire childhood (White House Conference on Children, 1970). Despite these statistics and the fact that children constitute one third of our population, only 1 out of 17 federal dollars for health care is spent on children (Keniston, 1977).

Immunization is an easily implemented element of well-child care. Despite our ability to eliminate infectious diseases through immunizations, epidemics continue to occur. The measles epidemics of 1969, 1971, and 1974 resulted from failure of nearly half of the children between the ages of 1 and 4 to get proper inoculations (Knowles, 1977). A recent immunization effort by the Surgeon General resulted in the inoculation of 90 percent of school-age children. However, 2 out of every 5 preschool children are still not immunized against childhood diseases (Edelman, 1980).

Childhood accidents constitute the single major cause of death among children between the ages of 9 and 14 (Furrow, Gruendel, and Zigler, 1979). Of the 22,539 children in this age range who died in 1975, nearly half were killed in accidents. Also in 1975, 28 million accidental injuries occurred among children aged 0 to 16 years. Among Western nations, the United States has the *second* highest rate of childhood deaths due to accidents and is ranked *first* in deaths caused by firearms and poisonings. Motor vehicle accidents are the leading type of accidental death for children of all ages. Yet, with the exception of a still not implemented accident prevention plan (Harmon, Furrow, and Zigler, 1980) approved recently by Dr. Julius Richmond, the Surgeon General, there are few preventive efforts to combat this number one killer and maimer of our young children.

Foster Care

Our complacency as a nation is most evident in the area of foster care. One of the basic tenets of the 1930 Bill of Rights for Children was that every child has a right to a permanent and loving home. Fifty years later we witness some 500,000 children adrift in the U.S. foster care system (Edelman, 1979). The foster care system, supposedly representing temporary care until decisions about permanent placement can be made, subjects children to the impermanency of being placed in one home after another for indefinite periods. In some states, the average time spent in foster care is nearly 5 years (Keniston, 1977). There are reports that 62 percent of children placed in foster care remain out of their own homes for their entire childhood. Only 15 to 25 percent of children placed in foster care return home. The number of children who eventually get adopted is even lower—less than 15 percent (Keniston, 1977).

Removing children from their homes is not necessarily the best solution, nor is it in the best interest of children. In fact, there is growing concern that children placed in foster care suffer permanent emotional damage, or worse. In a recent report in New York City, it was revealed that children in foster care have a death rate twice the national average. Some of the deaths are the result of abuse by foster parents (Lash, Sigal, and Dudzinski, 1980). However, federal dollars are available for a child's room and board away from home, but funds for supportive services such as homemakers or crisis counseling or day care, which could keep the family together and prevent the need for foster care placement, are scarce. With very little money directed at services which might facilitate family reunification or prevent family breakup, many of our children spend a painful journey being shuffled through the maze of our foster care system.

Child Abuse

The facts concerning child abuse and neglect are distressing. It is difficult to quote the exact number of cases of child abuse per year. The available estimates range from a conservative 500,000 (Light, 1973) to 4 million (Gil, 1970). According to the National Center on Child Abuse and Neglect, there are 1 million cases reported per year. Since even the definition of child abuse remains a controversial issue,[1] it comes as no surprise

---

1. The research literature on child abuse shows definitions ranging from an emphasis on serious physical abuse (Kempe, C. H., Silverman, F., Steele, B., Droegemueller, W., and

that estimated figures vary greatly. But there is one abusive act that may be measurable objectively—that is, the abusive act which results in the child's death. We can say this with certainty: nearly 2,000 children die each year as a result of abuse and neglect (Martinez, 1977).

Even more distressing are the facts concerning the instances of abuse that occur in America's public institutions—correctional settings, homes for the mentally retarded or otherwise handicapped, and the schools. Documentation of institutional abuse is noted by Blatt and his colleague (Blatt, in press; Blatt and Kaplan, 1966) and by Wooden (1976). Our nation is also supporting child abuse by allowing the barbaric practice of corporal punishment in the schools to continue. The figures of some of our large school systems—for example, Dallas—indicate that tens of thousands of children each year are subjected to physical punishment in the form of paddling (Anderson and Henry, 1976). This form of discipline gives implicit sanction to the use of physical violence within the family. Further, in what amounts to a legal mandate for child abuse, the Supreme Court, in a ruling on a case in which two junior high school students received severe beatings, upheld the use of corporal punishment in the schools (Ingraham vs. Wright, 1977). This ruling was made despite our knowledge that over half of child abuse incidents result from overzealous disciplinary actions by parents. If the highest court in the United States condones physical abuse of children, how are we to expect parents to reject this form of discipline?

Day Care

Child care in this nation is a source of a number of problems. The factors in the child care issue are related to both quantity and quality. At the 1970 White House Conference on Children, it was proclaimed that the number one priority for alleviating the problems faced by children and families was quality day care (White House Conference on Children, 1970). Despite this declaration, more than 10 years have passed and there continues to be a need for increased day care services. What is more, we seem unable to impress upon our nation's leaders that we not only need more day care facilities but that we must ensure that those facilities that are in existence provide adequate services.

The need for day care has increased substantially over the past decade as more women have entered the labor force. There are indications that

---

Silver, S. The battered child syndrome. *Journal of the American Medical Association*, 1962, *181*, 17–24) to a broader definition which emphasizes maltreatment (Fontana, V. J. *The Maltreated Child: The Maltreated Syndrome in Children* (2nd ed.). Springfield, IL: C. Thomas, 1970). K. T. Alvy, in "Preventing child abuse" (*American Psychologist*, 1975, *30*, 921–928) focuses on the fulfillment of the child's developmental needs.

this trend will continue at an even faster pace. The number of children under 6 years whose mothers are working—now 7,166,000—is expected to increase to well over 10 million by the end of this decade (Smith, 1979). In addition, the actual number of young children is expected to increase as the women born during the baby boom era (1946–1964) begin giving birth to their own babies during the next 10 years (Hofferth, 1979). It is estimated that over 50 percent of these mothers will be working by the time their children are 6 years old. A substantial number of them will opt to return to work within the first year after the birth of their infants.

Despite these facts and predictions, representatives of the Carter administration testified in 1979 that there was no need for increased day care services (Martinez, 1979). This statement was made in light of public acknowledgment of the U.S. Bureau of the Census statistic that every school day in this country, nearly 2 million children between the ages of 7 and 13 come home to an empty house (Congressional Record, 1979). These "latchkey" children, so called because they carry their house key on a string around their neck, are left to their own resources to suffer neglect during critical hours of the day. Reports of children encountering burglars or being victimized by molesters are not uncommon. And, in a recent study in Detroit, an investigator discovered that 1/6th of the fires in that city involved an unattended child (Smock, 1977).

While day care facilities are indeed in critically short supply, the quality of group child care in this nation leaves much to be desired. Not much is known about the kind of care children receive in day care since research tends to focus on high quality centers, the least common type of substitute care. However, in a study by the National Council of Jewish Women (Keyserling, 1972), 11 percent of all licensed nonprofit centers were rated as poor in quality; 51 percent were rated fair, 28 percent were rated good, and 9 percent were rated superior. Proprietary centers fared worse: 50 percent were considered poor, 35 percent were fair, 14 percent were good, and 1 percent were superior. In family day care homes, 14 percent were rated poor, 48 percent were rated fair, 31 percent good, and 7 percent were rated superior. These figures may not accurately describe the quality of day care in America since most care is provided in unlicensed homes that are not accountable to public authority. Yet unlicensed settings are not the only such settings that are unmonitored. Even among licensed centers, standards are often lax. Some states, such as New York and Connecticut, have reasonable day care standards that are enforced. But there are other states, for example, Florida and New Mexico, where it is permissible for one adult to take care of up to 10 infants. One has only to think of the difficulties of a mother of twins or triplets to

realize that this staff/child ratio is not only not conducive to optimal development, it is downright dangerous. In case of fire, how could one
caregiver bring 10 infants to safety?

Efforts to guarantee quality child care in centers across the nation and
to enforce uniform standards have been going on for over a decade. After
a lengthy moratorium on day care regulation and in the face of considerable opposition, Health and Human Services Secretary Patricia Harris had
the courage to approve the Federal Interagency Day Care Requirements
(FIDCR) (Federal Register, March 19, 1980). These requirements, representing the absolute minimum standards, imposed nothing on children
except protection from fires, nutritious meals, and the right to be cared
for by adults who are trained in the principles of child development and
recognized as competent caregivers. Yet, several weeks before these requirements were to take effect, their implementation was deferred for yet
another year, this time because of so-called budgetary restraints. The decision to defer the requirements was upheld despite a proposal by Senator
Cranston that made the budgetary impact of FIDCR negligible (Zigler
and Goodman, 1980).

Enforcement of federal day care standards is important in several aspects, especially as these relate to the training of caregivers of infants and
young children. The long-term consequences of day care, especially infant day care, are not yet known. Studies conducted over the past decade,
however, indicate that the single most important factor in determining
children's development is the quality of interaction that they have with
the adults in their lives. Children should be reared not only in a safe environment but also in a nurturant environment. We have developed the
means to assess caregiver competencies and to credential those caregivers
who are competent to take care of children in group situations.[2] But we
have yet to implement on a nationwide scale these assessment and credentialing procedures.

Social and Emotional Development

Children today spend less time with their parents or other adults than
they did several decades ago. In contrast to children of the 1950s, who
encountered a number of adults during the course of a day and who were
involved in community activities, many children during the 1970s reported spending most of their time, when not in school, alone or with

2. An assessment and credentialing procedure for child care workers has been established
by the Child Development Associate Consortium, Inc. (CDAC). CDAC is a nonprofit organization based in Washington, D.C. Since its establishment in 1972, over 7,000 child care
workers received the CDA credential, an award signifying competence in child care and
knowledge of basic principles of child development.

other children, mainly watching television, eating snacks, and fooling around (Boocock, 1977). Condry and Siman (1974) noted that children today show a greater dependency on their peers than they did a decade ago. They found that attachment to age mates was more influenced by a lack of attention and concern at home than by any positive attraction of the peer group (Condry and Siman, 1976).

What are some of the consequences of these trends? Siman (1973) noted that peer-oriented children have negative views of themselves and their friends, are pessimistic about the future, and are more likely to engage in antisocial behavior. Other investigators relate the rising rate of juvenile crime and the increase in the incidence of childhood depression to the changing way children are growing up. Since 1958, there has been a substantial increase in the number of children with criminal records. What is more, increasingly younger children are involved in serious crimes. In 1975, for example, larceny and burglary accounted for just under 40 percent of all arrests of children under 15; violent crime (aggravated assault, armed robbery, forcible rape, and murder) accounted for 3.3 percent of such arrests (Advisory Committee on Child Development, 1976).

Depression in young children is only now beginning to be recognized so that estimates are difficult to obtain. Kashani and Simonds (1979) estimate that the number of depressed children between the ages of 7 and 12 years in this country is over 400,000, or 1.9 percent of the total number of children in that age range. Albert and Beck (1975) estimate that 33 percent of the population of children between 11 and 15 years experience moderate to severe depression. Suicide may be another indicator of childhood depression. Between 1950 and 1975, the annual suicide rate of white youths between the ages of 15 and 19 increased 171 percent. No other age group had so high a rate of increase. During the same years, the overall white suicide rate increased by only 18 percent (Wynne, 1978).

Marital Disruption as a Stressor

Bernard L. Bloom

❖   A very large proportion of psychopathology, particularly the milder forms, seems to be brought about as a consequence of psychological rather than biological factors, and a variety of psychological strategies for preventing emotional disorders are currently being developed and tested. The efforts fall into two major categories. First, and most common, are efforts to decrease people's vulnerability to specific stresses; second, considerably less common, are efforts to reduce these stresses at their source.

❖   In 1975 more than three million persons were directly involved in a legally defined marital disruption in the United States. There were over one million divorces during this time period, and in each divorce an average of 1.22 children. Thus, two million adults and over one million children were affected by divorce in a single year, representing 1½ percent of the total United States population (Glick, 1975; U.S. Bureau of the Census, 1974; and U.S. Department of Health, Education, and Welfare, 1976).

These figures might have little interest to any group other than demographers were it not for the growing body of evidence that marital disruption often constitutes a severe stress, the consequences of which can be seen in a surprisingly wide variety of physical and emotional disorders. Persons undergoing marital disruption have been shown to be at excess risk for psychiatric disorders, suicide, homocide, motor vehicle accidents, and a variety of forms of disease morbidity and disease mortality (see Bachrach, 1975; Bloom, Asher, and White, Note 1).

❖   In considering the research studies linking marital disruption to physical and emotional disorders, it would be useful to keep in mind four general hypotheses that have been invoked to account for the obtained relationships. First, if physically or emotionally handicapped persons marry, their preexisting handicaps may reduce the likelihood that they will remain married. Second, physical or emotional disorders arising after marriage in either spouse may significantly reduce the likelihood that the marriage will continue. Third, the status of being married and living with one's spouse may reduce vulnerability to a wide variety of diseases or emotional disorders. Fourth, marital disruption may be a life stressor which can precipitate physical or emotional disorders in married people presumably already vulnerable to them but not yet affected. Since these hypotheses are not mutually exclusive, and in fact may all be true to some extent, it has been understandably difficult to develop research designs whose conclusions could support them differentially.

Of all the social variables whose relationships with the distribution of psychopathology in the population have been studied, none has been more consistently and powerfully associated with this distribution than marital status. Persons who are divorced or separated have been repeatedly found to be overrepresented among psychiatric patients, while married persons living with their spouses are underrepresented. In a recent review of eleven studies of marital status and the incidence of mental disorder reported during the past 35 years, Crago (1972) did not find a single exception to the following summary statement: admission rates into psychiatric facilities are lowest among the married, intermediate among widowed and never-married adults, and highest among the divorced and separated. The differential appears to be stable across different age groups (Adler, 1953), reasonably stable for each sex separately considered (Thomas and Locke, 1963; Malzberg, 1964), and as true for blacks as for whites (Malzberg, 1956).

Not only are highest admission rates reported for persons with disrupted marriages, but the differential between these rates and similarly calculated rates among the married is very substantial. In the most recent data available on a national level (for the year 1970), Redick and Johnson (1974) have shown that the ratio of admission rates for divorced and separated persons to those for married persons is around 18 to 1 for males and about 7 to 1 for females. In the case of admissions into public section outpatient clinics, admission rates are also substantially higher for persons with disrupted marraiges than for married persons—nearly 7 to 1 for males and 5 to 1 for females.

Another view of the magnitude of these differences can be seen from data we collected between 1969 and 1971 in the city of Pueblo, Colorado (Bloom, 1975). Data from public and private inpatient facilities were combined but analyzed separately by sex and by whether the patient was admitted for the first time or had a prior history of inpatient psychiatrric care. In all cases, admission rates are substantially higher for patients with disrupted marriages (divorced and separated patients combined) than for patients married and living with their spouses. Specifically, with first admissions, rates for males with disrupted marriages are nine times higher than for males with nondisrupted marriages; among the females, the difference is around three to one. Among patients with histories of prior psychiatric care the differentials by marital status are greater for both sexes: 16 to 1 for males and 6 to 1 for females.

Another way of viewing the Pueblo data is to note that while divorced and separated males constitute only 6.5 percent of ever-married males age 14 and above, they constitute 46 percent of evermarried patients of both sexes in the same age span. Similarly, divorced and separated females constitute 8 percent of ever-married females age 14 and above but 32 percent of all ever-married patients in this age span. More than 7 percent of males with disrupted marriages are hospitalized annually because of a psychiatric condition—indeed, a quiet epidemic.

Two important sources of data serve to link marital disruption and suicidal behavior. First, Schneidman and Farberow (1961) have compared some personal characteristics of attempted and committed suicides from the year 1957 in Los Angeles County.* Thirteen percent of committed suicides were divorced and 8 percent were separated. Both of these figures are more than double what would have been expected from the proportion of divorced and separated persons in the general population of Los Angeles County. Furthermore, while about the same proportion of attempted and committed suicides are married and while about twice as large a proportion of single persons attempt as commit suicide, the divorced, separated, and widowed are significantly overrepresented among those who commit suicide and significantly underrepresented among those who attempt it. Schneidman and

---

*Data regarding committed suicides were obtained from the Los Angeles coroner's office, and for attempted suicides from Los Angeles physicians, records of the Los Angeles County General Hospital, and records from the sixteen Los Angeles municipal emergency hospitals.

Farberow suggest that "it seems probable that the losses and disturbances in dyadic relationships occurring among the older groups, where more divorced, separated, and widowed appear, are also more likely to result in more lethal suicidal behavior" (p. 30). In a related study, Litman and Farberow (1961), proposing a strategy for undertaking emergency evaluations of self-destructive potentiality, note that "many suicide attempts, especially in young persons, occur after the separation from a spouse or loved one. . . . When there has been a definite loss of a loved person, such as a spouse, parent, child, lover, or mistress, within the previous year (by death, divorce, or separation), the potentiality for self-destruction is increased" (p. 51).

The second source of data linking suicide with marital status comes from the continuing reports of the National Center for Health Statistics. The most recent report (National Center for Health Statistics, 1970) covers the period 1959–61 and is based on an analysis of total U.S. mortality data. With particular reference to deaths from suicide, among white females the rate is higher among the divorced than any other marital status category and is more than three times the rate found in the married, while for white men it is also highest among the divorced and is more than four times as high as for married persons. For nonwhite females, the suicide rate is highest in the widowed and second highest in the divorced, where it is twice that of the married; and finally, among nonwhite males, it is highest in the divorced and is nearly two and one-half times as great as among the married.

The figures for deaths from homicide are even more striking. In both sexes and among both whites and nonwhites, risk of death by homicide is far higher for the divorced than for any other marital status group. With white women the risk is more than four times higher among the divorced than the married and with white men, more than seven times higher. Among nonwhites, the risk is twice as high among women and three times as high among men.

Two studies demonstrate excess vulnerability to motor vehicle accidents among the divorced. The analysis of total U.S. mortality data published by the National Center for Health Statistics (1970) shows that in both sexes and for whites and nonwhites alike, automobile fatality rates are higher among the divorced than among any other marital status group, averaging about three times as high as among the married. Second, a study by McMurray (1970) demonstrated that the accident rate of persons undergoing divorce doubled during the period between the six months before and the six months after the divorce date.

A variety of studies have attempted to link stress experiences to disease morbidity. Indeed, such linkages form the empirical basis of psychophysiological disease hypotheses. Holmes and Rahe (1967; also Rahe, McKean, and Arthur, 1967; Rahe, 1968; and Theorell and Rahe, 1970) have developed a measure of stressful life events based on the amount of readjustment required by each such event and have shown that this measure (in which marital disruption figures heavily) distinguishes persons likely to become ill from those not likely to become ill (see also Cline and Chesy, 1972).

Two recent studies suggest that alcoholism (both acute and chronic) is more prevalent among the divorced than among the married, a finding that corroborates much earlier literature. Wechsler, Thum, Demone, and Dwinnel (1972), studying the blood alcohol level of over 6,000 eligible consecutive admissions to the emergency service of Massachusetts General Hospital, found that "in both sexes, the divorced or separated had the highest proportion with positive Breathalyzer readings. . . . Divorced or separated men included 42 percent with positive alcohol readings" (p. 138). Widowers had the lowest proportion with positive readings (10 percent), and single (24 percent) and married (19 percent) men were intermediate. Rosenblatt, Gross, Malenowski, Broman, and Lewis (1971) contrasted first admissions with readmissions for alcoholism and concluded that their results "reveal a significant relationship between disrupted marriage and multiple hospitalizations for the acute alcoholic psychoses at ages below 45" (p. 1094); also see Woodruff, Guze, and Clayton, 1972).

Both the widowed and the divorced have higher age-adjusted death rates for all causes combined than do married persons of equivalent age, sex, and race. With respect to specific diseases, death rates from tuberculosis and cirrhosis of the liver are consistently higher among the divorced. Among white men and nonwhites of both sexes, death rate is higher among the divorced than among the married from malignant neoplasm of the respiratory system, and among nonwhite males it is higher among the divorced for diabetes mellitus and arteriosclerotic heart disease.

Finally, an extensive literature testifies to the generally negative consequences of marital disruption for the children in the disrupted family. While empirical studies are not numerous, there is some equivocal support for this general assertion, although few studies report data from control children in nondisrupted families, and many are based on a very limited number of cases.

❖   A review of the American literature suggests six specific stresses associated with marital separation. First, the psychological and emotional problems associated with a marriage breakup appear to be intense. The termination of a marriage is the death of a relationship, requiring constructive mourning and a coming to grips with the resulting sense of failure, shame, and low self-worth. Second, particularly among women, there often are stresses associated with the need to think about employment, career planning, or additional education preparatory to establishing an independent economic existence. Third, legal and financial problems often occur, creating additional stress. Separated women often find it impossible to get loans or establish charge accounts. Parental rights are often poorly understood. Fourth, with the change from a two-parent to a one-parent family setting, child-rearing problems frequently emerge. Fifth, particularly among men, problems regarding housing and homemaking appear. And sixth, for both men and women—particularly if they are beyond the early adult years—there are often serious difficulties in finding adequate social groups and experiences.

In spite of the fact that there is a large body of research and opinion regarding the stressful character of marital disruption, a careful search of the published literature of the past fifteen years has failed to uncover a single controlled study designed to reduce those stresses.

It is important to acknowledge at the outset that the concept of a "good divorce," that is, the idea of divorce counseling in contrast to marriage counseling, remains controversial in the literature. In fact, the existence of the controversy may help explain the lack of evaluated intervention programs for persons undergoing marital disruption. Basic to the anti-divorce counseling position is the fact that reconciliation is often seen as a far more desirable outcome to marital conflict than divorce. Rutledge (1963), for example, argues that "seldom does a divorce solve the fundamental personality problems resident in a marital situation" (p. 320), and Bodenheimer (1970) suggests that with the liberalization of divorce laws many couples turn to divorce rather than trying to rebuild their marriages. She urges that "care should be taken to avoid a complete swing of the pendulum from yesterday's marriage breakdown without recourse to divorce, to today's divorce without breakdown" (p. 219).

❖   It would now be appropriate to examine more closely the four hypotheses that have been advanced to account for the associations found between marital disruption on the one hand and various physical and emotional disorders on the other. First, it has been asserted that persons with physical or emotional disorders who marry will be less likely to maintain a successful marriage than persons without preexisting disabilities. Our review of the literature indicates that data have not been collected in such a way that the validity of this hypothesis can be distinguished from that of the second hypothesis, which proposes that marital disruption may be significantly increased as a consequence of disabilities arising after marriage. These hypotheses suggest that psychopathology is the cause and marital disruption the consequence.

Turner describes the hypothesized relationship linking emotional disorder with subsequent marital disruption in terms of the incipient character of psychopathology that "makes marriage less likely and, given marriage, is likely to speed divorce or separation" (1972, p. 365). Srole and his colleagues make a similar point when they indicate that "elements of mental health may be crucially involved in determining whether or not individuals choose to marry; if they do so choose, whether or not they are successful in finding a spouse; and, if they are successful in this respect, whether or not the marriage is subsequently broken by divorce" (1962, p. 175). Briscoe and his colleagues, interpreting findings in their research, suggest that "one of the implications of finding such a significant amount of psychiatric illness in a divorced population is that psychiatric illness is probably a significant cause of martial breakdown" (Briscoe et al., 1973, p. 125).

Crago, in her review of research studies linking marital disruption and psychopathology, raises the same possibility, stating: "Studies of hospitalization rates and marital status are sometimes criticized because the differences in rates may be due to effects of mental disorders on the marital status of individuals before they are admitted to a mental hospital. For example, if mental disorders tend to lead to divorce, this would boost the rate of mental disorders among the divorced and at the same time decrease the rate for married persons" (1972, p. 115).

These two hypotheses can be tested through a single prospective research design that would assess physical and psychological functioning in individuals as well as couples at the time of marriage. The first hypothesis could be evaluated by following such a cohort over a number of years, by means of an annual physical and psychological evaluation determining the relationship between pre-existing disability and marital adjustment and success. In addition, by identifying couples with postmarital onset of emotional or physical disability in a group judged healthy at the time of marriage, the second hypothesis could be evaluated. In this case one would need to examine the temporal relationships between disability onset after marriage and marital dissatisfaction or disruption. Undoubtedly, the cost and personal commitment required to complete a longitudinal study lasting perhaps a decade or longer have been a major reason why such studies have not been undertaken. Yet without them, it is possible neither to evaluate the hypotheses individually nor to differentiate between them.

The third hypothesis is that the status of being married reduces vulnerability to a wide variety of illnesses. Turner, for example, suggests that different marital statuses may place an individual in diffᵉrent social systems which may vary in their supportive character, and thus that the "marriage state . . . is seen as protective against hospitalization" (1972, p. 365). In an interesting report by Dupont, Ryder, and Grunebaum (1971) regarding their study of 44 married couples in which one spouse had been diagnosed as psychotic and hospitalized, a surprisingly large number of couples reported that the problems associated with coping with the psychosis strengthened their marriages.

Syme has recently reviewed the statistics linking disease mortality and marital status and has concluded:

> It may be instructive to recall the very wide range of conditions for which married people have lower mortality rates. The list of such conditions includes lower death rates for respiratory tuberculosis, stroke, influenza, pneumonia, and cancer of almost all sites including cancer of the buccal cavity and pharynx, the digestive organs, the respiratory system, the breast, and the urinary system. While the possibility cannot be ruled out, it is difficult to see how people who die of a stroke when

they are 70 or 80 years old were less likely to have gotten married 50 years earlier. Further, if the marital state provides an environment which reduces the risk of death from this long list of conditions, it must be that a very profound and important influence is at work which is certainly worthy of prompt and careful study. By such detailed study of marital status and its varied disease consequences, we may be able to develop a whole set of insights about social processes and health status. (1974, p. 1045)

The notion of the special protective power of being married suggests that never-married persons and divorced and separated persons matched for age and sex might have similar disease morbidity and mortality experiences. But the data clearly indicate that never-married persons are at lower risk for most disorders than persons undergoing marital disruption. Another hypothesis suggested by this explanatory concept is that in people equated for age, length of marriage might be inversely related to a variety of morbidity or mortality risks. To our knowledge, this hypothesis has not been definitely examined.

Research intended to examine the hypothesis that marriage is a special protective environment could be accomplished retrospectively and has in fact been done with respect to certain disorders. The Pueblo study (Bloom, 1975), for example, linked psychiatric admissions rates to marital history. What is significant about this research is that marital history data and not merely marital status data were collected at the time of admission, thus allowing analysis not only of the relationship of current marital status to a specific disorder (the approach taken in most of the available literature) but also of the effect of patterns of marital history on the evolution of a specific disorder. We found that six patterns were sufficient to identify the marital histories of 93 percent of ever-married psychiatric inpatients (1975, p. 223) and that first inpatient admissions and patients with prior histories of psychiatric inpatient care differed significantly in the distribution of these martial history patterns. Through an analysis of marital history it is possible to address the questions of whether the benefits of the protective power of being married are outweighed by the relative stress of separation and divorce and whether total length of marriages, or time since separation and divorce, are related to subsequent vulnerability to physical and emotional disorder.

The fourth hypothesis is that the marital disruption constitutes a significant stressor. This hypothesis can be viewed within the rubric of crisis theory (see Caplan, 1964; Parad, 1965) and, of course, it is this hypothesis that has the greatest implication for primary prevention. The national psychiatric admission rate statistics already cited, which show a substantially higher admission rate for separated persons than for divorced persons, support this hypothesis.

Perhaps, more generally, contemporary role theorists would look for stress associated with particular status assignments and would see being separated or divorced as having particularly stressful role attributes. In 1960, for example, national mental health service statistics indicated that married women had mental illness rates twice as high as those of married men. In contrast, there were no appreciable sex differences between the admission rates of divorced or separated men and women. Gove (1972) used these figures to postulate a special vulnerability associated with the role of married women in western society. More recent statistics suggest that his hypothesis may no longer be tenable. In admission rates reported since 1970, sex differences for married patients have disappeared and sex differences for separated and divorced persons have emerged, with the male admission rate far higher than the female. What has remained stable over this time period, however, is the excessive admission rate, in both sexes, of the separated and divorced when contrasted with admission rates among the married.

❖   Research in the area of marital disruption as a life stress has been further complicated by the fact that the data support the notion that marital disruption and physical and emotional disorders are clearly interactive, in the sense that each has the potential to influence the other. These interactions have yet to be explored empirically, not only because of the methodological difficulties but also, in part, because of the complexity of the task (see B. P. Dohrenwend, 1975). One needs to identify and follow a cohort of married persons who differ in marital satisfaction but not in psychological well-being to determine if differential rates of psychopathology are subsequently generated. In a companion research program one needs to identify and follow married psychiatric patients to determine how their psychopathology has a subsequent effect on marital adjustment and disruption. Improved measures of marital adjustment, marital satisfaction, and mental health need to be developed before these programs can be successfully mounted.

Perhaps the most appropriate interpretation of the research that has been reviewed is that an unequivocal association between marital disruption and physical and emotional disorder has been demonstrated and that this association probably includes at least two interdependent components: first, illness (physical or emotional) can precede and can help precipitate marital disruption; and second, marital disruption can serve to precipitate physical and psychiatric difficulties in some persons who might otherwise not have developed such problems. Conversations with newly separated persons leave no doubt that separation is an important stressor.

❖   When the history of twentieth-century efforts to control mental disorders is written, the great contribution of the last third of the century may well turn out to be the movement away from considering predisposing factors in mental illnesses toward concern with precipitating factors. This movement, away from a concern with the past and toward a concern with the present, has come about in part from a sense of frustration with our efforts at remediation. But in addition, a growing accumulation of empirical evidence has turned our attention away from the past. Kohlberg, LaCrosse, and Ricks (1972, p. 1233), for example, reviewing the literature linking childhood behavior and adult mental health, comment:

> To conscious experience, moods change, anxieties disappear, loves and hates fade, the emotion of yesterday is weak, and the emotion of today does not clearly build on the emotion of yesterday. The trauma theory of neurosis is dead; the evidence for irreversible effects of early-childhood trauma is extremely slight. Early-childhood maternal deprivation, parental mistreatment, separation, incest—all seem to have much slighter effects upon adult adjustment (unless supported by continuing deprivation and trauma throughout childhood) than anyone seemed to anticipate.

In our concern with the development of effective preventive intervention programs, we find ourselves inexorably drawn to the simple dictum of Barrington Moore (1970, p. 5): "Human society ought to be organized in such a way as to eliminate useless suffering."

REFERENCES

Adler, L. M. The relationship of marital status to incidence of and recovery from mental illness. *Social Forces*, 1953, *32*, 185–194.

Aponte, J. F., and Miller, F. T. Stress-related social events and psychological impairment. *Journal of Clinical Psychology*, 1972, *28*, 455–458.

Bachrach, L. L. Marital status and mental disorder: An analytical review. DHFW Publication No. (ADM) 75–217. Washington, D.C.: U.S. Government Printing Office, 1975.

Baguador, E. *Separation: Journal of a marriage*. New York: Simon and Schuster, 1972.

Bloom, B. L. The medical model, miasma theory, and community mental health. *Community Mental Health Journal*, 1965, *1*, 333–338.

Bloom, B. L. *Changing patterns of psychiatric care*. New York: Behavioral Publications, 1975.

Bloom, B. L., Asher, S. J., and White, S. W. Marital disruption as a stressor: A review and analysis. *Psychological Bulletin* (in press).

Bloom, B. L., Hodges, W. F., Caldwell, R. A., Systra, L., and Cedrone, A. R. Marital Separation: A Community Survey. *Journal of Divorce*, 1977, *1*, 7–19.

Bodenheimer, B. M. New approaches of psychiatry: Implications for divorce reform. *Utah Law Review*, 1970, 191–220.

Briscoe, C. W., Smith, J. B., Robins, E., Marton, S., and Gaskin, F. Divorce and psychiatric disease. *Archives of General Psychiatry*, 1973, *29*, 119–125.

Brown, G. W., Sklair, F., Harris, T. O., and Birley, J. L. T. Life events and psychiatric disorders: 1. Some methodological issues. *Psychological Medicine*, 1973, *3*, 159–176.

Caplan, G. *Principles of preventive psychiatry*. New York: Basic Books, 1964.

Cline, D. W., and Chesy, J. J. A perspective study of life changes and subsequent health changes. *Archives of General Psychiatry*, 1972, *27*, 51–53.

Cochrane, R., and Robertson, A. The life events inventory: A measure of the relative severity of psycho-social stressors. *Journal of Psychosomatic Research*, 1973, *17*, 135–139.

Crago, M. A. Psychopathology in married couples. *Psychological Bulletin*, 1972, *77*, 114–128.

Dohrenwend, B. P. Sociocultural and social-psychological factors in the genesis of mental disorders. *Journal of Health and Social Behavior*, 1975, *16*, 365–392.

Dohrenwend, B. P., and Dohrenwend, B. S. *Social status and psychological disorder: A causal inquiry*. New York: Wiley-Interscience, 1969.

Dohrenwend, B. P., and Dohrenwend, B. S. Social and cultural influences on psychopathology. *Annual Review of Psychology*, 1974, *25*, 417–452.

Dohrenwend, B. S. Life events as stressors: A methodological inquiry. *Journal of Health and Social Behavior*, 1973, *14*, 167–175. (a)

Dohrenwend, B. S. Social status and stressful life events. *Journal of Personality and Social Psychology*, 1973, *28*, 225–235. (b)

Dohrenwend, B. S., and Dohrenwend, B. P. *Stressful life events: Their nature and effects*. New York: Wiley and Sons, 1974.

Dupont, R. L., Ryder, R. G., and Grunebaum, H. U. An unexpected result of psychosis in marriage. *American Journal of Psychiatry*, 1971, *128*, 735–739.

Gardner, R. A. *The boys and girls book about divorce*. New York: Science House, Inc., 1970.

Glick, P. C. *Some recent changes in American families*. (Current Population Reports, Series P-23, No. 52. Bureau of the Census.) Washington, D.C.: U.S. Government Printing Office, 1975.

Gove, W. R. The relationship between sex roles, marital status, and mental illness. *Social Forces*, 1972, *51*, 34–44.

Holmes, T. H., and Rahe, R. H. The social readjustment rating scale. *Journal of Psychosomatic Research*, 1967, *11*, 213–218.

Hudgens, R. W., Robins, E., and Delong, W. B. The reporting of recent stress in the lives of psychiatric patients. *British Journal of Psychiatry*, 1970, *117*, 635–643.

Hunt, M. M. *The world of the formerly married*. New York: McGraw-Hill, 1966.

Hunt, M. M. Review of *Marital separation*, by R. S. Weiss. *New York Times Book Review*, Nov. 30, 1975, p. 4.

Kellam, S. G., Branch, J. D., Agrawal, K. C., and Ensminger, M. E. *Mental health and going to school: The Woodlawn program of assessment, early intervention, and evaluation*. Chicago: University of Chicago Press, 1975.

Klassen, D., Roth, A., and Hornstra, K. Perception of life events as gains or losses in a community survey. *Journal of Community Psychology*, 1974, *2*, 330–336.

Kohlberg, L., LaCrosse, J., and Ricks, D. The predictability of adult mental health from childhood behavior. In B. Wolman (Ed.), *Manual of child psychopathology*. New York: McGraw-Hill, 1972.

Krantzler, M. *Creative divorce: A new opportunity for personal growth*. New York: M. Evans and Co., 1973.

Lantz, H. R., and Snyder, E. C. *Marriage: An examination of the man-woman relationship* (2nd ed.). New York: Wiley and Sons, 1969.

Litman, R. E., and Farberow, N. L. Emergency evaluation of self destructive potentiality. In N. L. Farberow and E. S. Schneidman (Eds.), *The cry for help*. New York: McGraw-Hill, 1961.

Malzberg, B. Marital status and mental disease among Negroes in New York State. *Journal of Nervous and Mental Disease*, 1956, *123*, 457–465.

Malzberg, B. Marital status and the incidence of mental disease. *International Journal of Social Psychiatry*, 1964, *10*, 19–26.

McMurray, L. Emotional stress and driving performance: The effect of divorce. *Behavioral Research in Highway Safety*, 1970, *1*, 100–114.

Mindey, C. *The divorced mother: A guide to readjustment*. New York: McGraw-Hill, 1969.

Moore, B., Jr. *Reflections on the causes of human misery and upon certain proposals to eliminate them*. Boston: Beacon Press, 1970.

Morrison, J. R., Hudgens, R. W., and Brachha, R. G. Life events and psychiatric illness. *British Journal of Psychiatry*, 1968, *114*, 423–432.

National Center for Health Statistics. *Mortality from selected causes by marital status*. (Series 20, No. 8A and B. U.S. Department of Health, Education, and Welfare.) Washington, D.C.: U.S. Government Printing Office, 1970.

National Center for Health Statistics. *100 years of marriage and divorce statistics: United States, 1867-1967*. (Vital and Health Statistics, Series 21, No. 24. Washington, D.C.: U.S. Government Printing Office, 1973. (a)

National Center for Health Statistics. *Remarriages: United States*. (Vital and Health Statistics, Series 21, No. 25.) Washington, D.C.: U.S. Government Printing Office, 1973. (b)

Parad, H. J. (Ed.). *Crisis intervention: Selected readings*. New York: Family Service Association of America, 1965.

Prokopec, J., Dytrych, Z., and Schuller, V. Rozvodova chovani a manzelsky nesoulad (Divorce and marital discord). *Vyzkumny Ustav Psychiatricky Zpravy*, No. 31, 1973.

Rahe, R. H. Life-change measurement as a predictor of illness. *Proceedings of the Royal Society of Medicine*, 1968, *61*, 44–46.

Rahe, R. H., McKean, J. E., Jr., and Arthur, R. J. A longitudinal study of life-change and illness patterns. *Journal of Psychosomatic Research*, 1967, *10*, 355–366.

Redick, R. W., and Johnson, C. *Marital status, living arrangements and family characteristics of admissions to state and county mental hospitals and outpatients psychiatric clinics, United States 1970*. (Statistical Note 100, National Institute of Mental Health.) Washington, D.C.: U.S. Government Printing Office, 1974.

Reid, D. D. Precipitating proximal factors in the occurrence of mental disorders: Epidemiological evidence. In E. M. Gruenberg and M. Huxley (Eds.), *Causes of mental disorders: A review of epidemiological knowledge, 1959*. New York: Milbank Memorial Fund, 1961.

Rohner, L. *The divorcee's handbook*. Garden City: Doubleday, 1969.

Rosenblatt, S. M., Gross, M. M., Malenowski, B., Broman, M., and Lewis, E. Marital status and multiple psychiatric admissions for alcoholism: A cross-validation. *Quarterly Journal of Studies on Alcohol*, 1971, *32*, 1092–1096.

Rubin, Z., and Mitchell, C. Couples research as couples counseling: Some unintended effects of studying close relationships. *American Psychologist*, 1976, *31*, 17–25.

Rutledge, A. L. Should the marriage counselor ever recommend divorce? *Marriage and Family Living*, 1963, *25*, 319–325.

Schneidman, E. S., and Farberow, N. L. Statistical comparisons between attempted and committed suicides. In N. L. Farberow and E. S. Schneidman (Eds.), *The cry for help*. New York: McGraw-Hill, 1961.

Spanier, G. B. Further evidence on methodological weaknesses in the Locke-Wallace Marital Adjustment Scale and other measures of adjustment. *Journal of Marriage and the Family*, 1972, *34*, 403-404.

Srole, L., Langnor, T. S., Michael, S. T., Opler, M. K., and Rennie, T. A. C. Mental health in the metropolis: The midtown Manhattan study. New York: McGraw-Hill, 1962.

Stewart, C. W. Counseling the divorcee. *Pastoral Psychology*, 1963, *14*, 10-16.

Syme, S. L. Behavioral factors associated with the etiology of physical disease: A social epidemiological approach. *American Journal of Public Health*, 1974, *64*, 1043-1045.

Theorell, T., and Rahe, R. H. Life changes in relation to the onset of myocardial infarction. In T. Theorell (Ed.), *Psychosocial factors in relation to the onset of myocardial infarction and to some metabolic variables—a pilot study*. Stockholm, Sweden: Department of Medicine, Seraphimer Hospital, Karolinska Institutet, 1970.

Thomas, D. S., and Locke, B. Z. Marital status, education and occupational differentials in mental disease. *Milbank Memorial Fund Quarterly*, 1963, *41*, 145-160.

Turner, R. J. The epidemiological study of schizophrenia: A current appraisal. *Journal of Health and Social Behavior*, 1972, *13*, 360-369.

U.S. Bureau of the Census. *Current population reports, Series P-20, No. 271. Marital status and living arrangements: March, 1974*. Washington, D.C.: U.S. Government Printing Office, 1974.

U.S. Bureau of the Census. *Current population reports. Series P-20, No. 287. Marital status and living arrangements: March, 1975*. Washington, D.C.: U.S. Government Printing Office, 1975.

U.S. Department of Health, Education, and Welfare. Births, marriages, divorces, and deaths for 1975. *Monthly Vital Statistics Report*, 1976, *24*, (12), 1-8.

Vinokur, A., and Selzer, M. L. Life events, stress, and mental disorders. *Proceedings, 81st Annual Convention, American Psychological Association*, 1973, 329-330.

Wechsler, H., Thum, D., Demone, H. W., Jr., and Dwinnel, J. Social characteristics and blood alcohol level. *Quarterly Journal for the Study of Alcoholism*, 1972, *33*, 132-147.

Weiss, R. S. *Marital separation*. New York: Basic Books, 1975.

Weissman, M. M. The assessment of social adjustment. *Archives of General Psychiatry*, 1975, *32*, 357-365.

Woodruff, R. A., Jr., Guze, S. B., and Clayton, P. J. Divorce among psychiatric out-patients. *British Journal of Psychiatry*, 1972, *121*, 289-292.

Women and Sexuality

Julia R. Heiman

❖   Studies on how menstrual cycle changes affect sexual interest must address the cultural context. Menstruation has traditionally, in this society and many others, been surrounded with taboos. Its association with uncleanliness has historical and cultural roots. It is also connected with sexuality, another traditionally taboo topic. This negative context has two effects.

First, individual attitudes toward menstruation may influence sexual patterns in that many women and men will exclude the menstruation days as possible days to have sexual contact. Thus, the days before and the days after menses show more sexual behavior, though there is no physiological reason to avoid sex during menstruation. Furthermore, orgasm during menstruation decreases cramps for some women (Clifford, 1978a). However, social norms, combined with the physical discomfort a number of women feel at the onset of their periods, are enough to reduce sexual contact during menstruation (Kinsey et al., 1953).

The second effect of negative sociocultural attitudes toward menstruation is that researchers seem to spend more time and questionnaire space on the negative consequences than on the positive consequences of menstruation. Many researchers only look for pathology and neglect to evaluate possible positive concomitants of the menstrual phases. Moos's (1968) menstrual distress questionnaire, a widely used symptom questionnaire, is slightly more inclusive of positive factors and includes scales for evaluating water retention, pain, negative affect, behavior changes, concentration, autonomic revelations, control, and arousal. A study by Brooks, Ruble, and Clark (1977) found that out of a sample of 191 college women, 77 percent rated menstruation as a positive experience, 59 percent claimed it was bothersome, and 32 percent claimed it was psychologically and physically debilitating (women could respond to more than one factor, thus the total percentage exceeds 100 percent). The inclusion of a positive dimension to evaluate cycle changes would similarly benefit our understanding of sexual changes, since it would be more likely that women would be asked about their degree of enjoyment of general and genital physical touching, in addition to questions on desire and frequency.

❖ Menopause often results in various intensities of physical symptoms such as excessive fatigue, nervousness, irritability, headaches, flushing, or pelvic pain. These symptoms can last from several weeks to several years and can be alleviated by low doses of artificial hormones, though these preparations are currently under review. What must be kept in mind is that menopause has many of the complementary positive and negative psychological features that menarche does. Because menopause signals the end of the woman's fertility, it may be particularly difficult for a woman who has attached a great deal of her self-esteem to her image as a mother or sexually productive person. It also may be difficult for those women who were unable or elected not to have children. For some women, menopause may also signal the beginning of old age and the end of sexual attractiveness.

Alternatively, this period can be the start of a new phase. Free from concerns about pregnancy, and freer from the demands of children, the woman who passes 50 may be able at last to feel more sexually relaxed.

Menopause and sexuality in the advanced years is a fairly recent evolutionary phenomenon, particularly in humans. Most other species die before their reproductive abilities end. Yet, the slow social adjustment to the postreproductive period in women is difficult to see as purely a problem of recency. In our culture, women are viewed as most useful for their seductive or reproductive (including childrearing) capabilities. When those years have passed, women's roles and their value in our society have no clear definition. The social message is indeed a sexless one.

In summary, females are sexually responsive after menopause, and there is evidence to suggest that maintaining some kind of consistent sexual activity is more psychologically and physically healthy than abandoning sex. Furthermore, sex interest postmenopausally is best predicted by sex interest premenopausally (Kinsey et al., 1953). Sexual desire rarely stops or even experiences a sudden drop for either sex (George and Weiler, 1981). It remains to be seen if some of the negative attitudes toward age and sexuality can be constructively altered (see Hotvedt, in press, for an interesting review of this topic).

❖ During the 20th century, women in Western cultures have generally lived with a physical ideal image of female sexuality that equates sexual attractiveness with slender, youthful, sometimes pubescent, features.

Whether or not women intellectually "buy" this image, emotionally it does register. The cultural message of sexual beauty is difficult to resist. One outcome of this restricted sexual attraction criterion is that it furthers competition among women, adding to the distance between, rather than cooperation among, individuals who belong to a less powerful class (if we consider males to be the first and more powerful class, as does de Beauvoir, 1953). More directly relevant is the tendency for women to be in competition with themselves, fighting wrinkles, weight, age, and making their bodies their adversaries. Conflict results from battling one's body and, at the same time, expecting it to give sexual pleasure.

Such conflict can become expressed in a variety of sexual problems. It may create a discrepancy between what a woman thinks she wants sexually and what she can actually express, such as arousal and orgasm (Barbach, 1975; Heiman, LoPiccolo, and LoPiccolo, 1976). Or, a woman may take out her own perfectionistic demands on her partner by being critical of his body and by being suspicious and resentful of his sexual interests. In the latter situation, the woman may become disinterested in sex, since sex becomes defined as his lusty and indiscriminate arousal toward a physical self that she hates. For some women, a countercultural body appearance is safer than having to deal with sexuality and sexual attractiveness. To be svelte and sexually attractive in a conventional sense means being vulnerable to sexual advances.

References

Abraham, K. *On character and libido development.* New York: Basic Books, 1966.

Barbach, L. G. *For yourself: The fulfillment of female sexuality.* New York: Doubleday, 1975.

Barnett, M. C. Vaginal awareness in the infancy and childhood of girls. *Journal of the American Psychoanalytic Association,* 1966, *14,* 129-141.

Bateson, G., Jackson, D. D., Haley, J., and Weakland, J. H. Toward a theory of schizophrenia. *Behavioral Science,* 1956, *1,* 251-264.

Becker, E. *The denial of death.* New York: Free Press, 1973.

Benedek, T. Discussion of Sherfey's paper on female sexuality. *Journal of the American Psychoanalytic Association,* 1968, *16,* 424-448.

Benedek, T., and Rubenstein, B. The correlations between ovarian activity and psychodynamic processes: I. The ovulation phase. *Psychosomatic Medicine,* 1939, *1,* 245-270.

Bonaparte, M. *Female sexuality.* New York: International Universities Press, 1953.

Briffault, R. *The mothers.* New York: Atheneum, 1977.

Brooks, J., Ruble, D., and Clark, A. College women's attitudes and expectations concerning menstrual-related changes. *Psychosomatic Medicine,* 1977, *39,* 288-297.

Buckley, T. Doing your thinking. *Parabola,* 1979, *4,* 29-37.

Campbell, J. Joseph Campbell on the Great Goddess. *Parabola,* 1980, *5,* 74-85.

Clement, U., and Pfafflin, F. Changes in personality scores among couples subsequent to sex therapy. *Archives of Sexual Behavior,* 1980, *9,* 235-244.

Clifford, R. Development of masturbation in college women. *Archives of Sexual Behavior,* 1978, *7,* 559-573. (a)

Clifford, R. Subjective sexual experience in college women. *Archives of Sexual Behavior,* 1978, *7,* 183-197. (b)

Cornor, G. W. The events of the primate ovarian cycle. *British Medical Journal,* 1952, *2,* 403-409.

Dalton, K. *The premenstrual syndrome.* Springfield, Ill.: Charles C. Thomas, 1964.

Davis, K. B. *Factors in the sex life of twenty-two hundred women.* New York: Harper, 1929.

de Beauvoir, S. *The second sex.* New York: Alfred A. Knopf, 1953.

Derogatis, L. R., and Meyer, J. K. A psychological profile of the sexual dysfunctions. *Archives of Sexual Behavior,* 1979, *8,* 201-224.

Deutsch, H. *Psychology of women* (Vol. 1). New York: Grune and Stratton, 1944.

Dinnerstein, D. *The mermaid and the minotaur: Sexual arrangements and human malaise.* New York: Harper and Row, 1976.

Drellich, M. G., and Bieber, I. The psychologic importance of the uterus and its functions. *Journal of Nervous and Mental Disease,* 1958, *126,* 322-336.

Engel, R., and Hildebrandt, G. Rhythmic variations in reaction time, heart rate, and blood pressure at different durations of the menstrual cycle. In M. Farin, F. Halberg, R. Richart, and R. L. Van de Wiele (Eds.), *Biorhythms and human reproduction.* New York: John Wiley and Sons, 1974.

Fenichel, O. *The psychoanalytic theory of neurosis.* New York: W. W. Norton, 1945.

Fisher, S. *Body experience in fantasy and behavior.* New York: Appleton-Century-Crofts, 1970.

Fisher, S. *The female orgasm.* New York: Basic Books, 1973.

Fisher, S., and Cleveland, S. E. *Body image and personality.* New York: Dover Press, 1968.

Foucault, M. [*The history of sexuality*] (Vol. 1) (R. Hurley, Trans.). New York: Random House, 1979.

Frank, E., Anderson, C., and Rubinstein, D. Frequency of sexual dysfunction in "normal" couples. *New England Journal of Medicine,* 1978, *229,* 111-115.

Frank, E., Anderson, C., and Rubinstein, D. Marital role strain and sexual satisfaction. *Journal of Consulting and Clinical Psychology,* 1979, *47,* 1096-1103.

Freud, S. *Collected papers* (Vol. 5). J. Strachey (Ed. and trans.). New York: Basic Books, 1959.

Freud, S. *Three essays on the theory of sexuality.* New York: Basic Books, 1963. (Originally published, 1905.)

Fried, E. *The ego in love and sexuality.* New York: Grune and Stratton, 1960.

Gagnon, J., and Simon, W. *Sexual conduct: The social sources of human sexuality.* Chicago: Aldine, 1973.

George, L. K., and Weiler, S. Sexuality in middle and late life. *Archives of General Psychiatry,* 1981, *38,* 919-923.

Grimm, E. R. Psychological and social factors in pregnancy, delivery, and outcome. In S. A. Richardson and A. F. Guttmacher (Eds.), *Childbearing: Its social and psychological aspects.* Baltimore: Williams and Wilkins, 1967.

Heiman, J., LoPiccolo, L., and LoPiccolo, J. *Becoming orgasmic: A sexual growth program for women.* Englewood Cliffs, N.J.: Prentice-Hall, 1976.

Hite, S. *The Hite report.* New York: Macmillan, 1976.

Hoon, E. F., and Hoon, P. Styles of sexual expression in women: Clinical implications of multivariate analyses. *Archives of Sexual Behavior,* 1978, *7,* 105-116.

Horney, K. *Feminine psychology.* New York: W. W. Norton, 1967.

Hotvedt, M. The cross-cultural and historic context. In R. Weg (Ed.), *Sexuality in the later years.* New York: Academic Press, in press.

Hunt, M. *The natural history of love.* New York: Minerva Press, 1959.

Janeway, E. Who is Sylvia? On the loss of sexual paradigms. *Signs,* 1980, *5,* 573-589.

Jensen, M. D., Benson, R. C., and Bobak, I. M. *Maternity care: The nurse and the family.* St. Louis: C. V. Mosby, 1977.

Kaplan, H. *The new sex therapy.* New York: Brunner/Mazel, 1974.

Kinsey, A. C., Pomeroy, W. B., Martin, C. E., and Gebhard, P. H. *Sexual behavior in the human female.* Philadelphia: W. B. Saunders, 1953.

Korchin, S. J., and Heath, H. A. Somatic experience in the anxiety state: Some sex and personality correlates of "autonomic feedback." *Journal of Consulting Psychology,* 1961, *25,* 398-404.

Leroi-Gourhan, A. *Treasures of prehistoric art.* New York: H. N. Abrams, 1967.

Levi-Strauss, C. *Structural anthropology.* New York: Basic Books, 1958.

Lifton, R. J. *The broken connection.* New York: Simon and Schuster, 1979.

LoPiccolo, J., and Heiman, J. The role of cultural values in the prevention and treatment of sexual problems. In C. B. Qualls, J. Wincze, and D. Barlow (Eds.), *The prevention of sexual disorders: Issues and approaches.* New York: Plenum Press, 1978.

Luria, Z., and Rose, M. D. *Psychology of human sexuality.* New York: John Wiley and Sons, 1979.

Margueron, J. *Mesopotamia.* New York: World, 1965.

Masters, W. H., and Johnson, V. E. *Human sexual response.* Boston: Little, Brown, 1966.

Mead, M. *Male and female.* New York: William Morrow, 1949.

Melody, G. F. Behavioral implications of premenstrual tension. *Obstetrics and Gynecology,* 1961, *17,* 439-446.

Money, J., and Ehrhardt, A. *Man and woman: Boy and girl.* Baltimore: Johns Hopkins University Press, 1972.

Moos, R. H. The development of a menstrual distress questionnaire. *Psychosomatic Medicine,* 1968, *30,* 853-867.

Moos, R. H. Typology of menstrual cycle symptoms. *American Journal of Obstetrics and Gynecology,* 1969, *103,* 390-402.

Moos, R. H., Kopell, B. S., Melges, F. T., Yalem, I. O., Lunde, D. F., Clayton, R. B., and Hamburg, D. A. Fluctuations in symptoms and moods during the menstrual cycle. *Journal of Psychosomatic Research,* 1969, *13,* 37-44.

Moos, R. H., and Leiderman, D. B. Toward a menstrual cycle typology. *Journal of Psychosomatic Research,* 1978, *22,* 31-40.

Mordkoff, A. M. Some sex differences in personality correlates of "autonomic feedback." *Psychological Reports,* 1966, *18,* 511-518.

Naeye, R. L. Coitus and associated amniotic fluid infections. *New England Journal of Medicine,* 1979, *301,* 1198-1200.

Rossi, A. S., and Rossi, P. E. Body time and social time: Mood patterns by menstrual cycle phase and day of the week. *Social Science Research,* 1977, *6,* 273-308.

Sherfey, M. J. *The nature and evolution of female sexuality.* New York: Vintage Books, Random House, 1973.

Slater, P. *The pursuit of loneliness: American culture at the breaking point.* Boston: Beacon Press, 1970.

Symons, D. *The evolution of human sexuality.* New York: Oxford Press, 1979.

Terman, L. M. *Psychological factors in marital happiness.* New York: McGraw-Hill, 1938.

Thompson, W. I. *The time falling bodies take to light.* New York: St. Martin's Press, 1981.

Tooley, K. M. "Johnny, I hardly knew ye": Toward revision of the theory of male psychosexual development. *American Journal of Orthopsychiatry,* 1977, *47,* 184-195.

Travers, P. L. What the bees know. *Parabola,* 1981, *6,* 42-50.

Udry, J. R., and Morris, N. M. Distribution of coitus in the menstrual cycle. *Nature,* 1968, *220,* 593-596.

Zilboorg, G. Masculine and feminine: Some biological and cultural aspects. In J. Miller (Ed.), *Psychoanalysis and women.* Baltimore: Penguin Books, 1973.

Sexual Problems in Men

Joseph LoPiccolo

❖ The Role of Cultural and Religious Values

The Judeo-Christian ethic that shapes our culture's view of sexuality has remained remarkably consistent over the last 2,000 years. From the writings of the Apostle Paul, St. Augustine, and the 1976 Vatican Council statement on sexuality to Pope John Paul II's recent statements, the message has been clear: procreation, not pleasure, justifies sexuality; birth control, masturbation, premarital sex, and homosexuality are anathema (Taylor, 1970). Protestant views are generally similar, both Calvin and Luther argued that even marital sexuality was shameful, unclean, and sinful (Bailey, 1970).

These religiously based negative views of sexuality are especially severe in regard to women's sexuality. While the view of the good woman as asexual and virginal certainly creates dilemmas and problems for women, this view also has negative effects on men. Many men find it difficult to accept sexuality as part of the personality of the sort of woman that one loves, marries, and chooses as the mother of one's children. For these men, there is a dichotomy between good women and sexual women. This dichotomy is often referred to by clinicians as the "princess and the prostitute" syndrome.

The effects of this syndrome are disastrous for both men and women. One aspect of the syndrome is that the man gives subtle (and sometimes not so subtle) cues to the woman that he does not really want her to be too sexual. Thus the man who perhaps was initially attracted to his future wife at least partially by her sexual responsiveness, finds himself, after marriage, feeling uncomfortable with it. Alternatively, such a man, when seeking a future wife, chooses someone who is not particularly sexually responsive. Clinicians specializing in sexual dysfunction see many such cases: the complaint presented is that the wife is not very interested in sex, does not get very aroused or have orgasms during sex, and has a low desired

From Joseph LoPiccolo, "The Prevention of Sexual Problems in Men," in George W. Albee, Sol Gordon, and Harold Leitenberg (eds.) *Promoting Sexual Responsibility and Preventing Sexual Problems.* Copyright © 1983 by the Vermont Conference on the Primary Prevention of Psychopathology. Reprinted by permission.

frequency of sex. Often, the husband has convinced her to come to therapy by threats of divorce or having an affair if she does not change. In sex therapy, the positive benefits of sex for women are stressed, not as a way to please her husband, but as something highly pleasurable for herself that she is now missing. What we often see, if therapy is successful, is that as the woman becomes more sexually expressive and responsive, the male begins to undermine therapeutic progress. Although his stated reason for entering therapy was for his wife to enjoy sex more, once this begins to happen, he feels vaguely uneasy and uncomfortable. In some of these cases, the man refuses to find the time for the assigned sex therapy homework procedures. Other men become threatened if their wives now attempt to initiate sex with them, which, typically, was one of their pretherapy goals. As a more direct example of this ambivalence about female sexuality, one of our patients told his wife, after she had had a particularly intense orgasm, "I don't like it when you act that way."

In discussing this ambivalence about female sexuality with the male client, we try to reassure him that his wife will not have an affair, become promiscuous, or become insatiable as a result of discovering and expressing her own sexuality. Neither will she have a personality change and become a different sort of woman. In dealing with these fears, however, we are confronted with rather basic, powerful cultural and religious values about female sexuality that men have learned. Obviously, these sorts of profound changes in attitude are not easily produced, and prevention of the development of the negative attitudes would be worthwhile.

Another variation of the princess and the prostitute syndrome more directly affects the man's own sexuality. In this case, the man is unable to reconcile his feelings of love and respect for a woman with his sexual feelings for her, since, after all, decent women are not sexual. Such a man has no sexual difficulties in functioning adequately with prostitutes and other women that he does not love, respect, and value, but finds himself, to his bewilderment, unable to function with his wife. In one of our cases, the male had had intercourse with some 200 different women before his marriage at age 26. Most of these women had been prostitutes; the others he described variously as "whores, party girls, and one-night stands." He married a very attractive woman with whom he did not have intercourse before marriage. Actually, during one of their heavy petting sessions before marriage, she suggested they have intercourse, but he refused. He explained that, since her parents were being very good to them and helping them out financially, he "couldn't do that to them." Yet after marriage, his sex drive toward her actually declined, and he found himself unable to have an erection. At first this was attributed to financial pressures and other worries, and it was only in therapy that his difficulty in experiencing both love and sexual feelings toward the same woman became evident.

Another way in which our culture's religiously based view of sexuality causes problems for men concerns what might be called the "primacy of the penis." That is, since sex is only legitimized by procreation (and only then if you do not enjoy it too much), only penile-vaginal intercourse is truly legitimate. This value, of course, places considerable pressure on the man to have an erection sufficient for intromission and to ejaculate in the vagina. If he cannot accomplish either of these culturally prescribed (and religiously based) goals, he is a failure. Thus, in trying to treat men whose inability to get an erection or ejaculate in the vagina is caused at least in part by anxiety about failure, we run up against a culturally induced set of values that stresses that *real* sex *is* "penis in the vagina plus ejaculation." Furthermore, in working with physically disabled men who cannot attain these goals (men who are diabetic and cord injured), we find it difficult to convince them that other types of sexual expression can be equally valid and pleasurable. Again, our cultural and religious values block therapeutic progress.

In trying to treat the problems caused by these values, rather than to prevent them by changing the values, there are two common but different problems. One problem concerns the male patient whose religious values are central to his whole life. Any attempt to change his sexual values may be seen as an attack on his religion, and this will probably result in resistance to therapeutic suggestions and may even result in his leaving treatment. Obviously, it is presumptuous and intrusive for a therapist to try to change a patient's religious beliefs when the patient only contracted for help with his erection. Yet what is the clinician to do when it is the religious value that is contributing to the problem? Our treatment approach at Stony Brook is to attempt to separate for the patient—sometimes with pastoral assistance—religious views about sex in general from the particulars of the marital relationship and sexuality as an expression of love within marriage. Sometimes this works, but prevention would probably be more effective.

The second type of problem is more subtle. In these cases, the man has already, at a cognitive level, rejected what his religion taught him about sex. Yet emotional "gut level" changes do not come as easily, and an emotionally powerful residue of the values that were developed in childhood and adolescence remains. Such cases are especially difficult, as in the face of the patient's statement that his religious values are no longer active, it is hard to focus on the role of these values in causing his dysfunction.

A set of values that views sex positively is not necessarily incompatible with religion. As numerous religious scholars have pointed out, there is remarkably little in the Bible and other scriptures to justify the antisexual stand of the Judeo-Christian ethic (Taylor, 1970). This antisexual bias actually reflects the sexual values of the lower-middle-class society in which organized Christianity and Judaism developed, rather than being inherent in the religions themselves. Thus, a change in sexual values does not have to be at the expense of religion per se. There is nothing necessarily incompatible between a positive view of sexual expression and a belief in God.

Another concern about changing values to a sex positive ethic concerns the effect on society. From Freud (1930) to your local police chief, there is agreement that allowing unrestrained sexual expression leads to the downfall of civilization. This belief persists despite the existence of stable, family-centered cultures—for example, Mangaia, in the South Seas, as described by Marshall (1971)—that allow virtually total sexual freedom. Furthermore, cross-culturally, it has been found that the level of sexual permissiveness is uncorrelated with the amount of intra- or extracommunal violence present in a culture (McConahay and McConahay, 1977). In the absence of evidence that sexual permissiveness has negative effects on cultural stability, the viability of the family, or level of violence, perhaps advocating a change in cultural values is not such a terribly radical proposal.

The Male Sex Role: "My Only Sex Problem Is That I Can't Get Enough of It"

A comprehensive review of American sex role stereotypes and their psychological effects is provided by Hochschild (1973). In our American sex roles, women are put in a double-bind situation and are expected to be beautiful, sexy, and seductive, while remaining chaste, celibate, and preferably virginal until marriage. Men, on the other hand, do not have such a contradictory and confusing sex role model to follow. Our culture gives a clear and unambivalent message to men about sex, but it is a demanding one. The content of this message includes several directives that create problems for men, lead to development of dysfunctions, and interfere with the attainment of optimum sexual gratification for both men and women.

Bem (1972) has presented evidence that children have learned to behave in accordance with sex role stereotypes by the time they enter nursery school. The male role, in general, stresses achievement, power, skill, competitiveness, strength, endurance, aggression, and success, while devaluing vulnerability, emotional expressiveness, dependency, and affiliation (Goldfried and Friedman, in press). When carried into the sexual area, this role model creates a number of different problems for men, and problems in relationships between men and women (Zilbergeld, 1978).

One major problem is that the male sex role requires a man to want sex always, to seek it out actively, and to define his masculine worth in terms of sexual conquest. This "always on" role, of course, places enormous demands on men. Men are not allowed to have fatigue, worry, or physical discomfort interfere with their sexual drive and ability to perform. To illustrate how strong this expectation for a constantly high male sex drive is, one need only examine the content of sex jokes. For example, consider the large number of jokes that have as the punch line the woman refusing sex by saying, "Not tonight, dear, I have a headache." If one reverses the sexes in these jokes, so that the man is refusing, do the jokes make any psychological sense to us? Almost without exception, they do not. We are simply not programmed by our cultural sex role stereotypes to think of a man as not wanting sex and needing to find an excuse not to have it.

What this model suggests is that men often attempt to have sex when at some level they do not really feel like it. Male patients often report that their problems of erection began at a time of increased stress, worry, or depression when they continued attempting intercourse despite these interfering emotional factors. Similarly, in working with single men (often postdivorced or widowed males), it is surprising to discover how often these men initiate sex or respond to partner initiation when in actuality they are not sexually or emotionally attracted to the woman. Not surprisingly, under these circumstances, arousal, pleasure, and erection are absent.

If you ask these men why they initiated sex or accepted a partner's initiation when they really felt no desire, the common response is that men are supposed to want sex all the time, and the need to maintain this image (both in the partner's eyes and the man's own self-image) makes refusal impossible.

Another aspect of the male sex role that has negative consequences concerns the demand that a man be a skilled, highly experienced, and competent lover. In adolescent male culture, this ethic leads to a good deal of competitive boasting, most of which is usually highly exaggerated. For adult men, this role as the expert has three main negative effects.

First, this role perpetuates sexual ignorance. Since men are supposed to know everything about sex, they cannot bring themselves to buy books, attend classes, or expose themselves to any source of sexual information. After all, if you do so, you are admitting that you could learn something. As an example, in the author's several years of teaching a very large undergraduate course in human sexual behavior, the male-female sex ratio of enrollees was about 60 percent female, despite the fact that the overall university sex ratio was the opposite.

A second negative aspect of the expert role is that men are not comfortable discussing sex with their partners. Since the man knows all about sex, he cannot ask the woman what she enjoys and indeed may be threatened by her attempts to communicate to him what it is that she likes. Men supposedly know what women like, and the idea that there are individual differences in preferences between women that require the man to take the role of learner, rather than expert, is unsettling to the traditional male.

A third negative aspect of the male role as sex expert is that when a sexual problem occurs, men find it extraordinarily difficult to seek out help. Goodman (1960) has noted that among men, "To boast of actual or invented prowess is acceptable, but to speak soberly of a love affair or sexual problem in order to be understood is strictly taboo" (p. 124). This attitude keeps many men with dysfunctions from coming to therapy, or indeed from talking to anyone about their problem. Unfortunately, men's fears about the consequences of revealing their vulnerability are not totally groundless. A study by Derlega and Chaikin (1976) found that males who do not disclose any problems are rated by both men and women as better adjusted than males who do admit to the normal problems we all experience. The opposite pattern, interestingly enough, was found for disclosure of problems by women.

There are other damaging messages in our culture's role model for male sexuality. Another aspect of the male role is that the man must not be emotionally expressive, especially in regard to any tender, intimate, dependent, and therefore unmasculine feelings. The model for male sexuality is conquest, with orgasm, but with as little tenderness, intimacy, and emotionality as possible. Obviously, this lack of emotional expressiveness impoverishes the quality of the sexual relationships for both men and women. Fortunately, with the advent of the women's movement, fewer women are willing to accept this sort of sexual encounter as satisfying and are supplying both pressure and permission for men to drop this unemotional facade.

If the ideal male sex role stresses high drive, expertise, and the lack of emotional expression, it also demands that men function adequately. Lack of erection, on even one occasion, is an emotionally shattering experience for many men. The more strongly the culture values male sexual competence, of course, the more susceptible the man becomes to having his ability to have an erection blocked by anticipatory performance anxiety. There is nothing like worrying about getting an erection for interfering with arousal to the extent that erection becomes impossible. The clearest example of this syndrome occurs in the South Sea Island culture mentioned earlier, Mangaia (Marshall, 1971). Although this culture is extremely free and permissive with regard to sex, a man's social standing is determined not by his wealth or wisdom, but by his sexual prowess, his ability to attain erection. Not surprisingly, with these sorts of stakes on the outcome, the incidence of erectile problems on Mangaia is high. In our culture, the sanctions are more private and internal, yet the demand that a man *always* function perfectly is clearly an unrealistic and damaging aspect of the male sex role.

As one aspect of the double standard, male competence has traditionally been defined only as having an erection and ejaculating. With the women's movement, the acceptance of female sexuality, and the focus on women's needs for sexual satisfaction, another demand for sexual competence has been added to the male sex role. Now the male must not only have an erection and ejaculate, but he must also make sure his partner has at least one and preferably several orgasms. Thus we see patients who put enormous pressure on their female partners to have orgasms, to reassure themselves about their adequacy as males. Again, this sort of pressure is damaging for both men and women. Given these unrealistic demands that men must meet if they are to satisfy the male sex role, it is not surprising that some men find it all a bit overwhelming and prefer to drop out and leave the battlefield. The incidence of complaints of male lack of interest in sex seems to be rising across many different sex therapy programs around the country (Kaplan, 1979; Zilbergeld and Ellison, 1980). In our center, 39 recently completed cases included 27 with complaints of low sexual interest; in 17 (63 percent) of these cases, it was the male who had the lack of interest.

Obviously, a good deal of therapeutic time is currently spent trying to undo these four negative aspects of the male sex role: constant high drive, expertise, emotional inexpressiveness, and flawless functioning. It would certainly be a positive change, and one likely to effect primary prevention, if we could redefine the male role in our culture.

We must attribute major blame for the perpetuation of the current role to advertising, television, and the mass media. If we look at the type of male who is used as a status model to sell everything from cars to beer, he is clearly an achieving, strong, unemotional, expert, and highly competent man. Many of the male role models we see in novels and television similarly do not include men who cry, who are vulnerable, need help, and have egalitarian, communicative relationships with women, especially in regard to sex. Instead, we see the image of masculinity as extremely "macho," dominant, aggressive, or, in short, suffering from what might be called testosterone poisoning.

The Effects of Sex Laws: Inhibitions from Prohibitions

Laws regarding sexual conduct in the United States have been in a state of flux for many years. The Supreme Court continues to struggle with the problems of defining what is obscene or pornographic. In many states husbands and wives break the law if, in the privacy of their own bedroom, they engage in oral or anal sex. Rape laws in many jurisdictions punish the victim rather than the offender. Given our culture's basically antisexual bias, it is not surprising that our sex laws tend to prohibit behaviors that virtually everyone engages in (Kinsey, Pomeroy, and Martin, 1948; Kinsey, Pomeroy, Martin, and Gebhard, 1953), forbid access to erotica in the absence of any evidence of negative effects of exposure to erotica (*Report of the U.S. Commission on Obscenity and Pornography*, 1971), and are especially severe in regard to sexual behavior in adolescence and outside of marriage.

There are three ways in which our sex laws contribute to sexual problems. One major negative effect of censorship and antipornography laws is to limit access to educational material and contraceptive devices and to generate media material that contains a suggestive rather than an open and honest approach to sex. If access to educational material were easier, especially for adolescents, we presumably would see fewer sexual problems caused by ignorance about sexual physiology and sexual technique. Of course, even many small towns have their local "X-rated" bookshops and movie theaters, but such places do not really address the problem. For one thing, people under the ages of 18 or 21 are typically forbidden to patronize these shops and movies. Additionally, the adults who are so lacking in information that they could benefit are also, of course, those likely to be too embarrassed or inhibited to enter such establishments. The quality of material found in "X-rated" books and movies is also problematic, in that it is often factually inaccurate, exploitive of women, and depersonalizing and mechanical in its approach to sex.

What is needed is legislation that would allow sex to enter the mainstream of American literature, film, and television, so that sexually explicit material of good quality would become widely available. Such a change would also have the positive effect of eliminating the titillating and suggestive approach to sex now common in mainstream media productions, especially those on television. Presenting sex as something that is exciting but cannot be discussed openly or portrayed honestly on TV probably contributes to the development of negative or ambivalent attitudes about sexuality and, in particular, women's sexuality, that are common in men with sexual problems.

Someone has worked out that the average American child, by age 18, will have seen 15,000 explicit murders on television. How many explicit, caring, and tender instances of making love will this 18-year-old have seen on TV? This difference is especially remarkable when one remembers that we have recently had separate presidential commissions conduct massive amounts of research on the effects of televised violence and pornography on children. The results of this research demonstrated overwhelmingly that exposure to media violence was harmful in a number of ways and that there was no negative effect of exposure to implicit erotica (*Report of the U.S. Commission on Obscenity and Pornography*, 1971; *Report of the U.S. Commission on Effects of Television Violence*, 1974). Yet violence is allowed in the mainstream of American visual media, whereas erotica are forbidden.

A second problem with our current sex laws concerns the legislation against premarital sexual activity, especially among teenagers under the "age of consent," which ranges from 12 to 21 in various states. These laws, aside from being out of touch with reality, as evidenced by recent research on teenage sexual behavior (Chilman, 1979), serve to legitimize parental attempts to inhibit the expression of sexuality in adolescence, as well as to support police harassment of adolescents at the local parking spot. It is unreasonable to have a law that forbids sexual activity until a certain age, and then expect people to have positive and healthy attitudes about sex after reaching this magic, highly variable age.

The presumed intent of age-of-consent laws is to prevent statutory rape—sexual exploitation of children by adults—which is a worthwhile motive. To prevent these laws from being used in problematic ways, all that would be necessary would be to specify that statutory rape does not apply when the sexual act is between two persons of similar age.

A third negative aspect of our sex laws concerns the laws against sodomy, which in many states includes anything other than penile-vaginal intercourse, even between husband and wife. As previously discussed, the belief that "real" sex consists of getting an erection to put in the vagina places men under considerable pressure to perform and is an especially severe problem for men with physical disabilities or illnesses that interfere with erection. The sodomy laws and the values they reflect are also a problem for the elderly couples now being seen in increasing numbers in sex therapy. Although the aging changes in sexual response are relatively minor and nonproblematic, one change is that as the male ages, it typically takes more direct physical stimulation of the penis for longer periods of time to produce erection. Although this can be a positive change, especially for men who previously had a problem with rapid ejaculation, it is often distressing for elderly couples who have not been comfortable with engaging in lots of foreplay prior to coitus, especially manual or oral stimulation of the male's penis. Prior to entering therapy, these couples typically had a history of many years of adequate functioning, focused exclusively on penile-vaginal intercourse, until the man began to have erectile difficulties. In some cases, direct stimulation of the penis had never been part of their sexual repertoire, and in others it had occurred but was of only brief duration before beginning intercourse.

Suggestions by the therapist to restore sexual functioning by engaging in manual and oral stimulation of the penis and continuing this for some time, often raise concerns about sodomy. One patient, a 77-year-old woman, said, "I've never touched that thing or put it in my mouth in over 50 years of marriage, and I'm certainly not going to commit sodomy now." A similar reaction often occurs when the therapist suggests the man bring the woman to orgasm manually or orally, to reduce the pressure on him to get an erection. Of course, the therapist tries to deal with these negative attitudes by citing the incidence of manual and oral sex, discussing its normality, self-disclosure, and so forth. Yet the fact remains that in many states the therapist is advocating that the patient commit a felony, and the patient may well be aware of this. Adoption of the American Bar Association's model legal code, which decriminalizes all sexual activity performed in private between consenting adults, might help prevent this type of sexual problem.

References

Bailey, D. S. Sexual ethics in Christian tradition. In J. C. Wynn (Ed.), *Sexual ethics and Christian responsibility*. New York: Association Press, 1970.

Bem, S. L. *Psychology looks at sex roles: Where have all the androgynous people gone?* Paper presented at a symposium on women, University of California, Los Angeles, May 1972.

Bidgood, F. The effects of sex education. *SIECUS Report*, 1973, *1*, 11-14.

Calderone, M. S. Is sex education preventative? In C. B. Qualls, J. P. Wincze & D. H. Barlow (Eds.), *The prevention of sexual disorders*. New York: Plenum Press, 1978.

Carton, J., and Carton, J. Evaluation of a sex education program for children and their parents. *Family Coordinator*, 1971, *20*, 377-386.

Chilman, C. S. *Adolescent sexuality in a changing American society*. Washington, D.C.: U.S. Government Printing Office, 1979.

Comfort, A. *The joy of sex*. New York: Crown, 1972.

Crooks, R., and Bauer, P. *Our sexuality*. San Francisco: Benjamin Cummings, 1980.

de Beauvoir, S. *The mandarins: A novel*. New York: Penguin Books, 1956.

DePalma, R. G., Levine, S. B., and Feldman, S. Preservation of erectile function after aortoiliac reconstruction. *Archives of Surgery*, 1978, *113*, 958-963.

Derlega, V. J., and Chaikin, A. L. Norms affecting self-disclosure in men and women. *Journal of Consulting and Clinical Psychology*, 1976, *44*, 376-380.

Ellenberg, M. Impotence in diabetes: The neurologic factor. In J. LoPiccolo and L. LoPiccolo (Eds.), *Handbook of sex therapy*. New York: Plenum Press, 1978.

Ellenberg, M., and Weber, H. Retrograde ejaculation in diabetic neuropathy. *Annals of Internal Medicine*, 1966, *65*, 1237-1246.

Ellis, H. *Studies in the psychology of sex* (7 vols.). Philadelphia: F. A. Davis, 1899-1928.

Faerman, I., Glover, L., Fox, D., Jadzinsky, M. N., and Rapaport, M. Impotence and diabetes: Histological studies of the autonomic nervous fibers of the corpora cavernosa in impotent diabetic males. *Diabetes*, 1974, *23*, 971-976.

Fisher, S. *The female orgasm*. New York: Basic Books, 1973.

Ford, D., and Beach, F. *Patterns of sexual behavior*. New York: Harper and Row, 1951.

Forsberg, L., Gustavii, B. A., Hojerback, T., and Olsson, A. M. Impotence, smoking, and Beta-blocking drugs. *Fertility and Sterility*, 1979, *31*, 589-603.

Frank, E., Anderson, C., and Rubinstein, D. Frequency of sexual dysfunction in "normal" couples. *New England Journal of Medicine*, 1978, *299*, 111-115.

Freud, S. [*Civilization and its discontents*] (J. Riviere, Trans.). London: Hogarth Press, 1930.

Freud, S. [Some psychological consequences of the anatomical distinction between the sexes.] In J. Strachey (Ed. and trans.), *Sigmund Freud: Collected papers* (Vol. 5). New York: Basic Books, 1959. (Originally published, 1925.)

Freud, S. [*Three essays on the theory of sexuality.*] (J. Strachey, Ed. and trans.). New York: Basic Books, 1963. (Originally published, 1905.)

Friedman, J. M. Sexual adjustment of the postcoronary male. In J. LoPiccolo and L. LoPiccolo (Eds.), *Handbook of sex therapy*. New York: Plenum Press, 1978.

Goldfried, M. R., and Friedman, J. M. Clinical behavior therapy and the male sex role. In K. Solomon and N. B. Levy (Eds.), *Men and mental health: Changing male roles*. New York: Plenum Press, in press.

Goodman, P. *Growing up absurd*. New York: Random House, 1960.

Gordon, D. G. *Self-love*. Baltimore: Penguin Books, 1972.

Haller, J. S., and Haller, R. M. *The physician and sexuality in Victorian America*. New York: W. W. Norton, 1974.

Hart, M., Roback, H., Tittler, B., Weitz, L., Walston, B., and McKee, E. Psychological adjustment of nonpatient homosexuals: Critical review of the research literature. *Journal of Clinical Psychiatry*, 1978, *39*, 604-608.

Hochschild, A. R. A review of sex role research. *American Journal of Sociology*, 1973, *78*, 1011-1029.

Hogan, D. R. The effectiveness of sex therapy: A review of the literature. In J. LoPiccolo and L. LoPiccolo (Eds.), *Handbook of sex therapy*. New York: Plenum Press, 1978.

Jenkins, C. D. Recent evidence supporting ecologic and social risk factors for coronary disease. *New England Journal of Medicine*, 1976, *294*, 987-994, 1033-1038.

Kaplan, H. S. *Disorders of sexual desire*. New York: Brunner/Mazel, 1979.

Kempczinski, R. F. The role of the vascular diagnostic laboratory in the evaluation of male impotence. *American Journal of Surgery*, 1979, *138*, 278-282.

Kinsey, A. C., Pomeroy, W. B., and Martin, C. E. *Sexual behavior in the human male*. Philadelphia: W. B. Saunders, 1948.

Kinsey, A. C., Pomeroy, W. B., Martin, C. E., and Gebhard, P. H. *Sexual behavior in the human female*. Philadelphia: W. B. Saunders, 1953.

Kolodny, R. C., Masters, W. H., and Johnson, V. E. *Textbook of sexual medicine*. Boston: Little, Brown, 1979.

Krafft-Ebbing, R. von. *Psychopathia sexualis*. Brooklyn, N.Y.: Physicians and Surgeons Books, 1899.

Lemere, F., and Smith, J. W. Alcohol-induced sexual impotence. *American Journal of Psychiatry*, 1973, *130*, 212-213.

LoPiccolo, J., and Heiman, J. Cultural values and the therapeutic definition of sexual function and dysfunction. *Journal of Social Issues*, 1977, *33*, 166-183.

LoPiccolo, L. Low sexual desire. In L. A. Pervin and S. R. Leiblum (Eds.), *Principles and practice of sex therapy*. New York: Guilford Press, 1980.

Marshall, D. S. Sexual behavior on Mangaia. In D. S. Marshall and R. C. Suggs (Eds.), *Human sexual behavior: Variations in the ethnographic spectrum*. New York: Basic Books, 1971.

Masters, W. H., and Johnson, V. E. *Analysis of human sexual response*. Boston: Little, Brown, 1966.

Masters, W. H. and Johnson, V. E. *Human sexual inadequacy*. Boston: Little, Brown, 1970.

Master, W. H. and Johnson, V. E. *Homosexuality in perspective*. Boston: Little, Brown, 1979.

McConahay, S. A., and McConahay, J. B. Sexual permissiveness, sex role rigidity, and violence across cultures. *Journal of Social Issues*, 1977, *33*, 134-143.

Meiselman, K. C. *Incest*. San Francisco: Jossey-Bass, 1978.

Michal, V., Kramar, R., Pospichal, J., and Hejhal, L. Arterial epigastricocavernous anastomosis for the treatment of sexual impotence. *World Journal of Surgery*, 1977, *1*, 515-524.

Remes, K., Kuoppasalmi, K., and Adlercreuty, H. Effect of long-term physical training on plasma testosterone, adrostenedione, globulin capacity. *Scandinavian Journal of Clinical Laboratory Investigation*, 1979, *39*, 743-749.

Renshaw, D. C. Impotence in diabetes. In J. LoPiccolo and L. LoPiccolo (Eds.), *Handbook of sex therapy*. New York: Plenum Press, 1978.

Report of the U.S. commission on effects of television violence. Washington, D.C.: U.S. Government Printing Office, 1974.

Report of the U.S. commission on obscenity and pornography. Washington, D.C.: U.S. Government Printing Office, 1971.

Roseman, R. H., and Friedman, M. Neurogenic factors in pathogenesis of coronary heart disease. *Medical Clinics of North America*, 1974, *58*, 269-279.

Saxton, L. *The individual, marriage, and the family*. Belmont, Calif.: Wadsworth, 1968.

Sherfey, M. J. *The nature and evolution of female sexuality*. New York: Vintage Books, Random House, 1973.

Sorenson, R. *Adolescent sexuality in contemporary America*. New York: Vintage Books, Random House, 1973.

Taylor, G. R. *Sex in history*. New York: Harper and Row, 1970.

VanThiel, D. H., Sherins, R. H., and Lester, R. Mechanism of hypogonadism in alcoholic liver disease. *Gastroenterology*, 1973, *65*(A-50), 574. (Abstract)

Waldron, I. Why do women live longer than men? *Social Science and Medicine*, 1976, *10*, 349-362.

Waldron, I. The coronary-prone behavior pattern, blood pressure, employment, and socioeconomic status in women. *Journal of Psychosomatic Research*, 1978, *22*, 79-87.

Weichman, G. H., and Ellis, A. L. A study of the effects of sex education on premarital petting and coital behavior. *Family Coordinator,* 1969, *18,* 231-234.

Wilson, G. T. Alcohol and human sexual behavior. *Behavior Research and Therapy,* 1977, *15,* 239-252.

Wilson, W. C. Can pornography contribute to the prevention of sexual problems? In C. B. Qualls, J. P. Wincze, and D. H. Barlow (Eds.), *The prevention of sexual disorders.* New York: Plenum Press, 1978.

Zilbergeld, B. *Male sexuality.* Boston: Little, Brown, 1978.

Zilbergeld, B., and Ellison, C. R. Desire discrepancies and arousal problems in sex therapy. In L. A. Pervin and S. R. Leiblum (Eds.), *Principles and practice of sex therapy.* New York: Guilford Press, 1980.

Zorgniotti, A. W., Rossi, G., Padula, G., and Makovsky, R. D. Diagnosis and therapy of vasculogenic impotence. *Journal of Urology,* 1980, *123,* 674-677.

Men and Rape

Gene G. Abel

Rape, though it appears to be a chaotic act, an irrational act perpetrated for no apparent reason, can be understood. If we interview the men who rape and systematically investigate the antecendents to their violent crime, we discover consistent patterns that precede the act. Knowing the antecedents, we can change the pattern that leads to rape and can break that pattern before the actual rape. Although scientific studies have revealed these crucial patterns, our ability to intervene at an early developmental point is obstructed.

First, investigation of rapists' behavior prior to rape has been previously invalidated because investigators did not deal with the rapists' desires to keep their thoughts and activities secret for fear of prosecution. Useful investigation requires a methodology that allows rapists to reveal, without fear of incriminating themselves, what drives them to rape. This has been accomplished by research limited to rapists who are outside the legal system and who as out-patient volunteers have been given confidentiality.

Even when a rapist's confidentiality is fully protected, many rapists still will not or cannot reveal the truth. Their motives, drives, and ability to control their compulsive urges remain secret. To overcome this obstacle, a new system of evaluation was incorporated into the research methodology: Direct psychophysiologic assessment of the rapist's sexual arousal pattern. This new system allows objective assessment of rapists by quantifying the rapist's arousal to violent and nonviolent sexual themes.

This quantification in the laboratory allows experimental studies of fac-

From Gene G. Abel, "Preventing Men from Becoming Rapists," in George W. Albee, Sol Gordon, and Harold Leitenberg (eds.) *Promoting Sexual Responsibility and Preventing Sexual Problems.* Copyright © 1983 by the Vermont Conference on the Primary Prevention of Psychopathology. Reprinted by permission.

tors that may contribute to rape. These assessment methods have considerable face validity; these studies are of men who have actually raped and, before treatment, had a high likelihood of raping again; men who were assured absolute confidentiality; men whose self-reports were confirmed by psychophysiologic assessment (Abel, Barlow, Blanchard, and Guild, 1977; Abel, Blanchard, Barlow, and Mavissakalian, 1975; Abel, Blanchard, and Becker, 1978; Abel, Blanchard, Becker, and Djenderedjian, 1978; Barbaree, Marshall, and Lanthier, 1979).

Studies of rapists who have been assured of confidentiality and whose self-reports were confirmed by laboratory measurement of their sexual arousal, have given us valuable information about the antecedents to rape. The antecedents include: compulsive use of rape fantasies for sexual arousal; rapelike behavior; displaced anger toward women; and distorted cognitions about rape.

Before one examines the antecedent patterns to rape, one should have a clear definition of rape and an understanding of the two distinct types of rapists.

Defining Rape

There can be considerable variation in how rape is defined. At one extreme, some only consider an act to be rape when the perpetrator has physically penetrated an orifice of the victim with his penis and the victim's resistance has been so vigorous that she has been physically injured during the act. At the other extreme, some consider any form of verbal or physical intrusion upon the physical and /or emotional space of another as rape. For the purposes of this chapter, we will consider rape as a hands-on intrusion by the rapist of the victim, with the rapist having an explicit goal of attempting to commit a sexual act against the victim's will.

The relationship between the rapist and his victim is another complex dimension of rape. Some rapes occur between strangers; other rapes involve closer relationships between perpetrator and victim, such as acquaintance rapes, date rapes, spouse rapes, and incest. Since those who rape the greatest number of victims choose victims whom they barely know or do not know, this chapter will emphasize the prevention of rapes between strangers.

Categorizing Rapists

Men who rape victims unknown to them can be divided into two types. The first type, the antisocial, has a history replete with antisocial activities. He does not report having ongoing thoughts of rape or urges to commit rape. He is self-centered and hedonistic. His social and work relationships are poor, and beginning at an early age, he carries out a variety of antisocial activities such as robbery, assault, and larceny. When he does rape, which is infrequently, he rapes during the course of another crime. His victim and his decision to rape are unplanned. Because so few rapes are committed by the antisocial rapist, our focus will be on the second type, the psychological rapist.

The psychological rapist has repeated urges to rape. He has frequently had these urges since his mid-teens, when he begins to masturbate to fantasies of rape. His urges gradually become stronger, and he attempts to resist acting on them, realizing that rape is morally wrong. As he continues to use fantasies of rape during masturbation or orgasm, his arousal and urges to rape become progressively more powerful. As thoughts of rape become stronger, his other sexual thoughts gradually become weaker and may even disappear (Abel and Blanchard, 1976). Eventually the psychological rapist begins to act on his rape urges. His commission of rape is frequently followed by considerable anxiety, guilt, depression, and diminution of his rape urges. These emotional responses, however, are generally short-lived; his urges to rape once again reappear, and the rape cycle repeats itself.

The psychological rapist, unlike the antisocial rapist, may commit from 2 to 100 rapes. The act of forcing himself on a victim becomes more and more erotic, so that eventually, given the choice between sex with a partner by mutual consent and forcing himself on that same partner, he would prefer to use force (Abel et al., 1975). The characteristics of the psychological rapist's sex offenses are similar to those of exhibitionists, child molesters, and other paraphiliacs. Each of these sex offenders has recurrent urges to commit the sex crime; their control breaks down; they commit the crime; they feel temporary guilt and anxiety immediately afterwards; their urges temporarily diminish, only to recur, and the process repeats itself.

Although we can identify four distinct antecedents to rape, preventing men from becoming rapists requires recognition of these precursors and the ability to actually intervene at an early stage in this developmental pattern. Implementing this intervention is inhibited on all sides: by the professionals who are in contact with rapists, by the legal system that attempts to control the rapist, by the society's acceptance of the pre-rape behavior, and by the rapist himself. Not only must we identify the steps to the primary prevention of rape, but we must also be aware of the techniques that can be used to overcome the obstacles that stand in the way of primary prevention.

Arousal Patterns That Are Antecendent to Rape

Studies of the psychological rapist indicate that he has had fantasies of rape and violence long before becoming a rapist. Since the fantasies of rape always precede the actual act of rape, it would be quite possible to evaluate those men who compulsively use rape fantasies and treat those men who have the greatest probability of becoming rapists. Unfortunately, a number of obstacles prevent us from reaching these men.

First, our culture views the control of an individual's sexual urges as simply a problem of willpower. If a man finds himself with recurrent urges to rape, he usually assumes that he must control these fantasies himself, by relying on his strength of character. This belief gains credence because the consequences from the breakdown of one's willpower are usually incidental: if you eat more cake than you probably should have, if you watch television excessively, no one is significantly hurt. Losing control over urges to rape is quite another thing. Men need to understand that as the consequences of loss of control increase, so does the need for consultation and assistance in order to ensure that control is maintained and victimization is prevented. In order to cope with violent thoughts, a client needs a treatment program that combines a comprehensive assessment and a systematic treatment intervention in multiple areas (Abel, Blanchard, and Becker, 1978).

Second, not only does the general population lack an understanding of the relevance of rape thoughts and attraction to sexual violence, but professional helping agents likewise share much of the public's naiveté. Practitioners have not been taught how to question their clients about their proclivitis for sexual violence. They ignore the reality that rapes occur at a rate of 20-40 per 100,000 individuals at risk, and that someone must be committing these rapes. We justify not asking clients about their sexual fantasies and urges for sexual assault by rationalizing that the potential rapist is of a low socioeconomic group, of low moral character, and certainly not like any of the people we evaluate. However, rapists come from all economic, ethnic, educational, and religious backgrounds. The practitioner needs to relinquish some of his or her stereotypes of rapists and ask clients about this issue. To ensure that practitioners feel comfortable about asking such questions, professional education should include role-playing interview skills in the area of sexual violence. We should not expect practitioners to begin to ask about sexual violence until they have learned how to pose such questions appropriately. A practitioner must know how to ask questions about sexual aggression in a way that allows the client to answer truthfully and thereby gain access to treatment.

Third, most individuals view their sexual lives as a taboo topic, something that they should not discuss with others. When the individual's sexual urges are more deviant than the general population's, when he has obsessive fantasies of raping a woman or a child, he becomes even more reluctant to reveal such thoughts. The rapist usually concludes that if he does not think or talk about his rape fantasies, they will go away in some magical way. This misbelief probably evolves because of the manner in which deviant fantasies develop (Abel and Blanchard, 1975). During genital arousal, our fantasies become associated with the enjoyment from intercourse, masturbation, and orgasm. For the rapist, the use of rape fantasies during masturbation and orgasm has been associated with progressively greater arousal to rape stimuli. Since rape thoughts have become more powerful because he has thought of rape, not thinking of rape should logically reduce arousal.

Studies where paraphiliacs were satiated with their deviant fantasies (Abel, Becker, and Skinner, in press, Marshall and Barbaree, 1978; Marshall and Lippens, 1977), however, suggest just the opposite. Externalizing these fantasies to the point of satiation destroys their erotic punch and allows the rapist to gain control over his aggressive fantasies. We therefore need to break through the taboo of talking about sexual topics, including the urge to rape, so that treatment agents can openly discuss with such individuals the existence of the problem and what men with urges to rape need to do to prevent themselves from acting on their urges.

Fourth, the legal system's method of dealing with the rapist appears to propagate the maintenance of rape thoughts and urges. The rapist is told in prison that anything he communicates to others will become part of his official record. The rapist learns that if he talks about his rape(s), its characteristics, and his persistent urges to rape, these comments will appear in his record. When this record reveals that he still has desires to rape, there is a high likelihood that the rapist's sentence will be prolonged and that he will be passed over for parole, and further investigation may result in his being charged with additional sexual assaults. The rapist subsequently stops talking about his rapes and instead attempts to convince prison personnel that though he had these thoughts at one time, the trauma of arrest and incarceration has destroyed them and he is now repentant and no longer at risk. Since he is no longer at risk, no treatment is in order in prison. He is released, his urges to rape accelerated and the circle is completed when he begins to rape again.

To disrupt this dangerous cycle, a system of confidentiality for rapists and those working with them needs to be developed both inside and outside of prison settings, so that potential rapists can describe their rape-related activities without fear of repercussion. With such confidentiality safeguards, the sexual aggressive could more easily describe his treatment needs, and helping professionals, armed with this information, could develop appropriate treatment programs to eliminate these urges. To continue to block this avenue of assistance to the rapist places him in a untenable position. We need more treatment methods that prevent rape, not methods that conceal the potentiality for the crime.

A final factor that prevents treatment from reaching those men with urges to rape is that most people believe that the majority of rapists are caught and imprisoned. In reality, most men who rape are still on the streets. Interviews with rape victims indicate that anywhere from 2 to 10 rapes occur for each 1 reported to the police. Since the most common "treatment" for rapists is arrest, and arrest is only possible if rapes are reported, the current system has little applicability to the majority of rape cases. Even when arrest does occur, only 13 percent of those charged with rape are actually found guilty and incarcerated (Csida and Csida, 1974). Should conviction and incarceration occur, recidivism rates 5 years after release indicate that at least 35 percent of rapists have recommitted their crime (Frisbie and Dondis, 1965).

The evidence is quite clear that our present legal approach is not effective, and additional methods are needed to combat rape. The difficult task will be to point out that while the fear of incarceration is a somewhat effective deterrent, it is not sufficient to prevent sexual violence. Treatment methods that can prevent men from acting on their urges to rape for the

TABLE 1
Rapists' Additional Paraphilias

Diagnosis	Percentage with Diagnosis
Heterosexual pedophilia	24.1
Exhibitionism (adult female targets)	18.5
Voyeurism	16.7
Heterosexual incest	9.3
Sadism	9.3
Homosexual pedophilia	5.6
Exhibitionism (young female targets)	3.7
Other	12.8

first time as well as preventing known rapists from repeating this violent crime exist and must be added to the limited impact of incarceration.

Behavioral and Emotional Antecedents to Rape

Rape prevention can be more effective if greater attention is paid to the types of behaviors that frequently precede the rape. In our studies of rapists, 49 percent were found to have histories of other types of paraphilias, generally preceding the rape behavior. When 34 rapists were questioned, they reported a total of 54 paraphilias, for an average of 1.6 other paraphilias per rapist. Table 1 demonstrates that the most common additional diagnoses were heterosexual pedophilia, exhibitionism, voyeurism, heterosexual incest, and sadism. This is not to imply that all men with various paraphilias will develop into rapists, but it does suggest that when a client is identified as having one of the paraphilias frequently associated with rape, the client should be questioned thoroughly about possible urges to rape. Unfortunately, many practitioners fail to do this.

Rapists may not have other paraphilias but often carry out aggressive acts short of rape. Henry, for example, was evaluated after being charged with two rapes. His history reveals that for 3 years prior to his rapes, he had been assaulting women in parking lots. He would follow women as they went to their cars, and while they were rearranging their packages and reaching for their keys, he would grab their genital areas and then run away. This behavior persisted for over a year, eventually occurred in his high school, and led to his expulsion. Ignored, his grabbing of women persisted and eventually he followed women into office buildings and escalated his sexual behavior to rape. What is impressive about Henry's case is that his family and school officials did not respond to his early grabbing behavior, even though this behavior duplicated four of the aggressive aspects of rape: hands on victim, aggressive attacks, unconsenting victim, and repetition. His behavior differed in only one aspect: his immediate escape from his victim once she had been touched. In Henry's case those around him ignored a form of sexual aggression that was identical in most respects to rape. Everyone appeared to be waiting for Henry's problem to get serious, but his grabbing behavior was serious. When we wait until rape actually occurs, it is too late: too late in this case because two innocent victims had already suffered severe trauma, and too late for Henry because once he had been arrested for rape, the likelihood of his receiving treatment was extremely remote. Treatment offered in prison is usually identical to the treatment given those who steal cars, evade income tax, or rob. However, those who display the behavioral antecedents of rape need a specific treatment for that specific sexual behavior, and by the time the client is arrested for rape, he no longer has access to appropriate treatment.

In addition to behavioral antecedents, emotional conflicts frequently precede rape. A common emotional antecedent is anger: the potential rapist becomes angry with a woman, but is unable to express that anger directly to her; instead, he inappropriately expresses that anger to an innocent woman by raping her.

Jim, at age 22, married Mildred, 14 years his senior. Jim had been raised in a mining town, where he had developed a variety of stereotypic attitudes about the importance of men being in charge and making all decisions. While dating in high school he had always determined the where, when, and what of dating. When unable to control the dating situation he would have outbursts of anger and "slap his girlfriends around" until they complied with his demands.

Following his marriage, he found that Mildred was equally domineering. Her behavior made him feel she was intruding into his life: She demanded that he be home at specific times and did not allow him to go hunting with his friends. Conflicts arose early in their marriage and he was increasingly displeased with Mildred. When his family heard that he was no longer able to do what he wanted, they supported his increasing confrontations with Mildred. Fights ensued and Jim left home and drove to a motel to live temporarily. That night, on returning from a bar, he stopped to help a woman whose automobile had broken down. While pretending that he was driving her to the closest gas station, he stopped the car, tied her up, gagged and blindfolded her, and sadistically raped her. In Jim's case, there was a direct relationship between his inability to assert himself with Mildred, the development of angry feelings toward her, and the subsequent rape of an innocent victim.

Recent experimental studies in the laboratory have confirmed a direct relationship between anger and increased sexual arousal toward rape themes. Marshall (1981) measured normal subjects' arousal to rape stimuli before and after subjects were confronted by a hostile, angry female (who was actually a rsearcher feigning anger toward the subjects). Following this brief confrontation, subjects showed definite increases in their sexual arousal to descriptions of rape.

If the inappropriate expression of anger by males is so closely linked to less inhibition toward violence toward women, training in the appropriate expression of anger may serve as a preventative measure against rape. This training could take the form of assertiveness training, a relatively common clinical intervention used to teach others how to ask appropriately for behavioral change in others, and how to express various positive and negative feelings.

Cognitive Distortions Antecedent to Rape

When interviewing rapists, one is struck by the cognitive distortions men display about the rapes they have committed, their victim's responses, and the interaction that preceded the rape.

Steven was interviewed in jail following his first arrest for rape, but he reported at least 21 other occasions that the interviewer would have called rape. Typically, Steven would begin by talking to women in bars. He was convinced that any woman in a bar had gone there specifically to meet a man to have sex with. He would next ask her to go for a ride with him in his car. He believed that any woman who agreed to go with him was also agreeing to have intercourse with him, irrespective of what she said to him later on.

In a secluded area he would then attempt to have intercourse with the woman and if she resisted, he would tear her clothes off and slap her repeatedly. All of his victims initially resisted these physical attacks but eventually stopped resisting for fear of injury. When they stopped fighting, however, he failed to interpret this as fear. He interpreted their lack of extreme resistance as another way of saying yes, they wanted to have sex with him. Steven's criterion for rape was that if he attempted to have sex with a woman and she unceasingly fought him while he escalated his violent attack, only then would he classify his act as rape. If she fought until he injured her or she was terrified of being injured, he mistakenly categorized this as normal courtship behavior that is typical of most women. Steven, like many other rapists, believed that a large percentage of women wanted to be "roughed up" during sex, so that they could justify having intercourse with a man without feeling guilty later.

These cognitive distortions are psychologically helpful to the rapist. By accepting these distorted beliefs, he justifies his rape behavior: his acts are not rape; they are normal courtship behaviors. The potential rape victim, however, is in a no-win situation. If she is in the bar, he sees her as an appropriate target to attack. If she resists, it is permissable to "slap her around" since she needs to be convinced to have sex so she will not feel guilty afterwards. Irrespective of what the victim does, the rapist can justify his behavior; therefore there is no reason for him to become upset or feel guilty afterwards since it really was not rape.

Even more startling is that many of the rapist's cognitive beliefs about rape are shared to some degree by over 50 percent of the general population (Burt, 1980; Malamuth, Haber, and Feshbach, 1980). If half the population believes that roughing up women is acceptable and possibly even sexually stimulating to many women, if 50 percent believe that only women "who are asking for it" get raped, if 50 percent believe that it is physically impossible for a healthy woman to be raped against her will, then the world is a dangerous place for most women.

A number of steps must be taken to prevent the development of cognitive distortions that support rape behavior. First, potential rapists and potential rape victims must learn that actual rapes are not like their usual fantasies of rape. Rape is not the rough seduction of an ambivalent woman who becomes overwhelmed by her biological response to a penis in her vagina or mouth and ultimately orgasms from the experience. Only a minute number of women have ever reported that they would be aroused by being raped, and when this small group was questioned in detail (Malamuth et al., 1980), they reported that the rape they were thinking of was one in which they were in complete control, a rape they could terminate at any time. However, real rapes are just the opposite: rape victims feel a complete loss of control. Victims report no sense of being able to stop the assault, but instead believe they are at the mercy of the rapist. Potential rapists (generally young men, 15 to 25 years old) must be taught to view rape as it actually is: a violent, life-threatening attack by a male, who beats up the victim, penetrates her orifices with his penis, and irrationally demands that she report being sexually turned on.

Second, the systems that support these cognitive distortions must be dismantled. The most obvious of these are the media that support the image of man as the aggressor, woman as victim of that aggression, and rape as a seduction game that ends with orgasms for the rapist and the victim. Not only do such depictions provide models for males to become aggressive with women, but they also teach women that it is acceptable and expected that women should be victims of men's aggression. These cognitive distortions must be debunked. What we need to see are examples of mutual caring and respect between men and women in all types of interaction, sexual or nonsexual.

Third, the potential rapists (men) must be helped to understand that it is their attitudes toward women as sexual objects and property that allow them to ignore similar attitudes in other males, who act on them and become rapists. It is because our fellow man acts on his cognitive distortions that our wives, sisters, and daughters are raped. If any man doubts the prevalence of such beliefs, he might try walking 10 feet behind his wife, sister, or daughter down any major street in any city in the United States and observe the men nearby.

Finally, males must become involved in the struggle to eliminate rape. As long as men see rape as a problem outside of themselves, committed by strangers for reasons totally unrelated to themselves, men will not be motivated to change the male attitude that leads to rape. In actuality men must realize that their own whistles and leers on the street are part of the cognitive distortions which become magnified in the minds of other men who eventually rape.

❖   In summary, we must keep in mind that rape is not an innate behavior but a behavior that follows logically from a variety of antecedents. If we learn to recognize these antecedents, primary prevention can occur. Men who have compulsive psychological urges to rape can be distinguished from the general population and be taught to eliminate their urges to rape *before* they actually rape.

Currently this society's efforts to deal with rape occur almost exclusively *after* a woman has been victimized. No one wants rape victims. Effective primary prevention prevents two tragedies: men as rapists; women as rape victims.

References

Abel, G. G., Barlow, D. H., Blanchard, E. B., and Guild, D. The components of rapists' sexual arousal. *Archives of General Psychiatry*, 1977, *34*, 895-903.

Abel, G. G., Becker, J. V., and Skinner, L. J. Treatment of the violent sex offender. In L. Roth (Ed.), *Clinical treatment and management of the violent person.* Washington, D.C.: Crime and Delinquency Issues, United States Department of Health and Human Services, in press.

Abel, G. G., and Blanchard, E. B. The measurement and generation of sexual arousal. In M. Hersen, R. M. Eisler, and P. M. Miller (Eds.), *Progress in behavior modification* (Vol. 2). New York: Academic Press, 1976.

Abel, G. G., Blanchard, E. B., Barlow, D. H., and Mavissakalian, M. Identifying specific erotic cues in sexual deviation by audio-taped descriptions. *Journal of Applied Behavior Analysis*, 1975, *8*, 247-260.

Abel, G. G., Blanchard, E. B., and Becker, J. V. An integrated treatment program for rapists. In R. Rada (Ed.), *Clinical aspects of the rapist.* New York: Grune and Stratton, 1978.

Abel, G. G., Blanchard, E. B., Becker, J. V., and Djenderedjian, A. Differentiating sexual aggressives with penile measures. *Criminal Justice and Behavior*, 1978, *5*, 315-332.

Barbaree, H. E., Marshall, W. L., and Lanthier, R. D. Deviant sexual arousal in rapists. *Behavior Research and Therapy*, 1979, *17*, 252-259.

Burt, M. R. Cultural myths and supports for rape. *Journal of Personality and Social Psychology*, 1980, *38*, 217-230.

Csida, J. B., and Csida, J. *Rape: How to avoid it and what to do about it if you can't.* Chatsworth, Calif.: Books for Better Living, 1974.

Frisbie, L. V., and Dondis, E. H. *Recidivism among treated sex offenders.* California Mental Health Research Monograph No. 5, 1965.

Malamuth, N. M., Haber, S., and Feshbach, S. Testing hypothesis regarding rape: Exposure to sexual violence, sex differences, and the "normality" of rapists. *Journal of Research in Personality*, 1980, *14*, 121-137.

Marshall, W. L. *The evaluation of sexual aggressives.* Paper presented at the third annual Conference on the Evaluation and Treatment of Sexual Aggressives, San Luis Obispo, California, 1981.

Marshall, W. L., and Barbaree, H. E. The reduction of deviant arousal: Satiation treatment for sexual aggressors. *Criminal Justice and Behavior*, 1978, *5*, 294-303.

Marshall, W. L., and Lippens, K. The clinical value of boredom: A procedure for reducing inappropriate sexual interests. *Journal of Nervous and Mental Diseases*, 1977, *165*, 283-287.

A Typology of Risks and the Disabilities of Low Status

Elizabeth Taylor Vance

SOCIAL DISABILITY IN LOW STATUS INDIVIDUALS

I propose, in discussing the social disabilities that evolve in the context of low status, not to approach the subject from the perspective of what society does to certain of its members, but rather to examine such questions as why racism and sexism work. This is one of several possible approaches to identifying the most efficient point of intervention in any ecological risk.

Social Disability in Blacks and Females

In the last two years, while reviewing the developmental literature on women to prepare a book on lifespan development, I discovered that there are many similarities in being black and being female. At first my attention was caught by the risks of pathology in the two groups. But it has become more and more apparent to me that the issues I have been exploring are more fundamentally those of human development and human potential than of variations in clinical magnitudes of pathology. As I plan to illustrate, however, the two issues are inextricably related, as I think they are in all stabilized "ecosystem" problems.

The story that follows is not a straightforward one. Piecing it together hangs not on one crucial, well-designed study but on an integration of diverse sources of cumulative evidence. There are many gaps in the story, particularly with respect to the part played by the black experience. As a strategy for presenting a coherent picture, I therefore rely heavily at some points on

From Elizabeth Taylor Vance, "A Typology of Risks and the Disabilities of Low Status," in George W. Albee and Justin M. Joffe (eds.) *The Issues: An Overview of Primary Prevention.* Copyright © 1977 by the Vermont Conference on the Primary Prevention of Psychopathology. Reprinted by permission.

extrapolation to blacks from findings with women. The picture is suggestive. Verification of specific parts will require continued research.

I would like to begin by reviewing the findings on symptom variance and prevalence of disorder in blacks, females, and low socioeconomic groups generally. I repeat that the epidemiological knot with respect to ecological problems is a very tough one to unravel. Awareness that if one is poor one's chances of becoming hospitalized for an emotional disorder are 64 times what they are if one is not has unfortunately only served to stir up the old nature-nurture controversy. In a review of comparative studies of blacks and whites in the United States, Dreger and Miller (1968) suggested that the ideal experimental design for analyzing the complexities of epidemiological findings would be a multivariate analysis of variance with interactions reaching to the 25th order.*

In spite of the intimidating picture suggested by Dreger and Miller, I want to try to make some sense of the epidemiological findings. What is to follow are relevant findings on "true" prevalence rates—that is, estimates of pathology in the general population (Dohrenwend, 1974). Also discussed are patterns of symptom variance as observed in several studies conducted with hospitalized clinical groups.

(1) In "true" prevalence studies which include all analyses since 1969, the most consistent result reported is an inverse relationship between overall rates of psychopathology and socioeconomic status. (For example, of 33 communities studied, 28 yielded highest rates in the lowest classes.)

(2) The steepest part of the curve portraying the falloff for severe disorders occurs between the lowest status groups (those below the poverty line) and the working class. That is, the point in the socioeconomic structure which shows the greatest, most precipitous increase in serious pathology demarcates the worst levels of poverty in our culture.

(3) Personality disorders and schizophrenia represent the types of disorders showing the most consistent inverse relationship with economic and social status.

(4) Estimates of the prevalence of pathology among blacks and among white females have been conflicting. To date, Dohrenwend

*For an analysis of methodological issues and the current status of inter- pretations of epidemiological research, the reader should see Dohrenwend's 1974 review.

counts 16 studies in which men showed higher rates than women and 27 studies in which women show higher rates than men. In an analysis of prevalence rates in Baltimore, Pasamanick (1962) finds that state hospital rates for blacks (nonwhites) is 75 times that for whites. He nevertheless concludes from an analysis of all institutions (private, state, and federal) that there is no difference in prevalence of disorder for blacks and whites.

From a review of much of the literature, it seems reasonable to draw the following conclusions for the present about prevalence in blacks and in white females:

• With respect to women, there is no *overall* difference in "true" prevalence rates for all disorders when compared with males. There are consistent differences, however, in type and intensity of disorder and in the conditions under which these develop. Also, duration for certain types of disorder is higher among women—thus selectively raising prevalence rates.

• Black prevalence rates vary considerably from locale to locale, in some areas being equivalent to those of whites. In other places, however, particularly in urban high-stress areas, prevalence rates for blacks are as much as three to four times as great as white rates in the same locales. Thus, there is epidemiological evidence for a differential response to high stress.

• Although one reviewer (Malzberg, 1959) has concluded that there are no black-white differences in type of disorder, a comparison of symptom pattern indicates the type of disorder for both blacks and females differs in similar ways from that of white middle class males. The following is a summary of several findings on symptom variance for these groups.

(5) Rates of personality disorder are higher in males. There is, however, significant interaction with such other factors as socioeconomic status and race. Low socioeconomic status or being black account for a large portion of the variance among males.

(6) Neuroses among women are higher than among men in both rural and urban settings. Aside from depression, a large component of the symptom picture tends to be hysteriform in type (for example, conversions and somatization). In rural areas, female psychotics outnumber male psychotics; in urban areas, the reverse is true. (It is my impression that the difference in relative rates is accounted for not by a drop in women's rates for psychosis in

urban areas but by an increase in male rates, female rates being relatively constant across locales.)

(7) Among blacks, the largest portion of the difference in rates is accounted for by schizophrenia, which in one study in the New York area was found to be roughly 100 in 100,000, as compared to 33 in 100,000 for whites.

(8) A common description of behavioral differences between males and females given by investigators and clinicians alike is that women patients are much more frequently narcissistic, abandoned, and attacking than male patients (Raskin and Golob, 1966; Weich, 1968).

The following represent differences in characterics of male and female acutely disturbed patients in independent ratings of ward and group therapy behavior (Weich, 1968).

• Males are better organized, more responsive to instruction, more constrained, more intrapersonally and socially organized, less prone to acting out, less "sick," less inclined to scream and cry, less hostile, more inclined to clump in groups, less demanding, and more cooperative.

• Females are more explosive, more violent, more overtly homosexual and acting out, more hysterical, more exhibitionistic, characterized by more physical activity, more overtly hostile, more sexual, more seductive, manipulative, badgering, and talkative, less conventional toward the doctor; they "grab your hand more," do more disrobing, are sillier, are more expressive and more imploring, want more attention, show no "group spirit," exhibit wilder extremes of behavior, are more unkempt, and show more self-neglect. In therapy, the level of noise and activity in women's groups was markedly higher than in the male groups and there were more instances of striking the therapist and other patients.

(9) Remarkable similarities have been observed between the level and quality of symptoms found among women and those among black patients as a group. In a study by Schliefer, Derbyshire, and Brown (1964) in which black and white male and female patients were compared on admission and over the first three days of hospitalization, black patients were generally sicker on admission, with black males rated sickest and white males as least sick. "Sicker" in this study referred to a greater degree of disorientation, irrelevance in speech, and, to a lesser extent, hostility, activity,

appearance, and loudness and quantity of speech. At least 40 percent of the females, both black and white, showed symptoms of somatization; relatively few such symptoms were reported in male patients. The investigators noted a fact of particular interest: there appeared to be a faster reduction in symptoms in women than in men over the first three days. This turned out to be due almost entirely to a kind of suggestive hysterical pattern shown in the dramatic reduction in somatization during this period.

Certain findings concerning somatization in black males bearing on the ecology of this symptom are also relevant. There is an interesting reversal of sex differences with respect to somatization in black males and females in southern samples as measured on MMPI (Mosby, 1972). In the south, higher rates of somatization are found among black males than among black females. Northern black males, on the other hand, use this mechanism much less than northern black females—a pattern more common for the population as a whole.

Epidemiological findings indicate that somatization is a common mechanism in the pathology of immigrant and ethnic minorities. Is it reasonable at this point to raise the question of the relationship of status and power and coping mechanisms to these particular *symptom patterns?* Before pursuing that question, I would like to mention two other types of findings that are helpful in interpreting this material.

The first concerns the process-reactive distinction relative to these groups. The process-reactive distinction classifies the schizophrenic according to the level of social competence achieved prior to decompensation. Individuals are classified as process schizophrenic when they have exhibited a wide range of failures on developmental tasks—social development, school achievement, heterosexual relationships, work commitment—throughout the formative years. It is generally assumed that there has been some underlying morbid process present since childhood which has interfered with normal learning. The process does not ordinarily manifest itself in accessory symptoms until maturity. In contrast, individuals are classified as reactive schizophrenics when premorbid adjustment has been good by these standards but accessory symptoms develop suddenly and often in relation to some recognizable stress.

This distinction has been very powerful in that it has reduced some of the behavioral heterogeneity in the schizophrenic group and has also been found to correlate with severity of symptom (or degree of sickness) and length of hospitalization. The problem with the distinction is that it does not hold equally well for all social groups. A particularly consistent finding is that female schizophrenics as a group tend to achieve "healthier" premorbid levels of adjustment than their male counterparts. It is quite difficult to explain the level of decompensation in women on the basis of any simple relationship between degree of socialization and disposition to process pathology. In women, whatever the process is that leads to pathology in adulthood, it has not crippled social development as society defines it for women.

We are faced, on the contrary, with at least the tentative paradox that the behavioral characteristics underlying process decompensation may be the same ones that make women attractive to many males under favorable life circumstances. At the very least we are talking about developmental outcomes that are independent of success or failure in primary socialization or in moving through the few adult social roles available for women.

This fact is quite remarkable to me. I cannot emphasize it enough. It is at the root of the problem of ecological risk. Apparently quite acceptable levels of socialization can proceed as an overlay of a developing incapacity for lifetime growth and of a high vulnerability to stress. The relationship between premorbid ratings and morbid status for blacks is much more consistent with expectations; but this particular difference between black males and white females is only apparent. White females who later become schizophrenic are more successfully conforming to social expectations than are white males who later become schizophrenic. But then so are black males, in that the subcultural social norms of black males just happen to prescribe much of the behavior (narcissim, aggression directed outward) that helps define the process category. The behavior of low status black males is in many respects quite consistent with the pressures of their niche, just as is that of females.

❖   In general, the problematic findings with women schizophrenics underline discontinuity between apparent premorbid resources and morbidity—a discontinuity that does not hold for any other group. A second set of findings provides further support for this observation. There is a differential relationship between girls' and boys' early adjustment and later predictions of pathology. It is well known that girls as a group receive higher adjustment ratings than boys (Weinstein and Geisel, 1960). Rutter, nevertheless, has shown that girls' early adjustment histories do not predict adult adjustment, though certain symptoms in early history do predict for boys: Gardner (1967), for example, found that neurotic symptoms in boys usually predict adult pathology. No such relationship has been found for females. Predictors for girls are not early adjustment attributes at all but presence of pathology in the mother (Rutter, 1974). Rutter has proposed a genetic interpretation for his finding; but it is useful to compare the consistent findings of Heilbrun and others, using nonclinical samples, that when degree of sex role identification is used as a predictor of adjustment in adult males and females, high femininity is more often associated with poor adjustment than any other attribute measured (Heilbrun, 1968).

One other interesting set of findings bears on this story. Ego strength has long been considered among clinicians as a predictor of mental health and as a way of summarizing the potential for resistance to stress. Among other things, it is considered to include the capacity to delay gratification and to regulate and control reactivity, and is generally assumed to involve a high degree of perceptual-cognitive differentiation in the discrimination of external reality, self, and feelings. Using the field dependence technique as a measure of differentiation, Vaught (1965) found that high ego strength is always associated with a highly differentiated perceptual-cognitive system in men—that is, a highly differentiated discrimination and perception of reality. Males with low ego strength, regardless of sex role identification, show poor perceptual-cognitive differentiation. For women, however, there is no such relationship; rather, only masculine sex role identity predicts perceptual differentiation. Women with high ego strength who are also high masculine identifiers are highly differentiated and articulated cognitively. Women with high ego strength who are high feminine identifiers show poor cognitive differentiation. Apparently a behavioral and experiential identification in the masculine mode provides assimilations that lead to such cognitive schemata.

What does this mean about sex role, ego strength, and prediction of pathology? For one thing, it must mean that the structure of ego strength differs for males and females. Further, it would seem that the psychological loading of ego strength is greater for males than for females. Thus, as ego strength develops in women it may reflect little more than the resources required in assuming the feminine role. At the same time, as we have seen, feminine identification is related to poor adjustment. One interpretation of these observations is that ego strength in women is unrelated to quality of coping with stress outside the dictates of social role and bears only upon her comfort with and acceptance of the pressures of primary socialization—*the very factor which places her in great vulnerability for pathology.*

When these findings are combined with the paradoxical findings on premorbid-morbid characteristics, we might almost make the following startling predictions. In white middle-class males, a reasonable predictor of poor adjustment and potential pathology is the deficit in, or excessive demand on, the personal qualities and resources summarized in ego strength. For white females, a predictor of poor adjustment and potential pathology is the ecological fate of the degree to which she has made a feminine identification. Similarly, for black males, a predictor of potential pathology is the degree of assimilation of the social role status of black.

Social Disability and Ecological Risk

Now what is the nature of the interrelationships that define these problems as ecological risks? The common sociodevelopmental and intrapsychic problems of blacks (particularly black low-socioeconomic-status males) and females are rooted in an intricate combination of the power and status characteristics of their social roles and their developing dispositions. Subordinate roles and status are phenomena that are highly institutionalized for blacks and females. Their status, furthermore, is attached to each of their kinds of physical visibilities; therefore status is less negotiable from generation to generation than that of other low-status groups. History as well as ontological change is thus enlisted. But what makes the system work, ostensibly? And why are the risks we speak of so often obscured? Ecological risk refers, after all, to those problems in which vulnerable individuals complement the system's uses of their vulnerability. The answers to these questions lie, I think, in a combination of features that account for adaptation as well as social disability.

The following represents an attempt at a theoretical integration that may help to explain the paradoxes of ecosystem fit, social problems, and pathology. I have used the term social disability to classify a large group of seemingly disparate clinical and social disorders because it seems to me that the evidence strongly suggests they have a unitary ecological as well as developmental character. We must think in terms of some common sociopsychological mechanism, since the disorders are concentrated within the most socially and economically alienated and powerless groups in our society. This statement does not preclude heritability but assumes that the heritability operates—as does any polygenic influence— through the avenues available to it developmentally and through the filters and pressures of one's ecology.

In an earlier paper (Vance, 1973) I summarized the evidence for the relationship between environmental extremity and the development of effectance or competence—a position first formulated by Robert White (1959). Briefly, there is a close empirical and logical relationship between balance and imbalance in power between the child and the physical and social environment and the child's development of resources for dealing with the environment.

"Passivity" is the best term I can think of to summarize the consequences of an overpowering environment. Seligman (1970, 1975) has used the term "helplessness," but I wish to emphasize the perceptual-cognitive rather than the behavioral component. Perceptual-cognitive passivity may be the greatest single source of vulnerability to stress in man. In fact, at the risk of overstating the case, I would not be surprised if, with the fetalization of the brain during the evolution of the human species, an active perceptual-cognitive orientaton had become a major aspect in our survival as a species. Similarly, it has been said that the number of niches a species can fill (and thus by implication increase his survival potential) is a function of the diversity of roles he can actively master by means of his activity and creativity (Wallach, 1970).

The experimental variable *locus of control* (Rotter, 1966) refers to the relationship between the individual and an extreme environment. The variable has been demonstrated to have highly diverse effects in human functioning. I would like to summarize my interpretation of findings with respect to how this diversity of effects is accomplished. The locus of control refers to the belief most people seem to acquire that they can effect or initiate change in the environment. It also appears to be a measure of how much we tend to assume responsibility for the rewards and punishments we receive. Those who characteristically fail to perceive a relationship between their own activity and environmental events are described as "externals." Those for whom this relationship is well articulated are described as "internals."

The diverse behavioral and adaptive effects that have consistently emerged in studies of the locus of control suggest that it must serve as a threshold of some kind. I would guess that its greatest importance lies not in the confident sense of self it must provide but in the feedback it provides to cognition—in the relationship it establishes between the person and information, between the person and his own activity.

There are dimensions of reality that are available only where that feedback relationship exists. When beliefs of this kind are established very early, they sensitize us to information feedback and focus our attention on it. Feedback has turned out to be an extremely important phenomenon, whatever its object. The feedback about activity and inherent in activity provides the base for building differentiated cognitions that maximize the informational value of experience and provide the basis for the self-regulation of behavior.

The person who has no belief in internal causality, who is insensitive to feedback in his own activity and cannot perceive the link between his own behavior and events, is one for whom attention cannot be controlled by memories, images, or internal standards. Poor use of information is a necessary correlate, as is inadequacy in coping with novel, unstereotyped experiences and resolving conflict.

❖ One key to understanding the role played by these attributes in so many diverse morbid and premorbid pictures is that they are similar to the dissociative phenomena produced by any depressant drug. For example, animal subjects administered depressant drugs are incurious and incautious; they use problem-solving styles characterized by failure to alternate or withhold responses; they exhibit dissociation of learning; they rapidly learn instrumental and consummatory responses; they are insensitive to information and feedback; and they perform as though attention is poorly controlled by memory (Sachs, 1967). The evidence strongly suggests that underlying both the premorbid adaptations to stress and the morbid reactions to it are common behavioral and cognitive characteristics of this kind. Although symptoms may legitimately be viewed in many ways, the most useful view for understanding these problems is that the symptoms manifested under stress are related to the integrative state of the person. The integrative state of an externalizer is dissociative and basically passive (whether morbid or adjustive). The nature of symptoms-under-stress that express a dissociative and passive mode are exaggerated concreteness (since memory does not support inference), somatization, hysteriform modes of expressing tension, either lability or flatness of affect (depending upon conditioning history), openness to control by stimuli of all kinds, and, in severe decompensation, thought disorder exclusive of coherent delusions. Much of this syndrome is consistent with what is observed in process forms of schizophrenia.

On the other hand, in compensated levels of functioning I would expect a high susceptibility to the influence of whatever ecological niche the individual finds himself in. Thus we might expect a considerable range of adjustments by the standards of the larger society; that is, some of the life styles would be recognized as problems and some not. The life styles of many lower-class males are a case in point. Their life styles are quite compatible with their subcultural niches but are considered by the larger society to be maladjustive. We can imagine the social problems generated from niche sensitivities of this kind.

The adjustment of women is seen as much more generally desirable and benign to the society as a whole. A recent discussion of criteria of social competence by Anderson and Messick (1974), however, has suggested that some aspects of social competence must be assessed in terms of attributes that transcend limited niches. Thus, in spite of the differences in the way society views the adjustments and competence of black males and females, these adjustments have some important characteristics in common which in terms of the criteria of social competence reveal their vulnerability and risk. Blacks (males in particular) and white females are minimally distinguished by behaviors which in themselves are prized by "many segments of society and across a large number of situations." Their adaptations are significantly distinguished from those of middle-class males by the fact that they are characterized by behaviors less often universally admired in themselves and their resources are differentially appropriate to different situations.

Furthermore, findings are reasonably consistent that blacks and females and low socioeconomic status groups are external with respect to perceived power or control and that they are less well perceptually-cognitively differentiated than white middle-class males. Among other provocative and related findings are that information in instructions does not affect conditioning in women subjects though it does so for males (Berry and Martin, 1957). Another finding is that low socioeconomic status groups and women remain dominated by empathic identifications rather than cognitive mediations in their moral judgments (Kohlberg and Kramer, 1969; Boehm, 1962). With respect to women's performance on moral dilemma tasks, never at any age measured do women show the level of differentiated, principled thought involved in a generalized ethical orientation in relation to others that over 50 percent of middle-class males are able to exhibit by age 16!

The picture of development and adaptation is far from being as clearcut as this presentation might suggest. For example, achieving a capacity for advanced levels of principled thought and humanism does not seem to guarantee among males a like level of humanistic behavior in interpersonal relations (Kohlberg, 1974). On the other hand, when we consider all the meanings of passivity in women (as in a recent analysis of aggression, dominance, and passivity in males and females by Maccoby and Jacklin, 1974), it is clear that "passivity" in women is not only adaptive in many ways but may mediate some of the most desirable effects of primary and secondary socialization (see Lowenthal, 1971) when the mean level of the general social welfare within the social structure is regarded as the criterion.

❖   *ECOLOGICAL RISKS AND PRIMARY PREVENTION*

Is a society possible in which we can reduce the prevalence of such stabilized ecological risks as those related to social disability?

Are strategies of primary prevention—particularly social action that alters power relationships within groups and communities—the most appropriate and efficient way of making these very fundamental changes in society and in human beings? I do not pretend to answer those questions. One major barrier to significant change, however—at least for blacks and females—is the difficulty of incorporating an interaction perspective into a general strategy of interventions.

We cannot maximize human development and increase invulnerabilities to future stress by the elimination of poverty alone. Power, for example, is an element of the structure of all human and infrahuman relationships, deriving in part from the character of the organism in groups ranging all the way from dyads to communities. It is not simply asserted by certain kinds of societies, although unquestionably some types of societies thrive more on imbalances than others.

There are three sources of interactions involved in these social problems based in power imbalances: (1) the varying physical and social environmental parameters (for example, rates of environmental and social change; organization and consistency in the environment; power assertion strategies in families and institutions; (2) intra- and interindividual differences (which often translate into group differences); and (3) age changes. It is seldom that all of these sources of interaction can be incorporated into a single prevention plan.

Any group strategy based on the assumption that power imbalance leads to passive experiencing on the part of the "victim" will have to take into account individual differences and age changes in factors that influence the perception of stress and extremity. For this reason, I provide the following set of examples showing what information is needed about the individual to calibrate social interventions. In the first example I choose the trait reactivity because of what we have learned about the relationship between reactivity and perception. Autonomic reactivity mediates rapid social learning and, within limits, probably accounts for a great deal of developmental flexibility (Vance, 1973). Excess trait reactivity, however, is negatively related to discrimination and use of feedback (Levine, 1969; Denenberg, 1967; Gray, 1975).

There is much evidence for high trait reactivity among blacks, particularly black males (see review by Vance, 1973). If black males and white males differ on reactivity, and if environmental extremity and power imbalances should affect them in different ways, then the interaction between extremity and social disability may be accounted for by the extent to which the two groups are differently reactive.

In a recent study on socioecological stress involving power assertion environments, findings on race and blood pressure supported a hypothesis for an interaction between race, reactivity, and stress (Harburg et al., 1973). Comparing a sample of black and white married males in high-stress and low-stress areas in Detroit, the investigators found that suppressed hostility—a typical pattern for many males in both black and white high-stress areas—was related to high blood pressure levels and hypertension in both black and white males in both areas. Black high-stress males, however, showed significantly higher blood pressure levels and hypertension than any other group. Furthermore, reactivity was highest of all groups for dark-skinned, high-stress black males who suppressed hostility. Is it, then, high reactivity that makes black males particularly sensitive to the perception of extremity?

Reactivity is a survival mechanism which can be viewed as simplifying the discriminations that produce conflict and immobilization, increasing the disposition for physical action and aggressiveness in response to stress. The trait might be quite adaptive in some ecologies. It is relevant here not because of any absolute value of its adaptiveness but because it lowers a threshold for the kind of experience that seems to relate to passive perceptual modes and social disabilities. A similar disposition for white males may be activity level. High activity level, like reactivity, is also negatively related to finely tuned discriminations. Males —particularly white middle-class males—succumb to socialization pressures for modulating gross activity level relatively early in childhood. This fact may account for the finding that the relationship between boys and girls on perceptual-cognitive discrimination (girls exceeding boys in this development prior to four years of age) reverses itself in middle childhood (Coates, 1974).

Women comprise yet another pool of dispositions. There is only equivocal evidence for significant differences in total autonomic reactivity between males and females. If anything, males may be more autonomically reactive than females. But the physiological patterns of reactivity differ for the sexes fairly consistently in ways that suggest differences in perceptual modes for coping with reactivity. Males exhibit a more cortical orienting pattern and females a more cortical defensive pattern in which helplessness (a characteristic of anxiety) may be more acutely experienced (Neufeld and Davidson, 1974; Craig and Wood, 1971; Hare, 1971). Thus in women it may be that the form rather than the level of reactivity facilitates the experiencing of perceived extremity.

Finally, an example of an age-specific factor that can contribute to passive experiencing and trait development has to do with the relationship between sex, race, and the nature of the interpretations of the environment characteristic of the young child. Kohlberg theorizes that children take an active role in interpreting their environments. They attach sex role stereotypes to their own early, highly concrete cognitive categorizations, and for them the entire power dimension we have attached so much importance to *is related to body differences*. Children, then, derive their assumptions of social power from the physical power dimension. Before the age of four, size becomes the basic indicator for all important status differences like strength, knowledge, social power, and self-control. Stereotypes of masculine dominance and social power develop out of body stereotyping (Kohlberg, 1966).

For girls who do not identify with a perceived source of power as an intermediate step on the way to maturity, giving up the promises of power and settling for the perceived impotence in the feminine ideology must operate to obscure diverse and differentiating kinds of experiences as effectively as the extreme environments characterizing urban poverty.

I would also guess that some similar kind of perceptual considerations may operate for black children around color differences in a culture where power is easily perceived to accrue to the color dimension. Interestingly, one recent study tends to confirm the universality of physicalistic power perceptions in children while at the same time confirming the role of cultural specificity and shaping for other attributes of children's experiences—for example, nurturance (Gold and St. Ange, 1974).

This age-specific perceptual-cognitive style may account in part for recent observations that "spontaneous" and persistent traditional sex typing and differentiation appears to be continuing among children even in the face of changes in sex-typing norms by the society as awhole (Emmerich, 1973; Lynn, 1974, pp. 141–142).

It is highly desirable that conclusions following a discussion such as the one presented in this paper should set forth some usable generalizations. Yet generalizations are antithetical to the realities of interactions. Even so, some implications of this review for primary prevention can be noted. The general implications are two. For one, developmentalists have an important contribution to make in the primary prevention of social problems. Second, we must include at least first-order interactions in our prevention strategies. Specifically, we should be concerned with:

(1) *Universal human development.* Social disabilities and stabilized ecosystem problems are negatively related to social competence. Prevention efforts must therefore include knowledge about processes of human development. Furthermore, nothing short of the kind of change in both professional and social attitudes which would facilitate commitment to universal human development will lead to a significant reduction in the kinds of problems discussed in this paper.

(2) *Social competence as a developmental goal.* In most prevention efforts we tend to focus on the pathology we wish to avert. To prevent social problems produced by niche control, we must have a model of "man" that provides us with testable assumptions about social competence and the ecologies that facilitate its development. A good beginning is the recent attempt by a panel of experts under the auspices of the Office of Child Development to define the meaning of social competency (Anderson and Messick, 1974).

(3) *Individual differences.* Prevention strategies must be based on a recognition of the reliability and salience of the individual differences that contribute to developmental outcomes and the mediation of experiences in social contexts.

(4) *The structure of social institutions.* In an earlier paper I reviewed findings showing that various dimensions of poverty contribute to the experience of power imbalance and to social disability (Vance, 1973). The implication, of course, is that prevention requires the eradication of poverty. In this paper, however, we have discussed evidence for power imbalances that

are embedded in institutional structures and role relationships. In order to prevent what appears to be a disposition for perceptual-cognitive passivity and its sequelae among blacks and females, for example, there must be a metamorphosis of social institutions into fundamentally developmental institutions. Erik Erikson (1963) has proposed the concept of "mutual regulation" to describe the interdependency between the individual and the institutions of his society. According to Erikson, the structure as well as the content of the relationship between individual and society plays a large role in developing competence. It seems to me that the concept of mutual regulation provides an excellent basis for a model for prevention strategies requiring institutional change.

(5) *Age X institutional interactions.* Primary prevention efforts involving institutional change must focus on role relationships and communication patterns that facilitate effectance experiences in both children and socialization agents. This means designing social institutions of all kinds that will have enough structural flexibility to provide effectance experiences by different means depending on the characteristics of the different age levels with which the institution is in contact.

(6) *Person X institution interactions.* Institutions must also show enough structural flexibility to provide effectance experiences for different individuals or groups. A potential value of personality research is that it can provide information about personality variables that influence effectance experiences in the "interaction space" in person-situation interactions. As a general approach to identifying such variables, Vale and Vale (1969) have suggested that when we know we have something that represents an interaction, we should look for some third underlying variable that mimics the function between the behavior and the environmental variable. When such a variable relates similarly to different characteristics of different individuals, we can do some fine tuning of person-institution relationships. Very frequently, however, we will not have information about personal variables of this kind. For those circumstances, a prevention strategy is suggested by Atkinson and Paulson's (1972) concept of "response sensitive" treatments. Applied to the context of institution X person interactions, creating response-sensitive institutional structures would involve strategies for monitoring responses and roles of individuals

in institutional contexts and fine-tuning the roles and relationships according to the nature of the person processes that appear to be influencing the effectance experiences of the individual or group.

REFERENCES

Anderson, S., and Messick, S. Social competency in young children. *Developmental Psychology*, 1974, *10*, 282–293.

Anthony, E. J. A Risk-Vulnerability Intervention Model for children of psychotic parents. In E. J. Anthony and C. Koupernik (Eds.), *The child is his family: Children at psychiatric risk*. New York: Wiley, 1974. (a)

Anthony, E. J. The syndrome of the psychologically vulnerable child. In E. J. Anthony and C. Koupernik (Eds.), *The child in his family: Children at psychiatric risk*. New York: Wiley, 1974. (b)

Atkinson, R. C., and Paulson, J. A. An approach to the psychology of instruction. *Psychological Bulletin*, 1972, *78*, 49–61.

Berry, J. L., and Martin, B. GSR reactivity as a function of anxiety, instructions, and sex. *Journal of Abnormal and Social Psychology*, 1957, *54*, 9–12.

Boehm, L. The development of conscience: a comparison of American children and different mental and socioeconomic levels. *Child Development*, 1962, *33*, 575–590.

Coates, S. Sex differences in field dependence among preschool children. In Freidman, P. C., Richert, R. M., and Vance Wiele, R. L. (Eds.), *Sex differences in behavior*. New York: Wiley, 1974.

Craig, K. D., and Wood, K. Autonomic components of observers of pictures of homicide victims and nude females. *Journal of Experimental Research in Personality*, 1971, *5*, 305–309.

Cronbach, L. Beyond the two disciplines of scientific psychology. *American Psychologist*, 1975, *30*, 116–127.

Denenberg, V. H. Stimulation in infancy, emotional reactivity, and exploratory behavior. In D. C. Glass (Ed.), *Biology and behavior: Neurophysiology and emotion*. New York: Rockefeller University Press, Russel Sage Foundation, 1967.

DeWolf, A. S. Premorbid adjustment and the sex of the patient: implications of Phillips Scale ratings for male and female schizophrenics. *Journal of Community Psychology*, 1973, *1*, 63–65.

Dohrenwend, B. P., and Dohrenwend, B. S. Social and cultural influences on psychopathology. *Annual Review of Psychology*, 1974, *25*, 417–452.

Dreger, R. M., and Miller, K. S. Comparative psychological studies of negroes and whites in the United States: 1959–1965. *Psychological Bulletin Monograph Supplement*, 1968, *70*, 58.

Emmerich, W. Socialization and sex role development. In P. B. Baltes and K. W. Schaie (Eds.), *Life span developmental psychology: Personality and socialization*. New York: Academic Press, 1973.

Erikson, E. *Childhood and society*. New York, Norton, 1963.

Escalona, S. Intervention programs for children at psychiatric risk. The contribution of child psychology and developmental theory. In E. J. Anthony and C. Koupernik (Eds.), *The child in his family: Children at psychiatric risk*. New York: Wiley, 1974.

Fontana, A. F. Familial etiology of schizophrenia: Is a scientific methodology possible? *Psychological Bulletin*, 1966, *66*, 214–227.

Gardner, G. G. The relationship between childhood neurotic symptomatology and later schizophrenia in males and females. *Journal of Nervous and Mental Disease*, 1967, *144*, 97–100.

Garmezy, N. The study of competence in children at risk for severe psychopathology. In E. J. Anthony and C. Koupernik (Eds.), *The child in his family: Children at psychiatric risk*. New York: Wiley, 1974.

Gold, A. R., and St. Ange, M. Development of sex role stereotypes in black and white elementary school girls. *Developmental Psychology*, 1974, *10*, 461.

Gray, A. L. Autonomic correlates of chronic schizophrenia: a reaction time paradigm. *Journal of Abnormal Psychology*, 1975, *94*, 189–196.

Harburg, E., Erfurt, J. C., Hauenstein, L. S., Chape, C. A., Schull, W. J., and Schork, M. A. Socio-ecological stress, suppressed hostility, skin color, and black white male blood pressure: Detroit. *Psychosomatic Medicine*, 1973, *35*, 276–296.

Hare, R., Wood, K., Britain, S., and Frazelle, J. Autonomic responses to affective visual stimulation: Sex differences. *Journal of Experimental Research in Personality*, 1971, *5*, 14–22.

Heilbrun, A. B., Jr. Sex role, instrumental behavior and psychopathology in females. *Journal of Abnormal Psychology*, 1968, *73*, 131–316.

Hersov, L. Introduction: risk and mastery in children from the point of view of genetic and constitutional factors and early life experiences. In E. J. Anthony and C. Koupernik (Eds.), *The child in his family: Children at psychiatric risk*. New York: Wiley, 1974.

Hunt, J. McV. *Intelligence and experience*. New York: Ronald Press, 1961.

Hunt, J. McV. Parent and child centers: Their basis in the behavioral and educational sciences. *American Journal of Orthopsychiatry*, 1971, *41*, 13–38.

Irvine, E. E. The risks of the register: Or the management of expectation. In E. J. Anthony and C. Koupernik (Eds.), *The child in his family: Children at psychiatric risk*. New York: Wiley, 1974.

Jenkins, R. L. Psychiatric syndromes in children and their relation to family background. *American Journal of Orthopsychiatry*, 1966, *36*, 410–457.

Kelly, J. Toward an ecological conception of preventive interventions. In J. W. Carter, Jr. (Ed.), *Research contributions from psychology to community mental health*. New York: Behavioral Publications, 1968.

Kessler, M., and Albee, G. Primary prevention. *Annual Review of Psychology*, 1975, *26*, 557–592.

Kohlberg, L. A cognitive developmental analysis of children's sex-role concepts and attitudes. In E. E. Maccoby (Ed.), *The development of sex differences*. Stanford: Stanford University Press, 1966.

Kohlberg, L. Continuities in childhood and adult moral development revisited. In P. B. Baltes and K. W. Schaie (Eds.), *Life-Span developmental psychology: Personality and socialization.* New York: Academic Press, 1974, pp. 180-207.

Kohlberg, L., and Kramer, R. Continuities and discontinuities in childhood and adult moral development. *Human Development*, 1969, *12*, 93-120.

Lane, E. The influence of sex and race on process-reactive ratings of schizophrenics. *The Journal of Psychology*, 1968, *68*, 15-20.

Levine, S. An endocrine theory of infantile stimulation. In A. Ambrose (Ed.), *Stimulation in Early Infancy.* New York: Academic Press, 1969.

Lindon, R. L. Risk register. *Cerebral Palsy Bulletin*, 1961, *3*, 481-487.

Lowenthal, M. F. Intentionality: toward a framework for the study of adaptation in adulthood. *Aging and Human Development*, 1971, *2*, 79-95.

Lynn, D. *The father: His role in child development.* Monterey: Brooks/Cole, 1974.

Maccoby, E. E., and Jacklin, C. N. *The psychology of sex differences.* Stanford: Stanford University Press, 1974.

Malzberg, B. Mental disease among negroes: An analysis of first admissions in New York State, 1949-51. *Mental Hygiene*, 1959, *43*, 422-52.

Mosby, D. Toward a theory of the unique personality of blacks: a psychocultural assessment. In R. L. Jones (Ed.), *Black psychology.* New York: Harper and Row, 1972.

Neufeld, R. W. J., and Davidson, P. O. Sex differences in stress response: A multivariate analysis. *Journal of Abnormal Psychology*, 1974, *83*, 178-185.

Pasamanick, B. A survey of mental disease in an urban population: VII. An approach to total prevalence by diagnosis and sex. *American Journal of Psychiatry*, 1962, *119*, 299-305.

Raskin, A., and Golob, R. Occurrence of sex and social class differences in premorbid competence, symptom and outcome measures in acute schizophrenia. *Psychological Reports*, 1966, *18*, 11-22.

Rosenthal, D. Sex distribution and the severity of illness among samples of schizophrenic twins. *Journal of Psychiatric Research*, 1961, *1*, 26-36.

Rotter, J. B. Generalized expectancies for internal versus external control of reinforcement. *Psychological Monographs*, 1966, *80* (1, Whole No. 609).

Rutter, M. Epidemiological strategies and psychiatric concepts in research on the vulnerable child. In E. J. Anthony and C. Koupernik (Eds.), *The child in his family: Children at psychiatric risk.* New York: Wiley, 1974.

Ryan, W. *Blaming the victim.* New York: Random House, 1971.

Sachs, E. Dissociation of learning in rats and its similarities to dissociative states in man. In J. Zubin and H. F. Hunt (Eds.), *Comparative psychopathology.* New York: Grune and Stratton, 1967.

Schliefer, C., Derbyshire, R., and Brown, J. Symptoms and symptom change in hospitalized negro and white mental patients. *Journal of Human Relations*, 1964, *12*, 476-485.

Seligman, M. E. P. On the generality of the laws of learning. *Psychological Review*, 1970, *77*, 406-418.

Seligman, M. E. P. *Helplessness*. San Francisco: W. H. Freeman, 1975.

Vale, J. R., and Vale, C. A.   Individual differences and general laws in psychology. *American Psychologist*, 1969, *24*, 1093–1108.

Vance, E. T. Social disability. *American Psychologist*, 1973, *28*, 498–511.

Vaught, G. M. The relationship of role identification and ego strength to sex differences in the rod and frame test. *Journal of Personality*, 1965, *33*, 271–283.

Wallach, M. A. Creativity. In P. H. Mussen (Ed.), *Carmichael's Manual of child psychology*. New York: Wiley, 1970.

Weich, M. J. Behavioral differences between groups of acutely psychotic (schizophrenic) males and females. *Psychiatric Quarterly*, 1968, *42*, 107–22.

Weinstein, E. A., and Geisel, P. N. An analysis of sex differences in adjustment. *Child Development*, 1960, *31*, 721–728.

White, R. W. Motivation reconsidered: The concept of competence. *Psychological Review*, 1959, *66*, 297–333.

Wolff, S., and Acton, W. Characteristics of parents of disturbed children. *British Journal of Psychiatry*, 1968, *114*, 593–601.

Wynne, L. C., and Singer, M. T. Thought disorder and family relations of schizophrenics. I. A research strategy. *Archives of General Psychiatry*, 1963, *9*, 191–198. (a)

Wynne, L. C., and Singer, M. T. Thought disorder and family relations of schizophrenics. II. Classifications of forms of thinking. *Archives of General Psychiatry*, 1963, *9*, 199–206. (b)

III. Strategies of Empowerment: Programs for Individuals and Families

In this section, we present some illustrative program descriptions aimed at strengthening individuals and families—programs that help build resistance to the forces seeking to exploit and degrade women, adolescents, blacks, gays, and lesbians. Each program strikes at established social values that result in exploitation and damage to self-esteem. Each program represents an attempt to show individuals and families ways to cope, ways to flaunt the oppressors, ways to undermine exploitative power.

New Possibilities for Women

Betty Friedan

Ultimately I am going to hint at new patterns and problems and pleasures and possibilities in the relations of women and men, but having as-
siduously tried to do some research on your own experience of these
phenomena during the five days of this conference, I have decided that
we are not there yet. And that I had better spend most of the time giving
you concrete proof of primary prevention of psychopathology through
social change and political action as it really happened this last twenty
years in this country through the Women's Movement. I can bear witness
from my original training as a psychologist and from my nearly twenty
years as a social change agent, founding and leading that movement to
the complex interrelationship between psychology, social change, and
pathology that we mutually confront, dealing with the concrete human
being in the process of making and surviving the change, and evolving
strategies for the next stage of human liberation.

First I want to remind you, because a lot of you here are too young to
remember and others would just as soon forget, where we were twenty
years ago, when I, as a young housewife-mother guiltily hiding my free-
lance writing from my suburban neighbors like secret drinking, was
starting *The Feminine Mystique*. I want to remind you where we were vis-
à-vis psychology, psychopathology, and women. There was, if you will
remember, at that time, a single image of woman—the happy housewife-mother—who was always 25 with three children under six, who
was fulfilled as a wife and a mother solely through those emotions having to do with her sexuality, her husband, her children, her home: her
peak experience, her orgasm, was throwing the powder in the dish-
washer. The fact that so many women were already working outside of
the home did not affect that image. And it was, above all, in its per-
niciousness, a psychological image. Remember *Modern Woman, The Lost
Sex* (Farnham and Lundberg, 1947)? A whole slew of books had come
out using or twisting Freudian psychology to say that the previous cen-
tury-long battle for women's rights—the vote, careers, higher educa-

From Betty Friedan, "Women—New Patterns, Problems, Possibilities," in Justin M. Joffe and George W. Albee
(eds.) *Prevention Through Political Action and Social Change.* Copyright © 1981 by the Vermont Conference on
the Primary Prevention of Psychopathology. Reprinted by permission.

tion—had made modern women terribly neurotic, maladjusted in their proper role as women, which was to live passively, vicariously through men and children, through feminine fulfillment as a life-long housewife-mother. Heeding that message, younger women, 20 years ago, were happily marrying and being told to marry at 17, 18, 19, giving up their own education to put their husbands through, and making a career of three, four, five children—the new happy, happy housewives.

The fact that overwhelming fortunes were being made selling tranquilizer pills mainly to women; the fact that women made up the great majority of the patients in every doctor's office; and, of course, the clients of the burgeoning psychological industry was not supposed to belie that happiness. Further, if you read the magazines, if you listened carefully to the messages in the mass media, no matter how happy, happy, happy she was supposed to be, the woman was also suffused with life-long guilt because she was the culprit of every psychological case history. Something wrong with the children—what was wrong with the mother? Can this marriage be saved—adjust, the wife, adjust! The neurotic, frustrated American "mom" had been discovered as the massive cause of GI malfunction in World War II. But in this new image of woman, she was *fulfilled* as a housewife, totally fulfilled as a wife and mother.

Twenty years ago when I started interviewing suburban housewives, this image, which I called the "feminine mystique," was so pervasive in the mass media, in conventional sophisticated psychological and sociological thought, that there simply was no name for the malaise so many women suffered that did *not* have to do with children or husband. I called it "the problem that has no name," but every woman knew what I was talking about. Anything that had to do with the self of women was more repressed 20 years ago than sexuality had been repressed in the Victorian era.

The modern women's movement, as the history books say, began as a change of consciousness with my book, *The Feminine Mystique*. It made conscious the urgent need of women to break through that obsolete image that had confined their energies and kept them from facing their real problems and possibilities and opportunities in this changing world. You will remember or you will have heard from others, the relief it was to realize that you were not alone, that what you suffered was not necessarily your own personal sin or guilt to be confessed in the confessional, or on the couch, but a general social and political, economic and psychological condition that you shared with other women and that could be changed—that urgently had to be changed.

The modern women's movement had to happen when it did basically because of the evolution of human life. It was not an accident that when I began the change in consciousness I was in my mid-30s with my youngest child off to school . . . and over half of my life left ahead of me. With a life expectancy now of 81 years, there was no way that women could any longer define themselves as life-long mothers. They had to grow beyond the age-old practice of defining women through their child-bearing function. They had to move to a definition of themselves as persons. The post–World War II feminine mystique, misusing Freudian psychology and all the rest, was a last gasp of reaction that temporarily seduced women to evade the risks of personhood. The women's movement was a necessity in evolutionary terms, which I and others put into words. To remind you what happened, once we declared that women are people—no more, no less—then it was simply our American and human birthright—equality of opportunity, freedom, independence, our own voice in society. At first we followed the model of the Black movement, and made some mistakes by assuming too literal an analogy with it and with the labor movement. The modern women's movement began, above all, as an American movement. Its ideology was simply that of American democracy, the respect for the individual, human dignity, human freedom, equal opportunity, the right to fulfill your potential, the right to have a voice in your destiny. They said it was a movement without an ideology, but then I think they mistook what the ideology was.

The real ideology of the women's movement was simply the values of democracy applied to women, not a 10 percent minority, but a 52 percent majority. But when have the values of this, or any revolution been applied in the unique way that came from women's experience, not as an abstract doctrine, but concretely, to the dailiness of human life as it is lived in the home, in the bedroom, in the kitchen, in the office, hospital, classroom, and, therefore, immediately affecting everyone, changing everybody's life. It spread faster than could be believed, faster than any organization could contain. There was never any money. It was a miracle, and perhaps a paradigm of a new kind of human politics. All right. From 1966 to the present, a dozen years or so, there has been this movement, which used laws, which used the methods of the Civil Rights movement and then invented methods of its own, raising the consciousness of women, confronting the barriers of society. We got the laws and imperfectly got them enforced—against sex discrimination in education, employment, and credit. And enormous changes began to happen.

You are witness to these changes. The massive increase in the number of women who for economic reasons have to work outside the home now have a new sense of possibilities. In law schools and medical schools, women are no longer one, two, three percent of the class, but 30 percent and more. Every profession is now open to women. Sports are no longer just for boys, from the Little League up to national basketball. The breakthroughs against sex discrimination in employment are real breakthroughs, not just tokenism. But for many women now going to work as mothers after years at home, the only jobs·they can get are low-paying sales or clerical jobs, which are paid less because they have been held primarily by women. So in average wages, it looks like women are getting paid *less* in comparison with men than before. That obscures the movement of younger women to equal opportunity, and the whole new consciousness of sex discrimination, sexism, in every profession. And the new expectation of equality in marriage and the family.

The psychological effects of all of this may be quite different, in reality, from the doom and gloom predictions of reactionary social biologists or the simplistic preconceptions of radical feminists. Those who proclaim the natural inevitability of patriarchy are sure that equal opportunity for women will destroy culture itself. Certain sociologists say that the family is a disappearing species because of these selfish women that want to do other things with their lives than stay home all the time with their children. Certain psychologists proclaim widespread male impotence because of the new aggressiveness of women. The rising divorce rate and every other psychologically bad thing that is happening to people today is blamed on the women's movement. But the women who have moved know in their hearts, know in their guts, the rightness, the urgency, the life-opening exhilaration of their own moving.

As I go around this country, lecturing, every year more women of all ages come up and say, "It changed my life, it changed my whole life." (That's the title of my second book; *It Changed My Life: Writings on the Women's Movement.*) When I ask one of these women "What are you doing now?" she starts telling me the new problems: juggling work, her job, and the housework, the children, putting it all together with Band-Aids. New problems of divorce or husbands being threatened, economic problems, time problems; cheerfully, cheerfully, she tells me about all these new problems. "Sometimes it seems like the problems increase geometrically." But I never hear recriminations, regrets. I ask, "Would you go back where it was simpler, more secure?" And she says, "Are you kidding?" No woman would go back, despite the many new problems that women have today. It is better to be a woman today. You feel better being a woman today. You might have *more problems* being a woman today, but you are more alive. And the new problems are much more interesting than the old problems.

I could be accused of being prejudiced, self-serving in this proclamation so, therefore, I want to give you some new national statistics gathered by psychologists that confirm my personal experience and observations. Before I wrote *The Feminine Mystique*, I was in my late 30s and I felt old. I felt like it was all going to be downhill. When I look back, I felt older at 38 than I felt at 48 and a lot older than I feel now at 58. I noticed something interesting when I began looking for women that were moving beyond the feminine mystique. In the mid-60s, right after my book came out, I went around the country, much as I went around this conference, looking for new patterns. It was before we even had a women's movement, and of course, I did not find any new patterns. It was too soon. I did find some individual women who were putting their lives together in new ways, and they had a lot of problems because there were no social patterns, not in this country yet. One thing I did notice about those women—they looked vital, they looked alive. They tended to be a little older than the suburban housewives I had interviewed for *The Feminine Mystique* because this was a time when women in their 20s, in their 30s, were all home with kids. (Only the exceptional one was out there, then, and she might not even have kids.) The few women that had been combining marriage and motherhood and profession were in their menopausal years. But they looked and sounded more vibrant, vital, than the younger trapped housewives I had been interviewing who had all these vague syndromes and symptoms. They might not even wear as much make-up but their skin looked younger!

I started asking them about the menopause and they'd say, "Oh, I don't remember." or "I haven't had it." And I'd say, "What do you mean, you haven't had it?" I would figure out the woman was 50 or whatever. She did not remember when she stopped menstruation because she actually had not experienced the symptoms, traumas, and depression that were supposed to characterize menopause. In other words, menopause was a syndrome that did not exist for such women. What they experienced was a vitality, as if they were growing again.

Then, the women's movement really took off, and women in great numbers began to go back to school, go to work. And even if they continued to write "housewife" on the census blank, they began to feel differently about themselves. It was like a phenomenon you do not even notice because it is so large—that women after 40, after women's life was supposed to be over and downhill, were growing and moving with incredible zest and vitality. Recently, the various fashion magazines showed women now in their 40s and 50s against pictures of themselves in their 30s, and commented that the women really did look younger now. And it was not just a question of the styles that used to make women try to look younger. This was something different.

I began to ask a lot of questions about this "x" that was making some women experience menopause differently, women growing instead of deteriorating with age. I did not know how pervasive it was. Coincidentally, just in time for this conference, some figures were released that are really mind boggling. A repeat was done of the classic midtown Manhattan study (Srole, 1975), which in 1954 showed mental health impairment increasing with successive age groups, and women much worse off than men. In this and another comparable study by the National Center for Health Statistics, women were so much worse off than men for every possible index that could be associated with mental health, from insomnia and fainting to inertia, depression, and feeling about to have a nervous breakdown, that Jessie Bernard wrote a book dooming the future of marriage because she concluded that while marriage seemed to be okay for a man, it was driving women crazy.

The men and women originally studied were aged 20 to 59. At each 10-year interval their rate of impairment had increased: mental health deteriorated with age, and more acutely for women. They repeated the Midtown study in 1975, 20 years later. Instead of finding the expected increase in impairment, to their utter amazement, it looked as if mental health had stopped getting worse with age. After 20 years of wear and tear of living, the deterioration of mental health that had been expected had not taken place. They could not believe it. Then they began to analyze the statistics more carefully to see what had happened. The impression that mental health no longer deteriorated with age had come completely from *a massive improvement in the last 20 years in the mental health of women over 40* (Srole, 1975).

Whereas in 1954, 21 percent of women 40–49 had shown what they called impairment of mental health, compared with 9 percent of men, by 1974 the women who had been 20–29 or 39 in the first study, showed no worse mental health, or slightly better, at 40–49. Furthermore, the women now 40–49 showed enormous improvement in mental health compared with the women 20 years ago aged 40–49. Only 8 percent of women were now impaired compared with the 21 percent in 1954. In other words, the women had caught up to the men. They showed, in fact, less impairment of mental health with age than the men. The psychologists who analyzed these statistics concluded that something really massive must have been happening to women in the last 20 years that was not happening to men.

❖ All right. What does all this mean? Now I am drawing on my participant-observer knowledge, and from my own interviews of women over the years. It has been good for women to have more self-respect and independence as people, more freedom and options to move on their own in society. It has been good for women to get out the aggression that they used to turn against themselves in self-hate and self-denigration, in masochism, the impotent rage they used to vent on their own minds and bodies. It has been good for women, psychologically, economically— and economics is the bottom line in this. I cannot possibly stress too much the importance of having some independence and ability to support themselves. It has been good for women to come out of those tight, confining masks and be who they really are, to let it all hang out. It has been good for women to be part of a movement, to feel that they are supported by a great movement of other women, even to be able to share feelings without necessarily paying $50 to $100 an hour to do so. It has been good for women not only to be able to assert the self but to be a part, as many have been in one way or another, of a movement beyond the self. It has been good for women, finding the power to change their own lives and recognizing their power to change society.

It is already visibly good for women to have new options, but we are only beginning to know something about the potentials of human growth in females, about the healthy, active, fully grown personhood of women. At this time, certain transitional phenomena can obscure some of this. For instance, you have to be careful to distinguish in your own clinical work, or sociological or psychological analysis, phenomena of reaction, of defensive reaction, and understand that these may be temporary way stations to the real human autonomy and self-definition that women are seeking. Some of the extreme hostility against men that gave a bad image to "women's lib," which is a term I myself do not use, is not liberation, though the rage may be a real and even necessary stage in liberation. Some of that hostility and its acting out or the rhetoric that expresses it came from an ideological mistake, reducing the relationship of woman and man with its complex biological, psychological, social, and sexual dynamic by too literal an analogy to the relationship of worker and boss, or black and white. The separatism that resulted is not synonymous with liberation. To deny the psychological and biological and human interconnectedness of woman and man, to deny all the feelings that women have had about men, love, children, and home is to deny a part of woman's own nature.

It was reaction; women had to get their anger out; better than taking it out on the self. But an excess of that reaction is very similar to machismo. It hides enormous insecurity. Woman's worst problem today is the lack of confidence in herself. Having seen, maybe in your mother or your sister, that powerlessness, that trapped-housewife desperation, being afraid, still, that you might be pinched back into it, being unsure, still of your own ability to move in this complex society, in panicky defense you want to throw out all of the things that characterized woman in the past. Women are afraid of the softness; to hide their own inadmissible need for dependence, now they have to be more independent than any man. Be tough! Tough! Or we risk losing this hard-won autonomy.

But the more the woman moves, the more sure she is of her ability, the more she can afford to also admit her vulnerabilities and her weaknesses. And the more real she becomes. So you must not confuse the reaction, which is another kind of mask, with her real self that is not yet fully liberated. You must look for female machismo, as well as male machismo, and for what is hidden behind that facade.

In the discussions at the conference, I was a little disturbed (as I see that others of my generation are) by the seemingly utter preoccupation with the self, the selfishness, of some of the young women. They are choosing not to have children. They are only concerned with their careers, or they are only concerned with themselves. Now, a certain amount of selfishness is healthy for women. As one of the first woman theologians said, the sin of woman has been selflessness, too much selflessness, evasion of the risks of self by living through others. That can be a sin, you know. In my own origins there is a wonderful saying, "If I am not for myself, who will be for me? But if I am only for myself, what am I?" Woman has to be for herself, or she cannot really be for anyone else. You know from the psychopathology that you used to deal with, and may still be dealing with, what happens to the children when the woman has to use them for her own self-aggrandizement or to fulfill her own needs. She had to be for herself to really be there for her children.

Young women share with the young men today a loss of faith in institutions. When the politics of nation and profession seem irrelevant or utterly cynical and the dollar isn't worth much, when the old religion seems hypocritical, or denies women's reality and the new religion is not yet firm, in what institution can she find meaning? Can we blame the young for the so-called age of narcissism, after the politics of Watergate and Three Mile Island? I hope this is also a transitional stage. Women's rights is not the only issue that has concerned me in my lifetime. But in recent years the only politics where I did not feel like I was wasting my time was the women's movement because this really was changing our lives. And it is confronting the system in subtle ways. Since I do not see any other system giving the answers, I see my responsibility to change my own system. And the women's movement is doing that in ways that are not at first apparent.

Some of you have worried that this negotiating of contracts about who is going to do the housework is taking all the spontaneity out of love and marriage. I will tell you something about this. When you do not negotiate, when the woman is the resentful martyr and feels like a service station as the women that I interviewed 20 years ago used to put it . . . that is really bad for the spontaneity of love and marriage. Why in those years did so many books become best sellers that sold "88 New Ways to Make the Act of Love More Endurable"? Why did the vibrator seem for a while to be more titillating for some women than the human penis? It was not good for love, marriage, spontaneity of sex for women to feel like a service station. The negotiation is an improvement.

I discovered some interesting things in my new interviewing of young women in Vermont and elsewhere. They had been through these knock-down-drag-out fights every time the garbage had to be taken out or dinner cooked: Why should I do it. . . . You've got to do it equally. He won't do his share. Or he wouldn't do it right, and so on and so forth. Until, she tells me, "I suddenly realized that I still was the one really running the house. Maybe I didn't want to give up that power. But in order to do my other work, I simply couldn't be the one that was responsible for it any longer. I couldn't be the only one that everyone would look to. I really had to give up that power. And once I gave it up, then we were able to negotiate." She goes on: "Negotiate, we don't even negotiate any more. It flows. Whoever is able to do it at that time does it, and half the time we don't even bother to negotiate."

In other words, the psychology of power. In recompense for the lack of power in society, women had to have this absolute domination in the home. And that was the American "mom," and you are still dealing with the effects of that in psychopathology. In the last decade, research began to show that when women worked from choice and not from absolute, dire desertion of the husband or whatever, their husbands had more decision-making power in their own homes, compared with the husbands of full-time housewives. In the new families that may evolve as women begin to move to a more equal role in society, carrying a greater share of the economic burden, the power of the woman in the home will be less destructive. As many young men are now finding, sharing the intimate, active life and nurturing of the home and children has its own power and rewards. There may be a virtual disappearance of certain kinds of psychopathology that resulted from the powerlessness (power lust) of women and the absent, passive father. (Incidentally, *Time* magazine a few months ago ran a cover story called the depression of psychiatry. The psychiatry business is evidently down. Most of the patients used to be women. In addition to inflation, the gurus, and disillusionment with the psychological panaceas, have you ever thought that the women's movement itself is helping to put psychiatry out of business?)

I will tell you a new problem I worry about: the conscious or not conscious conflict or choice not to have children at all that may be one cause of the stress for the younger women. "Up Against the Clock," a new study that has come out of the University of California at Santa Cruz (Fabe and Winkler, 1979), shows women, in agonizing conflict over the choice as they approach 35 whether to have a baby or not. I do not want to go back to a mystique, and I do not think that a human being has instincts the same way that animals do, but I do not want to see women choosing not to have children for the wrong reasons. I want them to have the choice. I do not want them to have to have children to justify their existence. But I think there is a powerful generative need or impulse, in women and in men, that is not lightly denied.

I am not even talking now about reproducing the human race or deploring a situation in which the best or the brightest are not having children. I am talking about the woman herself and the woman's total personhood, which surely includes that powerful generativeness. I do not like the discussions in some of the feminist psychotherapy in which the self is defined apart from love, from nurturing, as if the self for woman were only the career, or only the work. As if the self were not also defined in the nurturing of the children, the intimate relationship with the man, whoever. Because if it was denying a part of the personhood of woman when she had to deny those human assertive needs to grow and act and have a voice and use the abilities that she shared with men, it is also perhaps denying a part of the personhood of woman if she denies the powerful needs and abilities and fulfillment of mothering. Motherhood is more than a mystique. But I am not blaming the victim here.

If you believe what you say about primary prevention of psychopathology, if you understand how liberating all that has happened has been for women's mental health, then, for instance, we have to get the Constitutional underpinning so it can not be taken away. We have to get the Equal Rights Amendment ratified. It is your obligation as people concerned with mental health to help do that. It is a mental health question as well as a question of economic and political justice. Then, we have to demand restructuring of institutions, more flexible hours of work, really good child care programs, so that women do not have to make either/or choices.

And we have to have education of men as well as women, not just women's studies, for equality to be livable, and workable, and possible to love in. Unless men change their roles and really begin to do equal parenting, unless we get professions restructured along more human lines by and for men and women (which is the only way it will happen), this will end up with a lot of tired women. Women are getting very tired, the way it is now. To the perfectionist demand on women to be perfect mothers is now added the demand to be perfect career women. Women are now even falling into some traps that men are climbing out of. I was appalled to hear from one of you that young girls are smoking while young boys have stopped smoking.

I am leery of the *mea culpa* kind of men's liberation. I do not think that men are going to do an awful lot to change, just to please the women. They will do some things to please the women. They will have to. But that is patronizing in a way. Let the men change because they need to change, to live their own lives well. Again going back to biological statistics, it is not good that men are dying 10 years younger than women of their age group, that the age discrepancy of men and women at death is widening, that men did not show that great improvement in mental health in this 20-year period. Men have got to make a breakthrough comparable to women's. It is not the same one, it will not have the same confrontational aspects. Men have got to break through the machismo, the competitiveness, the denial of their own real feelings and fears, and they are beginning to do it.

I think you may get shorter and more flexible working hours and less slavery to the corporation—not necessarily because of women moving into corporations, because a lot of women think they have to do it better than the man at this point. But because men, liberated from the whole earning burden and expected to share the parenting, are beginning to say their own "no" to living a whole life just for the corporation. Men's mid-life crisis—there is fire underneath all that smoke. There is a value change taking place among men. The next step of human liberation will be made by men.

Finally, I want to say just one word about feminist psychotherapy. I am a feminist. I was originally trained as a psychologist. I think that any good psychotherapist today must in a certain sense be a feminist, but what that means is simply this: that we listen very, very carefully and sensitively to the woman where she is now. To the woman, herself, whether or not she fits Freudian or feminist book definitions, with respect for her own authenticity or integrity. Taking her seriously, her totality as a person, a woman, and realizing that we do not know all the answers yet, that she is still *evolving*, that we have not even seen yet the limits of women's possibility, but we must respect the reality of her life, here and now.

And if you are a good feminist psychotherapist, you also have to look and listen with the same sensitivity to men, to men where they are now. Realizing that men also have been oppressed, truncated, by sex roles and obsolete definitions of masculinity, that men have all kinds of human potential, similar to women, that they have not been allowed to express or experience. And if you are also committed to the family, as the ground soil, the nutrient for mental health, then you have to realize that your commitment is to the evolving family. That there is no way to go back to the mom-the-housewife, dad-the-breadwinner, Junior-and-Janie-for-ever-children, Good-Housekeeping-seal-of-approval family that only 7 percent of Americans now live in. That we have to look with respect and sensitivity at all the ways that people are moving to live together, to meet their needs for intimacy and mutual support, in all the stages and the new length and complexity of the life span. There are old value judgments having to do with marriage, with divorce, with all sorts of things that were good and that were bad, which we have to hold in abeyance in order to understand where women, men, and the family really are, here and now, and where they are moving. It is going to require every bit of our ability, everything that has been learned in all times to really under-stand this fast-evolving reality—the changing woman, the changing man, the changing family.

I welcome this community of psychotherapists that were part of the problem 20 years ago, that helped perpetrate the mystique that kept women down. I welcome your embrace of the great human movement of social change, of the women's movement as a primary prevention of psychopathology.

References

Bernard, J. *The future of marriage.* New York: World Publishers, 1972.

Bird, C. The best years of a woman's life. *Psychology Today,* 1979, *13,* 20–26.

Fabe, M., and Winkler, N. *Up against the clock.* New York: Random House, 1979.

Friedan, B. *The feminine mystique.* New York: W. W. Norton & Co., 1963.

Friedan, B. *It changed my life: Writings on the women's movement.* New York: Random House, 1976.

Lundberg, F. G., and Farnham, M. F. *Modern woman: The lost sex.* Philadelphia, Penn.: Richard West, 1947.

Singer, E., Garfinkel, R., Cohen, S. M., and Srole, L. Mortality and mental health: Evidence from the Midtown Manhattan restudy. *Social Sciences and Medicine,* 1977, *10,* 517–525.

Srole, L. Measurement and classification in socio-psychiatric epidemiology: Midtown Manhattan study (1954) and Midtown Manhattan restudy (1974). *Journal of Health and Social Behavior,* 1975, *16,* 347–364.

Sex Education for Women

Paula Brown Doress and
Wendy Coppedge Sanford

We are two members of an 11-member group which has been meeting, writing, teaching, and strategizing around women's health issues for 12 years. We wrote the books *Our Bodies, Ourselves* (1979) and *Ourselves and Our Children* (1978), and recently some of us collaborated on *Changing Bodies, Changing Lives* (1980), a book for teens about sex and relationships. We meet weekly as a personal as well as a work group and are committed to trying for that important balance between working hard together and sharing from our personal lives. Our observations in this paper will reflect our professional experiences in sexuality workshops, interviews, and outreach which have let us hear from thousands of women. They will also reflect our personal experience in the close and trusting circle of the 11 of us in our group, as we listen, support each other, and strive for better understandings of our own sexuality.

Because we put "feminist" in the title of our paper, we want to give you our definition of feminism, which is so often distorted by the media. To us, feminism is an attitude held by women and men. A feminist takes women seriously as whole human beings with a right to full participation in all aspects of public life and full equality in private life. Our feminism does not simply seek to enter women into the world of men's institutions: we see tremendous potential for beneficial change in our social and political institutions as feminist women move into them, asking questions, in particular, about the use and abuse of power.

In writing this paper we considered what our group and the women's movement in general have to offer as preventive mental health measures for sexual problems. We want to address three themes: the crucial interconnections between the personal and political where sex is concerned, the movement toward a more inclusive definition of sexuality, and the power of shared information. We will also outline some of our group's encounters with the new right in the struggle over freedom of access to all kinds of sex education.

❖ The Personal Is Political

We have titled our paper "Reclaiming Our Bodies," a phrase which rings of possession, property, and politics. There are so many examples of men or male-dominated institutions laying claim to women's bodies: fathers, husbands, obstetricians, drug companies, hospitals, the advertising industry, legislators, and priests. The motive is sometimes profit, sometimes the need to control women, often both. As women begin to say no to this male ownership and control, we begin to experience our sexuality differently.

It is often in consciousness-raising groups that women first begin to make connections between our personal stories and the wider political scene. (A consciousness-raising group is composed of eight to ten women without professional leadership who are committed to talking honestly about their lives and to helping each other build solutions that are not just individual.) We begin to see that many of the things we suffer over and blame ourselves for in private turn out, once we speak up about them, to be experienced by many. We find that they are caused in large part by the social, political, and economic context in which we are living our lives.

Let us use this political or personal lens to look at sex. Often a woman will say, usually apologetically, "I just don't enjoy sex much, and my husband is getting more and more frustrated. There must be something wrong with me." To know what is going on, we have to look beyond her marriage bed, past whatever techniques they may or may not be using, past even the particulars of their relationship, to the social and political roots of their situation. We see the lack of sex education in the schools she and her husband attended, the absence of any legitimized setting in which sexual feelings and issues could have been discussed. We see sex role stereotypes that make her too shy to assert her need for pleasure. We see an institutionalized heterosexuality that has perhaps thrust them together without a knowledge of alternatives. We see social and economic inequalities: she earns, statistically, 59¢ for every dollar he earns, and the leaders in their society are almost exclusively men. As our first newsprint edition of *Our Bodies, Ourselves* declared in 1969, "There's no reason to expect the sense of inferiority and inadequacy to go away between the sheets!" This is still true. And she wonders whether there is something wrong with her!

In the public domain, sex is used to sell products. It becomes, like rape, an expression of hatred and domination. In the media it is interwoven with violence. When a man and woman go to bed together, no matter how much they love each other, these social and public meanings of sex creep in under the bedroom door to distort what they are doing. The media's efforts can convince them that her body is not good enough and that he should know all the moves. With violence toward women a daily reality, how can he express and she enjoy the full vigor of his passion? With sex so acutely depersonalized in public, can they re-own it in service of intimacy with any real sense of trust? External cultural factors can and do poison our intimate relationships and severely damage the role sex plays in re-creation and bonding between people.

Sex role stereotypes, heterosexism, and the double standard require us to fit our sexual feelings into a prescribed mold. When the fit is not right, we are encouraged to blame ourselves. Professionally, we see the results of this cruel syndrome. As a group of professionals and lay people exploring the prevention of sexual problems, we need to open our eyes to the ways in which social institutions and attitudes reach into the bedroom. In our work as counselors and educators, we can no longer look merely to personal solutions or to improving technique. More and more often we will encourage people who have individual sexual problems to join with others in order to grow in personal understanding, to mobilize and work for change in ways that are impossible alone. We ourselves will inevitably become advocates for certain kinds of social change. We will see women's sexuality in particular as existing in the context of reproductive rights; that is, in order to be able to express her sexuality freely and with love, a woman must have full access to birth control information and abortion services and to good prenatal care, all at prices she can afford. We must draw our circle of concern more widely.

From Personal Experience to Political Vision

Linking the personal and the political also encourages us to look into our personal lives for images of how our society might be different. When we feel safe enough to talk honestly with others about our explorations in intimacy, we can let our personal experience point toward a new politics.

What elements are you exploring in your lives which may have relevance for the wider society? Take lovemaking, for example: sexual intimacy has for so long been a reenactment of the power relationships in society: more crudely, man on top and woman beneath. Today many couples are trying to move beyond this picture. They seek to meet as two equal human beings who love each other, to bring their sexual feelings to each other as offerings and not demands, to let feelings draw them together, to touch each other with respect. Women explore initiating and men receptivity. Then, in turn, men may reexplore aggressive modes and women their more passive fantasies, on a new basis of equality and consensus between them. Positions for making love are arrived at in concert or spontaneously; for heterosexual couples, penis-in-vagina thrusting becomes only one of the things they might do, not the prescribed culmination.

Mutuality is the word that comes to mind. In sex as in other areas, like shared income-earning and shared parenting, couples are exploring a love grounded in equality, not hierarchy: in common experience, not separate worlds. The kind of mutuality we are discovering—in many cases struggling to achieve—has a value we need to integrate into our society. We would do well to carry this vision of mutuality into our public as well as our private lives.

Another personal experience which extends beyond itself belongs perhaps more particularly to men: the admission of vulnerability. In men's discussion groups and in sexual relationships based on a growing mutuality, men have been discovering how boxed in they have been by their need to appear strong, invulnerable, and all-knowing. They are finding deep feeling and experience possible only after they unlock their vulnerabilities, express their softer sides. It is risky, of course, but that is inevitable. Women, too, are taking risks to discover their powerful, autonomous selves. As we break through the double standard and rigid gender stereotypes in our personal relationships, we begin to see the possibility of a public life, a national life, which is not posited on tough, macho, super self-reliant male aggressiveness juxtaposed with female passivity and martyrdom.

We end this section by quoting a writer (Anonymous, 1981) who focuses the political/personal lens on her changing sexual experience. The passage is from an article in *Second Wave*, a women's journal published yearly in Boston. The writer has recently become a lesbian, which puts her outside the direct experience of some of us here, yet she expresses thoughts and feelings we will all recognize. Her words are a good example of what we are calling a feminist experience in sex education.

My relationship to myself is different in loving a woman, this woman. Sex was where I noticed it first. With men I always felt guilty when I didn't want sex. Even with a man who wasn't particularly pushy for sex, I always knew he'd want it again sooner or later, and so I'd watch my urges, hoping they'd rise in time. Rarely did a man hold off from sex long enough for me to feel my own desires move me. I got freer about saying "No, not right now," or "Let's just hold each other," but there was always the edge of apprehension, the sense that I'd better enjoy this moratorium while it lasted.

Underlying all this was the assumption that my body somehow belonged to him, not me. I thought I owed my partner my sexuality and should muster it up for him when he wanted or needed it....Whether or not he thought I owed him my sexuality was irrelevant, because the assumption that I did was deep in the culture and deep in my own sense of myself....

With my lover now I feel more consistently erotic than I ever have with men....But I remember the first night I didn't feel like making love when I thought she probably did, and my sudden surprising attack of guilt and awkwardness. There was a lot on my mind that week, and my erotic energy had vanished somewhere. So I went to sleep on "my" side of the bed and slept poorly, as I often had with men after an evening of turning away from sex: would she "want it" in the morning, and would I "have it" to give? Before dawn I woke her up to talk about it, heart in my mouth; it was such an old and potent guilt. What became clear for us was that while she would have liked to make love, she didn't "have to have it." The absence of my erotic energy didn't feel like a rejection; what she wanted more was my honesty, the truth of my feelings, and this I had given her. "Sex is only one part of our relationship," she reminded me. What a relief! Only then did I see what a betrayal of myself it was ever to have apologized to anyone for not wanting to make love.

We have begun to see our sexual desire as a gift which comes to us, not a product which can be mustered up or manipulated at will. I think this marks an important shift in our relationship to our bodies and feelings. Owing our bodies to no one, our role is to be with the sexual feelings when they come, and to let them lead us into connection with each other. Freed of ownership and obligation, sexuality *is* a gift; the ebb and flow of it, respected as a life-rhythm, not only nourishes our loving but also fills us with energy for the work we want to do in the world.

Radical feminists suggest that sexuality as patriarchally defined has been used to colonize woman's body and psyche. As I admitted the guilt feelings, heard my lover's response, and let go of the sense of owing my sexuality to her, I experienced a major step in *de*colonization: I was re-owning my body. I believe this step may be easier between lesbians (and perhaps gay men), because the politics between us are less loaded in terms of history, social expectations, and the realities of power in a sexist patriarchal society. But it also happens between men and women lovers who struggle toward mutuality; that is, toward self-respecting and other-respecting love. Couples like these challenge the patriarchy as deeply as anyone does. Whenever people facilitate such a decolonization in each other, such a re-owning of self— especially if they are able to see the wider politics of it—I think it is a step towards a world in which ownership of others no longer operates as the central metaphor for human relations. (Anonymous, 1981, pp. 25-26)

Making Our Definitions of Sexuality More Inclusive

Our cultural images of sexual people tend to portray the able-bodied, the affluent, the heterosexual, and people within the limited age range of 20 to 45. Although every human being is sexual, the conventional sexual images in our culture narrow our ideas about who can be sexual and work to make substantial groups in the population feel that their sexual options are severely restricted. This narrow definition of so-called normal sexuality hurts both the people who do not fit it and in more subtle and equally destructive ways hurts all of us by making us repress in ourselves what does not fit. We are all aware of the distortions which occur in the media, but we, as sex educators, must be attentive not only to the words we use but to the graphics in our work, making sure that they are inclusive of a wide range of body types, ages, and forms of expressing sexuality.

The women's movement has expanded women's sexual options. Today, women have alternatives to the traditional life-style which include relationships with younger men, childfree marriage, living together without marriage, and relationships with women. Yet the inequalities between women and men persist and continue to limit the options that women have in all spheres of life, including the sexual.

Aging and Changes in Sexual Needs and Opportunities

Women over 40 are bombarded with messages that they must protect themselves against the fading of their sexual appeal, as if women's sexuality is a fragile flower that briefly blossoms, then fades away. Aging is differentially evaluated in women and men: Women are wrinkled, men are craggy; women are matronly, men are distinguished.

Part of the oppression experienced by middle-aged women today is the steadily decreasing age of the cultural prototypes of sexual women. The use of very young women and even children as sexual objects may be part of the backlash against the greater freedom and increased sexual options women have begun to enjoy. By portraying the ideal sexual female as a girl—childlike, pliable, and nonthreatening to the male ego—the mature woman is dismissed as overly demanding, scary, and therefore sexless. In this way, sexism and agism combine to invalidate older women's sexuality.

We must resist the pronatalist ideology that sex exists mainly in the service of reproduction. Such expressions as "over the hill" and "past her prime" equate women's sexuality with reproductive capacity. Yet, as Rosetta Reitz (1979) so clearly demonstrates in her groundbreaking work on menopause, many older women enjoy sex more. Here are some excerpts from a chapter called "Sex Is Better When You're Older":

Ellen, 51: Not worrying about getting pregnant—that did it for me, that turned everything around. The same sex is different, it's better....

Maggie, 49: Once I decided the rest of my life is for me, I was shocked how easy it became to get what I want. There's hardly a thing I can think of sexually that I want to experience that I can't. I'm amazed and wonder why it took me so long not to be afraid to ask....

Deborah, 56: When I was younger, I used to feel that eventually we'll get used to each other, which meant I let [a new partner] do what he wanted—but I don't anymore. The first encounter has got to count. I say "be gentle," at the start....If they don't oblige, there's nothing to get used to, that's it for me. (1979, pp. 151, 153, 155.)

Although women with advancing age gain in their capacity for sexual arousal and orgasm (Sherfey, 1972), men during this same period may worry about a decline in sexual interest. A man in his 50s told us:

We've had a good marriage with lots of good sex. Now we have all the kids out of the house and we travel a lot and have fun together. But I just don't want sex as often as Liz does and it's really hard to tell her that.

Some men, like this one, may be pretty clear that they are the ones who are changing. Others who feel they must live up to a performance standard of male sexuality may choose to blame their wives. For the older woman, the culturally induced fears of losing her sexual attractiveness may seem to be confirmed by her man's decreasing sexual interest.

While we want to recognize that everyone is sexual, we must also be aware that not everyone has the same sexual options or interest. As health professionals concerned with openness toward sexuality we may have gone so far in our efforts to combat the old notion of sex as dirty or bad or harmful that we have put in its place an ethos of sex as "healthy," a prescriptive notion that a healthy person must be sexually active. For those whose sexual opportunities are restricted or who simply do not care to have sex much, this view may prove almost as oppressive as the old restrictions. People may wonder, "What's wrong with me if I'm not sexually active?" It is important for people to hear from health professionals that being in a relationship is not the only thing that makes a person sexual.

Divorce and Relearning Skills

As we expand our notions of "normal" sexuality, we find ourselves going beyond the concept of a linear development of sexuality and sexual skills. With one in two marriages ending in divorce and one-sixth of these occurring among those over 45, many people find themselves back at square one in terms of sex. Many experience something like a second adolescence, having to relearn ways of initiating a sexual relationship or living with periods of celibacy. A divorced woman in her 40s told us:

One of the first social events for single people that I went to after getting separated was a brunch for single and divorced professional people. I couldn't get over the way people interacted with each other. Here were all these mature adults standing around looking like wallflowers waiting for someone to talk to them, especially the men. They looked terrified. Thrown back on my teenage resources, I picked out the best-looking man in the room and started talking to him. I felt as though I had passed some test.

A divorced man told us:

When my wife moved out I felt sexually and emotionally numb. I just had no interest in anyone because I was completely preoccupied with my own pain. Then I started seeing a woman I'd met, and my sexual feelings took me by surprise. One day for the first time in years and years, I spent a whole afternoon making love.

As we look at the sexual lives of divorced women and men, a feminist perspective helps us examine the political, economic, and social factors that may be influencing their choices. The father who does not have custody of his children may lose out on the familiar and homey side of his life, but he has more freedom to explore this second adolescence without the encumbrances of seeking babysitters, explaining every lover to the children (or the children to the lover). The woman who has custody of her children finds her chances to meet new people limited by the wish to protect the children from disruptions of their accustomed routine. Moreover, we must not underestimate the impact of economic constraints on the social life of single mothers. Although alimony has gone out of style, the income gap continues to grow. Large numbers of divorced fathers fail to meet their child support obligations. One woman told us:

It's hard to feel up to going out to meet someone when your clothes are all worn and out of style, all your pantyhose have runs in them, and you've barely scraped together the money for the next month's rent. It's hard to feel sexy when you can't afford to get your teeth fixed.

This woman may want to expand her experience of sexuality, but her circumstances are not giving her a chance. The women's movement with its emphasis on women supporting one another can be a tremendous source of strength and resilience for women in this situation.

The Disabled as Sexual Beings

One group beginning to move beyond limiting stereotypes of "normal" sexuality is the physically disabled. Although feminists discovered early how crucial it is to learn to affirm diversity—racial, ethnic, and class diversity were what we became aware of first—it has taken us years to open our new understandings of sexuality to the voices and experiences of disabled women. Ideally, a feminist sex education would affirm the sexual feelings and special concerns of disabled people, but the 1976 edition of Our Bodies, Ourselves contains very little of this. Ignorance of, prejudices toward, and awkwardness around physical disability run deep in all of us, based mainly on a vicious cycle of fear for ourselves and lack of contact with those who are physically different. (The lack of contact, of course, comes from enforced isolation of disabled people, which then leads to more fear and prejudice.)

In the May 1981 issue of Off Our Backs, a monthly women's news journal from Washington, D.C., disabled women have spoken up in a way that invites each of us to change how we see them and how we see ourselves. Here are a few excerpts ("Women and Disability," 1981). From a woman with muscular dystrophy:

In terms of sexual independence, I never saw my vulva, because my mother dressed and bathed me and I couldn't get a mirror. Just remember that a disabled woman may not be as aware of her body because of problems like this. She may have little privacy so can't even get to masturbate alone. A disabled woman is apt to be ashamed of her body anyway. People look at you, stare, avoid looking, so there is a lot of inhibition to get rid of. (p.4)

The same woman goes on to talk about the isolation:

Some...are uncomfortable just being around a disabled woman, others are comfortable with being a friend, but can't consider a sexual relationship....People have often believed that if you are with a [disabled person] you can catch "it". . . . We are not allowed to be sexual beings. (p. 4)

An able-bodied woman whose lover is disabled speaks movingly about what they have learned:

My lover has been disabled since she was a baby....Health care professionals have handled her body again and again, without allowing her control over the process. So obviously it is difficult for her to let go of the control over her body and to entrust her lover with this control. I need to honor her experience, and to know that it is not my fault or my inadequacy as a lover, or hers. We have discovered that honest and loving communication, with no blame or criticism, leads us to finding...ways to experience sexual pleasure with each other. (p. 20)

She finished with an insight for all of us:

I find that I need to change my basic conceptualizations, beginning with the linking of "healthy" and "disabled" as opposites. It's oppressive, and not even true, that a person who is disabled cannot be healthy. My lover is filled with light and wisdom. (p. 20)

A male friend of ours who was disabled by polio at 15 has found where the stereotypes do not fit (Zola, in press):

There is the absence of a certain spontaneity in my sexual courting. There's simply no sexy, subtle, or even fast way for me to remove my braces and get undressed. And though I've often fantasized about having someone disrobe me, I've never been able in real life to do it very easily.

He goes on to say:

The women's movement with its emphasis on greater mutuality in sex has removed some of this burden....I'm also benefitting from women's lib since a lot more women seem to enjoy being on top and in many ways (given some of the residuals of my polio) that's easiest for me.

He is able to point out to all of us the limitations in our performance-oriented approach to sex:

Society has focused on sex as capacity and instrumentality. We have located far too much of our identity in our sexual organs....Where the chronically disabled are concerned, professionals search for compensatory techniques, devices, or symbols to reclaim the lost ability. [I suggest instead we look for] ways to reclaim the lost warmth, wholeness, and sense of being.

As we who are able-bodied listen to these women and this man, we are challenged to alter both how we respond to disabled persons and how we experience our own physical limitations. As a woman disabled from infancy by polio wrote, "Our society creates an ideal model of the physically perfect person unencumbered by weakness, loss or pain." Madison Avenue would have all of us find our bodies inadequate and buy expensive products to try to "improve" them. Hearing from disabled women and men as they seek ways to affirm and express their sexuality helps us find ways we could be less bullied by these cultural images of what an ideal body should look like, and of what ideal sex should be like. We are invited to focus less on capacity and technique and genitals, and more on loving. The courage of our disabled sisters and brothers helps us accept who we are and helps us let our sexual lives flow from that self-acceptance.

Including Homosexuality
Literally hundreds of lesbians and gay men have spoken up over the past decade to expand further our notions of what is "normal" sexuality. They challenge us to look at our homophobia (the irrational fear and hatred of homosexuals taught to nearly every child growing up in this country). They invite us to come to terms with our own sexual feelings for people of our same sex, to own and even enjoy those feelings whether or not we choose to act on them. They point to possibilities of mutuality and a freedom from power politics and role playing between lovers that many heterosexual couples would like to learn from. Most exciting, some homosexuals who are aware of the politics of their sexual preference urge us to look at our own heterosexual preference with new eyes.

Adrienne Rich (1980) puts this challenge to us in an important article called "Compulsory Heterosexuality and Lesbian Experience." Rich points to the many ways that heterosexual marriage has through the centuries been made the only possible choice for women: heterosexuality has been enforced by women's economic disadvantages, by the fear of rape, by child marriage, by the chastity belt, by erasure of lesbian existence in art and history. Rich gives the ugly facts:

Attacks on unmarried women have ranged from aspersion and mockery to deliberate gynocide, including the burning and torturing of millions of widows and spinsters during the witch persecutions of the fifteenth, sixteenth, and seventeenth centuries in Europe, and the practice of suttee of widows in India. (p. 635)

She suggests that it is important for all of us to question the assumption that most women are innately heterosexual:

To acknowledge that for women heterosexuality may not be a "preference" at all but something that has had to be imposed, managed, organized, propagandized, and maintained by force, is an immense step to take if you consider yourself freely and "innately" heterosexual. Yet the failure to examine heterosexuality as a [political] institution is like failing to admit that the economic system called capitalism or the caste system of racism is maintained by a variety of forces, including both physical violence and false consciousness. (p. 618)

Rich proposes that the "lie" of compulsory heterosexuality distorts love relationships between women and men. According to her, "The absence of choice remains the great unacknowledged reality" (p. 657). She leads us to ask what it would mean for women and men who love each other to see their coupling as possible but not inevitable, as choice and not institution. This would free up a kind of creativity in loving that would be scary and risky but refreshing. Rich extends her promise and challenge to women, but in this final statement she could be speaking to men as well:

To take the step of questioning heterosexuality as a "preference" or "choice" for women—and to do the intellectual and emotional work that follows—will call for a special quality of courage in heterosexually identified feminists, but I think the rewards will be great: a freeing-up of thinking, the exploring of new paths, the shattering of another great silence, new clarity in personal relationships. (p. 648)

Some of the most creative thinking today about sexuality and relationships is coming from homosexual people and from the physically disabled. Living on the edge, they are led to question our long-held assumptions and expectations about what loving should look like. Letting ourselves be educated and enriched by their insights is one of the benefits of the feminist attempt to define sexuality more inclusively.

Information as Power

At age 26 I walked into a roomful of 50 women talking about sex. It was the early women's movement, and I was totally new to such a scene. When they started talking about masturbation, I was spellbound. I had never even heard the word spoken aloud. Going home after the meeting, my friend awkwardly ventured, "That's the first time I've heard masturbation...talked about....Yet I do it." I gulped. "So do I." The silence was broken, and neither of us would ever be quite the same. I had masturbated and felt guilty about it since I was a child. To hear women speaking so openly about it started me on a process of self-acceptance which took me, some years later, to my first experiences of masturbation without that rush of guilt and shame next to the pleasure. I was beginnning to accept myself as a sexual person. (Unpublished material).

We have something to learn from this early women's movement success story. Information is crucial, it is healing, it prevents distress. *How* we get information is important, too. This woman learned about masturbation in the context of a group of informed women speaking honestly from their own experiences. Learning such things so personally, in a way that no textbook alone could ever convey, makes the information accessible in a different way: it becomes a tool for use in one's life. Our appreciation for this learning process shaped how we wrote *Our Bodies, Ourselves*, always interweaving the facts with the voices of women talking about their lives.

The story also raises the important question of "What information are we dealing with, anyway?" Who decides what the "facts" are? With masturbation, a generation of doctors and parents passed on the "fact" that masturbation hurts you and ruins you for adult sexual functioning. Women's ovaries and clitorises were surgically removed in the 19th century in order to prevent this and other forms of "unruliness." With female orgasm, psychologists and gynecologists argued as "fact" that mature women had orgasms vaginally. What we discovered finally in our women's groups was that these facts did not fit. We began to help each other to trust our own experiences.

In this new light, research itself got redefined. Innovative and courageous women began to pioneer a new kind of research: Betty Dodson (1974) wrote *Liberating Masturbation*; Mary Jane Sherfey (1972), *The Nature and Evolution of Female Sexuality*; Shere Hite (1977), *The Hite Report*. Women in the women's self-help movement all over the country started with the women themselves—ourselves—looking, touching, tasting, listening, to build up a more accurate set of "facts" about women's sexual patterns and possibilities. As Shere Hite declared, "Researchers must stop telling women what they *should* feel sexually and start asking them what they *do* feel sexually" (p. 60).

This new kind of research revealed masturbation as a consistently satisfying act of self-pleasure and self-exploration, which deepens women's understanding of their own sexual responses and affirms their sexuality whether or not they are in a relationship with someone else. Intercourse, too, took on a new look. Shere Hite found that a full 70 percent of her 3,000 women respondents never experienced orgasm through intercourse alone, though many of these did experience orgasm quickly in masturbation. This led Hite to challenge the male experts' definition of satisfactory intercourse, with its emphasis on penile penetration. She questioned whether intercourse was ever meant to produce orgasm for women and cited the awkward language Masters and Johnson had to use in their attempt to reaffirm penile intercourse by showing that the clitoris gets enough stimulation through the tugging of the labia. She challenged the labels of frigid and dysfunctional used on women who do not experience orgasm that way. Feminist research on female orgasm has freed women from self-blame and opened us to a new sense of activity and entitlement in sex. Feminists are now demystifying older women's sexuality as well, through menopause self-help groups and pioneers like Rosetta Reitz.

Thus the very "facts" about sex are in flux, and necessarily so. Getting them out in an accessible way gives people the power to take charge of important parts of their lives, from the simple control of pregnancy to the more complex emotional growth brought by self-acceptance and self-pride in a part of our life that has for generations been considered shameful.

Teenagers and the Power of Shared Information

In working on the sexuality sections of the new book for teens, *Changing Bodies, Changing Lives* (Bell et al., 1980), I was reminded that teenagers are prime targets for the worst kinds of misinformation about sex. Concerned parents will sometimes say, "My child isn't ready for the sex information in your book." But if that child is over 9 years old and has eyes and ears, chances are she or he is getting sex information all the time—from TV, disco lyrics, movies, jokes at school, porno magazines on the racks in local variety stores, and the ads which use sex to sell everything from cars and liquor to home insurance. These parents have to decide not "Will my child get a sex education?" but "What kind?" Those who try to counteract all this misinformation and attitude warping with silence are not helping their kids. Often they are the very ones who will find their teenage daughters pregnant—the daughters who say, "I thought I couldn't get pregnant if I didn't have my period yet...if I did it during my period...if we did it standing up."

We would probably all agree that kids need sex education early, that they need to know it is a safe topic to talk about at home. We would agree, too, that the facts alone are not enough, that kids need frequent chances to talk over the feelings and pressures in a safe and trusting atmosphere. We would also probably agree that it does not help to tell teenagers that *all* premarital sex is bad. Not only does prohibition not work in helping them set their limits, it even damages their ability to take responsibility for what they *do* do.

Let us look at how prohibition cuts down on responsibility. Despite being bombarded with sex by the media, most kids are given almost no clear, useful information about sex at home or in school or at church. Parents and teachers say they fear that if you tell teens about sex they will go out and "do it." Even parents who do not say don't often keep a silence around the topic which gives the same message. Yet here teenagers are with changing bodies, skyrocketing hormones, burgeoning sexual feelings, a growing capacity for real caring about another person, and abundant messages from the media that sex is cool, so *of course* many of them start exploring sex, no matter what their parents have said. We know that by age 19, 69 percent of all metropolitan area teens are sexually active (Kantner and Zelnik, 1978).

In talking about having intercourse, teens use images which express their overpowering feelings: feeling such a rush that you could not stop to think about birth control, so swept away that you could not help yourself or think about the consequences. Drugs and alcohol play into this scenario beautifully. People conclude that teens are too immature to think about the consequences of their sexual actions. Yet during these same years most teenagers are also working hard on their values. "What is a good friend?" they are asking. "Am I loyal to my friends? What causes do I believe in? How do I want to treat other people? Be treated by them?" By our massive, institutionalized disapproval of teen sexuality, combined with our shameless exploitation of sex in the media, we rob them of a chance to let their sexual actions be guided by the same kind of values that they are working on in other areas of their life. You cannot plan for something you are not supposed to be doing. You cannot ask yourself what your and the other person's true needs are when sexual impulses themselves are hidden in a cloud of guilt.

If sex education at home and in school can bring sexual feelings into the light of acceptance and self-acceptance, of honesty and humor, then teens' decisions about sex will at least have as fair a chance of being value centered as their decisions about how they treat their family and friends. Speaking openly about sex in this way will not totally eliminate the hurts or the unplanned pregnancies or the spread of sexually transmitted diseases (STDs) among teens, because these years will always be a time of experimentation and learning from mistakes. But it could reduce these greatly and have some psychological benefits as well.

It was with this aim in mind that we included a section in the teen book on making love making better. This is the part of the book we are always advised not to mention on TV or radio. Certain more liberal parents will say to themselves, "Okay, they're doing it, so we'd better give them the facts so they don't get into trouble." But even these would probably draw the line at increasing their kids' enjoyment of sex; many parents are uneasy even about their own sexual enjoyment. The bottom line is, then, that teens shouldn't be "doing it," that teen sex is an unavoidable evil to be dealt with but certainly not nurtured. This attitude communicates itself to the teenagers, and it backfires.

We chose to write in our book about getting privacy, learning how to talk with your partner about sex, getting used to being naked together, what to do if you do not have an orgasm and want to, how to cope with premature ejaculation. We included these as an act of respect for the teens as whole sexual beings and as an invitation to their self-respect. Once a young couple has decided to make love, they deserve to enjoy it. Part of that enjoyment comes from knowing you are protected against pregnancy.

Teenagers' enjoyment of sex is important in both the long and short term. Many of us know the distressing long-term consequences of early sex that we did not enjoy. We know the patterns of anxiety, defense, self-distrust, exploitation, guilt, self-protection, which reach years later into our loving relationships to distort our sexual relationships. We would like to help spare today's teenagers from some of that later suffering.

In the short term, being encouraged to consider their mutual enjoyment as something they can learn and plan for will help teenagers feel more self-respecting in sex and more respectful of it. Sex is not just something you fumble around with in the back of a car and then get your clothes together and pretend nothing happened. Something did happen, something that can be a source of energy, joy, pleasure, and human connection. Affirming this will help teenagers do all those things we so desperately hope they will do: use birth control, say no when they do not want to go any further, protect themselves against STDs. If you are encouraged to see your sexual relating as part of your whole self, you are more able to be responsible about it to yourself and to others.

For teenagers, then, as for all of us, information about sex is power—power to make choices, to take charge, to grow.

The Political Gets Personal: Keeping the New Right out of Our Bedrooms and Our Wombs

We are not the only ones who know that information is power. The right knows it, too. During the past several years we have seen an all-out attack on U.S. citizens' access to sex information and to the medical services which allow us to control our reproductive and sexual lives. If we learned in the early days of the women's movement that the personal is political, we are now dismayed to discover that the political has become personal in a way that threatens to turn the clock back on all our advances toward sexual equality and reproductive freedom.

We are seeing a massive effort by right-wing groups to enforce their rigid prescriptive views of sexuality on all of us, through legislation, court decisions, and/or a constitutional amendment. Here are some of the kinds of laws which have been proposed and even passed in some states:

Laws which would limit teenagers' access to information about birth control and sexually transmitted diseases;

Laws which would prohibit abortion or require consent of both parents or of a judge or of the spouse;

Laws which so define the beginning of life that abortion would be considered murder and certain forms of birth control would be outlawed;

Laws which would criminalize sexual intercourse between two consenting minors and would require a physician to report to a teenager's parents if she or he came in for birth control, or to report to the parents any reason to suspect sexual activity;

Laws which would infringe upon the civil rights of homosexuals and prohibit them from practicing certain professions;

Laws which would require mothers receiving welfare to submit to sterilization in order to receive their checks or to answer personal questions regarding where and with whom and when they had sex.

Listening to this list of proposed and incipient legislation, you can see again why we called our paper "Reclaiming Our Bodies." As one woman we know suggested, the right claims it is trying to get government off our backs, while it is actually working to insinuate government into our bedrooms and our wombs.

As counselors and as teachers and human service workers, we are going to see a lot of distress as these kinds of laws are enacted. As human beings who want to love and be loved freely in our own intimate relationships, we will face larger and larger obstacles.

This attack on sexual freedom goes hand in hand with an overall assault on women's new roles in the world of work. The so-called Moral Majority speaks openly about its goal of sending women back into the home. At the same time, the right wing's fiscal program cuts budgets for community services of many kinds. The sectors of the economy being cut back are those which offer some professional mobility for numbers of employed women. The despair of being out of work, out of money, and unable to use one's professional skills may propel many women back into traditional roles.

Each of us is affected on several levels by this monolithic backlash. We need a broad coalition of feminists, social service professionals, and clients. Many of us find ourselves in all three of these categories. We must respond to any attack on all of these levels. When a school system we teach in is threatened, we must respond as parents and as citizens and as teachers. When a community sex education program is threatened, we must respond not only as professionals about to lose our jobs, but as human beings who know the value of sexuality counseling to people's lives. As feminists we must be deeply concerned about attacks on particular sectors of the economy that employ large numbers of women or that primarily serve women and children.

The Moral Majority has mounted a well-financed campaign to force their particular view of religion and morality on the rest of us. Senators and members of Congress with long records of support for civil liberties and for human needs have been defeated by the single-issue campaigning of the right-to-life movement, so that today the configuration in Congress provides the numbers to pass a human life statute. The strength amassed by this movement comes from their grass-roots organizing which brings together an army of housewives frightened by social changes that seem to threaten their way of life. The strength and fanaticism of this well-organized minority now poses a threat to our work. We must respond quickly and effectively. We can no longer afford to think of sex education and counseling as occurring in a friendly climate or in a political vacuum.

Censorship is one of the right's primary weapons. The attacks on our reproductive freedoms are coupled with attacks on our rights to speak, to teach, to write. It is no coincidence that since the election of Ronald Reagan, banning efforts against public libraries have risen fivefold (*New York Times*, December 8, 1980, p. 1). As an ACLU regional counsel commented, "This is getting out of hand. Pretty soon we're going to have some very small libraries" (Cimons, 1981).

In our work as coauthors of *Our Bodies, Ourselves*, we have been directly affected by this movement toward censorship. We would like to share some of that history with you, because we have firsthand knowledge of it and we think it provides a way to track the gradual buildup of the strength of right-wing forces in this country.

Our Bodies, Ourselves has become a prime target of right-wing censorship activity. Paradoxically this began when, in 1976, the Young Adult Division of the American Library Association selected *Our Bodies, Ourselves* as one of their "best books for young adults." Since librarians around the country frequently use this list as a guide in selecting books, *Our Bodies, Ourselves* made its way into libraries in many small towns and semirural areas, where it attracted the notice of conservative groups such as the Eagle Forum and, more recently, the Moral Majority.

By 1977 we began to hear of banning attempts in small town high schools and libraries scattered through the Midwest, the South, and rural New England. Gradually a pattern emerged in that the Eagle Forum seemed to be involved in many of these banning campaigns which continued through 1978. The Eagle Forum even attacked the use of *Our Bodies, Ourselves* in a course for adult women given at a YWCA in Rockford, Illinois. They demanded that the course be dropped on the grounds that it was not consistent with Christian values and that another course, called "One Nation under God" be substituted.

The tactics employed by right-wing groups have ranged from quoting material out of context and making personal slurs against the authors to individual actions such as withdrawing books from libraries and refusing to return them. One parent argued that her local library should not be allowed to stock any material which she would not be willing to have in her own home! A minister demanded that his local library furnish him with the names of all persons who had withdrawn certain books in order to check the list for minors.

The 1980 campaign spearheaded by the Moral Majority has moved beyond the small towns of America to the big city dailies and the TV networks. Jerry Falwell targeted *Our Bodies, Ourselves* in a major fundraising letter, asking, "Do you want your children or the children of your loved ones reading this type of immoral trash? This is out and out humanistic garbage!" Falwell's instigation has stepped up the pace of banning efforts in local high schools and libraries. The Planned Parenthood Federation of America has informed us of numerous attempts to get the book out of their clinics and of a rash of phone calls to members of Congress requesting "obscenity hearings" to stop the purchase of *Our Bodies, Ourselves* with federal funds for agencies and clinics.

We have been heartened to hear of spontaneous defense groups arising in some communities. In Helena, Montana, an ad hoc coalition, Helena Citizens for Freedom of Expression, organized a defense in collaboration with the ACLU, which has been most helpful in many of these incidents. In Muskegon, Wisconsin, the local chapter of NOW defended attacks on *Our Bodies, Ourselves*. In Belfast, Maine, the school committee voted seven to three to keep *Our Bodies, Ourselves* in the school library despite a strong banning attempt by a local clergyman. These expressions of support signal the presence of a largely untapped core of progressives who will struggle with us for the preservation of choice and freedom in all our lives. We urge you to seek out such pockets of support in the communities where you work.

As a collective, our response to these attacks has been to step up our efforts to get information out to the people who need it. We are actively fundraising to be able to do this better; if you have any ideas, please let us know. To those resisting local attempts to ban *Our Bodies, Ourselves*, we have put together a packet of letters of endorsement from professionals who use our book in their work with adolescents and young adults, along with a list of localities that we know about where other banning attempts have taken place and news clippings of these episodes. You can order these materials from us.

As the campaign against *Our Bodies, Ourselves* escalates, we have been considering a more direct response to the Moral Majority. We welcome your ideas and support.

The new right is a grass-roots movement. It musters mailing lists, volunteers, and phone chains which reach literally millions of people. These are the ones our legislators are hearing from. Many of us in the prochoice, prosex education movement have lost the feel of this kind of grass-roots work. After the Supreme Court abortion decision in 1973, we hoped we would never need to do it again. But we do.

We feel saddened that we must take the time in which we could be learning from one another, advancing our knowledge of how to help ourselves and others, in order to sound the alarm and devise a strategy to fight back. But if we were to pinpoint the one thing we could do that would have the greatest effect in preventing sexual problems and promoting sexual responsibility in the next generation, it would be just this: to devise a strategy to defeat the Moral Majority and to prevent them from imposing their ideology on our communities and our nation. We must thoughtfully and energetically confront these reckless attacks on our freedom to provide sex information and resources. If we fail to do this, the risk is great that we may never meet as a conference of sex educators and family planners again.

References

Anonymous. Notes from just over the edge: A new lesbian speaks out. *Second Wave*, Summer 1981, *6*, 20-26.

Bell, R. et al. *Changing bodies, changing lives: A book for teens on sex and relationships.* New York: Random House, 1980.

Boston Women's Health Book Collective. *Our bodies, ourselves: A book by and for women* (Rev. ed.). New York: Simon and Schuster, 1979.

Boston Women's Health Book Collective. *Ourselves and our children: A book by and for parents.* New York: Random House, 1978.

Cimons, M. Feminist health book comes under Moral Majority's fire. *Los Angeles Times*, March 20, 1981.

Dodson, B. *Liberating masturbation: A meditation on self-love.* New York: Bodysex Designs, 1974. (Available from Bodysex Designs, P.O. Box 1933, New York, N.Y. 10001; $4.00.)

Hite, S. *The Hite report.* New York: MacMillan, 1976.

Kantner, J., and Zelnik, M. Contraceptive patterns and premarital pregnancy among women aged 15-19 in 1976. *Family Planning Perspectives*, May-June 1978, *10*, 135-142.

Reitz, R. *Menopause: A positive approach* (Rev. ed.). Radnor, Pa.: Chilton Books, 1977; New York: Penguin Books, 1979.

Rich, A. Compulsory heterosexuality and lesbian experience. *Signs*, Summer 1980, *5*, 631-660.

Sherfey, M. J. *The nature and evolution of female sexuality.* New York: Vintage Books, Random House, 1972.

Women and disability. *Off Our Backs*, May 1981, p. 11.

Zola, I. *Missing pieces: Chronicle of living with a disability.* Philadelphia: Temple University Press, in press.

Appendix A

Recommended Reading

Barbach, L., and Levine, L. *Shared intimacies: Women's sexual experiences.* Garden City, N.Y.: Anchor Books, Doubleday, 1980.

Boston Women's Health Book Collective, and ISIS. *International women and health resource guide.* Boston: Boston Women's Health Book Collective, 1980. (Available from Boston Women's Health Book Collective, P. O. Box 192, W. Somerville, Mass. 02144-0192; $5.00 [surface mail], $8.00 [air mail].

Corea, G. *The hidden malpractice: How American medicine mistreats women.* New York: Harcourt Brace Jovanovich, 1978.

Ehrenreich, B., and English, D. *Witches, midwives, and nurses: A history of women healers.* Old Westbury, N.Y.: Feminist Press, 1972.

Ehrenreich, B., and English, D. *For her own good: 150 years of the experts' advice to women.* New York: Anchor Books, Doubleday, 1978.

Gordon, L. *Woman's body, woman's right: A social history of birth control in America.* New York: Penguin Books, 1977.

Hite, S. *Hite report on male sexuality.* New York: Alfred A. Knopf, 1981.

Oakley, A. *Women confined: Towards a sociology of childbirth.* New York: Schocken Books, 1980.

Scully, D. *Men who control women's health: The miseducation of obstetrician-gynecologists.* Boston: Houghton Mifflin, 1980.

Seaman, B. *The doctors' case against the pill* (Rev. ed.). New York: Doubleday, 1980.

Zilbergeld, B. *Male sexuality.* New York: Bantam Books, 1978.

Appendix B

Following our presentation at the conference, an ad hoc meeting was called to discuss a response to the Moral Majority and other right-wing groups. The following resolution was developed for use with our professional constituencies and was passed by acclamation at the meeting of the whole conference the following morning.

As a group of 200 women and men who are mental health professionals, health educators, and teachers, we stand committed to continued work for free access to the information, sex education and medical and mental health services which enable all persons to express their sexuality in whatever nonexploitative ways they choose. We affirm our right to teach, to write, to speak, to learn from one another and to encourage people to grow.

We deplore the goals and tactics of a vocal right-wing minority to impose their narrow, prescriptive views of religion and sexuality on all the citizens of our country. We find the policies of this movement to be anti-life in the most profound ways.

We affirm parenthood by choice.

We oppose enforced parenthood, which has been proven to result in a dramatic rise in child abuse.

We affirm a full range of birth control choices

We oppose the prohibition of certain crucial methods of birth control like the low estrogen pill and the IUD.

We affirm the need for adequate food, shelter, health education, and social services for everyone.

We oppose cutbacks in critical human services.

We affirm a woman's freedom to choose abortion when necessary.

We oppose criminal penalties for women who have abortions. When legal abortion is not available, women seek illegal abortions, and many die.

We affirm our commitment to a society which nourishes and protects our diversity.

We oppose a rise in sexism, racism, anti-semitism and homophobia.

We affirm our inherent right to liberty in our personal and family life.

We oppose invasion of the most private aspects of personal and family life.

We pledge ourselves as individuals and professionals to a renewed grass-roots effort to mobilize the *real* majority of responsible citizens who believe in democracy and freedom as best expressed in the Constitution of the United States of America.

Sex Education in the Community

Nancy R. Hamlin

❖ Sex education has become a political issue. Anti-abortionists have without fanfare won several key positions in the Reagan administration and launched efforts to alter federal policy not just on abortion, but on sex education, family planning, and world population control. Headlines are filled with news on the subjects of abortion, birth control, and the so-called Moral Majority's attacks on women's rights.

❖   ...Human sexuality should not be a political issue. It is unfortunate that the personal has become the political. People must have control over their bodies and their destinies. There is a desperate need for community-based human sexuality programs for all people. Regardless of moral views or political affiliations, there are programs which are helpful and informative in meeting basic human needs. It is essential to remember that these programs must match the political, social, and cultural belief systems of the community, and that there must be community involvement and ownership in all aspects of the programs.

In planning sexuality programs, a 3-point design is used. The overall program is divided into the following categories: life-span approach, special population, and life stress or trauma points. In the life-span approach, life transition periods such as adolescence, young adulthood, middle years, pre- and post-menopause and old age are the key areas for program development. Special population groups include the physically handicapped, the mentally retarded, and the mentally ill. Childbirth, divorce, death of a loved one, abortion, rape, and birth of a handicapped child are examples of life stress or trauma points. Specific, targeted, time-limited primary prevention programs are needed for the special population groups and the population affected by life stress or trauma points.

Sexuality, its myths and realities, is not understood by the majority of our people. Sexual problems are found throughout the population as a result of the lack of available and appropriate information. From youth

From Nancy R. Hamlin, "Planning and Politics of Community-Based Human Sexuality Programs," in George W. Albee, Sol Gordon, and Harold Leitenberg (eds.) *Promoting Sexual Responsibility and Preventing Sexual Problems.* Cooypright © 1983 by the Vermont Conference on the Primary Prevention of Psychopathology. Reprinted by permission.

to old age, there appears to be a consistent lack of directed information and education on human sexuality.

Although birth control and abortions are more available today than ever before, teenage pregnancy and venereal disease are in epidemic proportion. The National Center for Health Statistics reports the number of out-of-wedlock births doubled in the U.S. during the period from 1970 to 1976. There are now about one million unmarried teenagers giving birth each year with 9 out of 10 of them keeping their babies (Out-of-Wedlock Births Doubled, 1980). One study showed that even today, 85 to 95 percent of all parents with children under 11 years old have never discussed sexual behavior. Another study found that one-third of mothers and teenage daughters do not discuss sex or birth control with any regularity. Our sex-indulging and sex-denying society lacks adequate sex education programs.

Current literature supports the need for continued sex education, family planning, and human sexuality programs. A recent report based on a long-term study of the New York state experience with legalized abortion presents some interesting and impressive facts. The Alan Guttmacher Institute's report of the state's 10-year experience with legalized abortion showed that abortions improved the health of mothers, babies, and the general populace. Illegal abortions have been virtually eliminated, with the associated death rate dropping from 6.7 per million to .8 per million. Yet, more than 75 percent of all U.S. counties currently have no abortion services. The imminent passage of new federal legislation to restrict all abortion services will leave few states with any hope of New York's achievement (Decade of Legal Abortions in New York, 1980).

Despite the United State's high standard of living, advanced medical technology, and sophisticated health services, the country ranks 14th internationally in terms of the infant mortality rate. Infant mortality is defined as the number of infants dying after birth and before reaching the age of 1 year. A startling statistic is the horrendous gap between the infant mortality rate of nonwhites and whites. It is 24.9 per 1,000 for nonwhites and 14.8 per 1,000 for whites (Wheeler, 1980).

The federal government is involved in family planning, at least for the moment. In 1980, the Office of Family Planning spent about 160 million dollars to finance 5,100 family planning clinics around the country to serve 4 million women of all ages. Another 7.5 million dollars was spent on programs to counsel pregnant teenagers. In addition, contraceptives are routinely purchased through Medicaid (The Feds and the Family, 1981).

Although progress has been made over the last decade, few programs exist to meet the special needs of the mentally ill, the mentally retarded, or the physically handicapped. The general population appears to fare no better. The future of sex education seems to be linked to the politics of our times.

I will discuss programs, paradigms, and strategies which have been used to develop community-based human sexuality programs and present a model which suggests strategies for bringing about change in communities and in institutions. It emphasizes that change is a slow, planned, and sometimes irrational process.

❖ Program Definition and Development

The planning and promotion of community-based human sexuality programs are complex. The planners and advocacy groups constantly change, whereas the professional medical opposition remains constant and persistent.

I am defining human sexuality programs in an educational context. Sex is a fundamental dimension of human awareness and development. It is innately a part of the ever present desire for personal expression and satisfaction. Life-styles reflect the manner in which individuals attempt to accomplish this goal, as well as the developmental stages at which people are functioning. Sex education takes into consideration that sex is at the base of our personality and identity. It incorporates our gender, anatomy, and physiology (Schiller, 1977, p. 133).

Human sexuality programs are needed throughout our life-span. Programs are essential for children, adolescents, adults, and the elderly. In planning human sexuality programs, this three-pronged scheme provides a conceptual framework:

life-span approach

special population groups

points of strees and/or trauma

Life-Span Approach

The task and scope of sex education are to develop the ability of the child, adolescent, and adult to cope with their individual sexuality. One often hears the term "sex education" and immediately focuses on the much needed and infrequently present school-based sex education program. However, human sexuality programs are needed throughout one's life-span. Programs are needed before, during, and after childbirth. Pregnant women and new mothers are plagued with myths and questions about their sexuality. How may times have you heard the myth that "women cannot get pregnant while breast-feeding" and that "having intercourse will bring on labor."

In 1972, a group of committed volunteers and I founded People's Education Organization for Prepared Life Experience (PEOPLE). The following is the mission statement:

> Project PEOPLE, People's Educational Organization for Prepared Life Experiences, was developed by myself and a group of professional and lay people to offer free quality education to all people, particularly those of low socioeconomic circumstances in the greater Lynn area. It was felt that many people are not meeting life's experiences with the aid of information and support that would increase the probability of a happy, fulfilled life. Project PEOPLE is a group of concerned and dedicated individuals who have volunteered their time to offer seminars, workshops, and rap sessions in the areas of (1) childbirth education, (2) sex education, (3) early childhood education, (4) human growth and development, and (5) drug education, so that individuals would have the choice of planning and participating in the educational program.

PEOPLE'S classes were located at community schools and the Community Health Center, and the Lynn Girl's Club (Hamlin, 1972).

The purposes of the organization were:

> to help unwed women and married couples attain a better understanding of childbirth and early parenthood in the belief that prepared, well-informed mothers can best experience the birth of a baby as one of the most meaningful and inspiring moments of life. Unwed mothers and expectant parents that participate actively in this program have an opportunity to have the optimum maternity experience;

> to insure support for mothers who choose to breast-feed by the establishment of a Nursing Mothers' Telephone Council;

to provide essential information on the intellectual, social, emotional, and physical development of young children;

to offer people birth control and family planning information;

to help people understand drugs, their use, and their effects;

to provide all people, especially low-income people, with free, quality family life education;

to refer individuals in need of additional information or help to the proper agency.

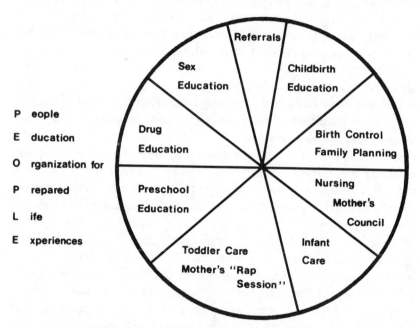

Figure 1. Project PEOPLE's Organizational Model.

The program was explained by viewing life as a continuum with sexuality, childbirth, and human growth and developmental issues integrated into the cycle. The following circle represents the PEOPLE model.

Project PEOPLE, which is free and nondiscriminatory, is a unique model for prepared family life experiences. The family or single parent began with prepared childbirth classes. Following the child's birth, the parents and child were invited to join a postpartum group to discuss the physical, psychological, and intellectual developments faced by the new mother. To give support to women who chose to breast-feed their child, a nursing mothers' telephone council was established which had an obstetrical nurse, a social worker, and a trained nursing mother on call. Birth control and family planning seminars were also given. A workshop in early childhood behavior was established to discuss topics such as discipline, behavior, toys, creative arts, planning and evaluation of preschool programs. Parents of preschool-age children had the choice of attending a child study "rap session" in which the group found its own subject focus. The goal of the sex education segment of PEOPLE was to provide parents and young people with an understanding of human reproduction and to encourage open discussion of sex. *Our Bodies, Ourselves* was both the name of the discussion group and the title of a handbook written by the Boston Women's Health Book Collective. The drug education component of the program was directed toward understanding the effect drugs have on the body as well as on the unborn fetus.

Community involvement was essential to the success of this program. From the outset, it was apparent that to succeed PEOPLE needed to reach individuals in need of services and insure their participation in the program. Equally important was an awareness and understanding of the needs of the community and of the learning process. Community people initiated the concept of PEOPLE and participated in all aspects of its development. In order to try to insure the continuance of PEOPLE, an interested community person, an "assistant," shared the responsibility with each group leader in the goal that each "assistant" would become the instructor.

Project PEOPLE had as its basic premise that parents were by far the most important positive influence in helping a child become socially, emotionally, physically, and intellectually mature. PEOPLE's position was that well-informed mothers would best experience the birth of a baby as one of the most meaningful and inspiring moments of life. Project PEOPLE hoped to begin a cycle that would produce informed, happy parents who would raise informed, happy children.

For 2 years, I coordinated project PEOPLE with all volunteers, teaching classes and training assistants. Ultimately funding was received from the Massachusetts Office for Children and then the Department of Public Welfare.

❖ Special Populations and Sex Education

For the last 5 years, I have shared friendship and office with the founder of the Handicapped Peoples' Support Program (HPSP). This volunteer program based on the self-help philosophy believes that people who have successfully adjusted to their own disabilities are better qualified in relating to and understanding what the special needs are of others with similar handicaps. HPSP focuses on the social and psychological needs of people with physical handicaps through a threefold model of working with physical medicine, mental health, and peer counselors. This "triage" approach is followed by participation in mutual support groups. A readjustment to personal sexuality is integrated into the context of the program.

Attending a recent Boston conference on "Sexuality and the Handicapped," one of the HPSP volunteers, an amputee, stressed the importance of peer counseling in sexuality. She spoke of the intense feelings and anxieties which she experienced reengaging in sex after her operation and her need to have peer support.

Human sexuality programs are not limited to the needs of the "normal" population. Special human sexuality programs for institutionalized, mentally ill, and retarded patients are essential. For these patients, the problem of living in an institutional setting must be taken into account. From my own observations, even in the finest institutional settings for retarded citizens, the bathroom is sometimes the only place where a resident can find privacy.

Deinstitutionalization brought with it a whole host of exciting challenges. In Lynn, the Greater Lynn Mental Health and Mental Retardation Association addressed the issues of sex education and retarded citizens by offering a 3-day training program for parents and professionals. This program was followed by years of planning, involving parents, community agencies, and consultants. The outcome is an agency, community, family, and individualized approach to human sexuality including policies, programs, privacy, and respect for the basic needs and human rights of retarded citizens.

The program consists of educational groups, birth control counseling, and parental involvement. The groups are composed of seven clients and are run by cotrainers for 7-week periods. Client selection is based on the client's functional level of retardation, whether they are mildly or severely retarded. The curriculum depends on the level of the group. A well-functioning group may discuss feelings, relationship issues, and sexual intercourse. A less well-functioning group may focus on friendship, the parts of the body, how to avoid being taken advantage of and/or violation in the community. Since clients are at different levels of sexual development, birth control and family planning counseling are individualized. Clients are taught individual responsibility within the family, and agency staff reinforce the prescribed plan. Women are frequently counseled to use birth control pills or an IUD. The men are taught to take responsibility by using condoms.

The profoundly, severely retarded are not forgotten. A special consultant works with these clients in body movement, verbal and nonverbal communication, and getting in touch with their bodies.

Parents are an integral part of the program. They are invited to attend the groups and meet with the family planning counselor. Parents are encouraged to see their children's sexuality in developmental, chronological, and physiological terms, not simply in terms of the child's mental age. The philosophy of the program is not to foster or to discourage sexual activity, but to understand that sexuality can be expressed by retarded people. The goal is to help clients express their sexuality in positive, healthy ways. Parental consent is mandatory for participation, and the success of the program depends on parental involvement. When clients are living in group community-based facilities, it is essential to involve residential staff and case managers, who are seen in the surrogate parent role. Parents and community staff attend the program with clients. It does absolutely no good to train the mentally retarded client if parents and staff are not involved. Some parents enter a "Train the Trainer" program and are taught to help other parents. They often become cotrainers in the group. It is found that parents of mentally retarded people relate better to other parents.

Life Stress/Trauma Points

Divorce Education
Life is a developmental process. If we accept the notion that sexuality is at the core of this development, then all aspects of human life must be reexamined with our sexuality in mind. For example, with one out of two

marriages ending in divorce, divorce groups and seminars must present people with an understanding of the changes brought about by new feelings, behaviors, and social mores. This knowledge can be catalogued under "anticipatory preventive education."

The Newport, Rhode Island, Divorce and Mediation Resource Center offers community forums, educational support groups, assertiveness training, and social effectiveness groups for the divorced and separated. Popular topics included in the community forums are: dating, being single in a couple's world, new relationships, and dealing with loneliness. (Sullivan, 1980).

An 8-week educational group provides time for members to establish peer support and work through the mourning process in which they are involved. The topics are similar to those of the community forum, but more specific and comprehensive. The curriculum includes:

introduction to the divorce process;

coping with loneliness and ambivalence;

handling guilt and feelings of failure;

children and divorce;

alternative ways of handling anger;

looking at emotional patterns;

new relationships;

saying goodbye and looking ahead.

Support groups are held in participants' homes.

Assertiveness training offers practice in communication skills to help divorced and separated people increase their effectiveness in new social, work, and family situations.

The social effectiveness training program is directed toward divorced, separated, widowed, and single adults. The purpose of the series is to help people meet affiliation needs. Many adults, after years of marriage, are anxious and ill at ease relating to the opposite sex in the single world. Some people marry early in life and never develop these skills. Skill training in this area is a preventative service which helps single people recognize the problem and develop strategies to handle it rather than withdrawing into further isolation.

Childbirth and Family Life Education

Family life education is a polite term coined to mean sex education, child-birth education, family planning programs, exercise classes, preparation for childbirth, and nutrition and postpartum education. All of these issues are either emotionally or politically charged. Sex educators working in schools are plagued with the nagging question of whether responsibility lies with the home or with the school. Many progressive parents would welcome the opportunity to discuss sexuality with their teenagers but need support and guidance.

Childbirth is often the first crisis one encounters in adulthood. If home birth and prepared childbirth offer the opportunity to promote self-help, self-care, and primary prevention medicine, then this life crisis allows for a key opportunity to affect a person's coping skills throughout life. The impact of this experience has ramifications on all aspects of both parents' and children's lives.

In the medical community, childbirth education has been controversial. It brings into play complex medical, ethical, and legal questions for prac-ticing physicians and, to a lesser extent, for hospitals. The prepared child-birth movement of the 1950s, 1960s and early 1970s, whose goal was to bring fathers and significant others into the labor and delivery rooms and provide women with the opportunity to have natural childbirth, was followed by the home birth movement of the 1970s and 1980s.

Through the 1970s, I saw the prepared childbirth movement grow. I saw hospitals rapidly convert to family-centered maternity units with hospital-based classes. Some childbirth educators describe the 1970s as the "co-optation of the prepared childbirth movement." Childbirth classes became increasingly hospital-based. The philosophy focused on teaching women to be "good patients" who would accept the fetal monitor, med-ication, induced labor, unnecessary Caesarean section, intravenous feeding, and episiotomy.

In the mid-1970s, the home birth movement gained momentum. In Mas-sachusetts, the Boston Health Planning Council and the North Shore Health Planning Council both grappled with this major political issue of home births. Many physicians flatly resisted the notion of individuals and phy-sicians attending home births. On the North Shore there was discussion of outlawing home births because there was no emergency back-up system available. The compromise was that one out-of-hospital birth center was set up in a cottage next to the Beverly Hospital. The North Shore Birthing Center is staffed by nurse midwives, who are supervised by a physician. Women are screened carefully and only low-risk women are accepted. Emergency equipment is available, but out of sight. The hospital is present for any crisis.

Different models are needed to meet the needs of high-risk and low-risk births. Currently, many systems, as promulgated in state and national guidelines are based on a monolithic model of regional maternity centers. From a quality of care point of view, it is often argued that a sufficient volume of patients or procedures is necessary for staff to maintain a high level of proficiency. A single study by the American College of Obstetricians and Gynecologists (1971) suggested that units with less than 500 deliveries per year often lacked personnel, services, and equipment necessary for adequate maternity and newborn care. As a result of this one inadequate study, the quality of care is presumed related to the volume of service provided.

Results of recent studies show there is no basis in terms of quality care and the outcome for the arbitrary figures assigned as minimum numbers of annual births. Further research has also shown that there are no supporting data available which show the actual cost, much less the cost effectiveness of this system of care. Such figures as available are based on 1973 data from a Level 2 hospital in New Jersey. The figures are cited in Appendix C of a well-known document, "Toward Improving the Outcome of Pregnancy," which has been used widely in maternity care planning. According to Norma Swenson, founder of the Boston Association of Childbirth Education (BACE), past president of International Childbirth Education Association and coauthor of Our Bodies, Ourselves, there is no evidence which proves that a regional system of childbirth will improve the quality of the childbirth experience. In fact, low-risk mothers do not need the sophisticated technology of hospitals and highly trained obstetrical staff. They are well served by an out-of-hospital birthing center or a nurse midwife in the home with an emergency back-up system. It is a far more humane and cost effective approach. The North Shore Birthing Center's total fee is $800 as compared with the $2,300 fee for an inpatient maternity stay. If a woman is covered under comprehensive maternity benefits, Blue Cross-Blue Shield pays for either service (Cramer, 1981).

High-risk mothers tend to be poor; they receive late prenatal care and are nutritionally deficient. They need high technology care only because they do not receive proper care in pregnancy. These women are better served by a familiar, accessible community-based hospital, staffed by nurse midwives and physicians. Nurse midwives follow the pregnant woman prenatally in the home and hospital. This model can frequently change her status from high to low risk. A program model designed for high-risk mothers needs to include:

a nutrition program;

nurse midwives who follow the pregnant women prenatally in the home and hospital;

a team of nurse midwives and doctors working together;

prenatal and postnatal educational groups;

staff which is representative of the ethnic composition of the community.

The nutrition and outreach program will identify high-risk mothers early in their pregnancy. Prenatal care will begin earlier in order to prevent and reduce complications at birth.

Maternal and newborn services need to be reconceptualized and reorganized with the greatest emphasis on preventative primary ambulatory care utilizing nurse midwives, and implementing substantial food, nutrition, and outreach programs for high-risk mothers. This will reduce costs for all maternity patients. Prompt attention must be paid to the proliferation and expansion of high technology centers, and the development of birth centers must continue.

Birth has become a political issue because it involves money, and large amounts of money. If birth is treated as a normal, natural, and nonpathological experience, many people will stay out of the hospital, they will not use drugs, and will not bottlefeed their babies; altogether this will mean a loss of millions of dollars for the medical and baby industries.

The most important challenges facing childbirth in the 1980s is to help make it a creative growth experience for parents. Childbirth between now and the year 2000 must involve:

the development of out-of-hospital birth centers;

acceptance of home births and midwives;

establishment of community-based birth centers;

mutual support groups for pregnant women and new mothers;

greater cooperation between doctors and midwives;

food and nutrition programs for high-risk mothers.

Issues in Planning

Strategies for Bringing About Change

There are three strategies for bring about change. In creating new programs, organizers must remember that planned change is conscious, deliberate, and intended. Planned change utilizes knowledge as a tool for modifying patterns and institutions.

First, the *empirical rational strategy* assumes people are rational and will follow their rational self-interest once this is revealed to them. A change is proposed by some person or group which knows of a situation that is desirable, effective and in line with the self-interest of the person, group, organization, or community that will be affected by the change. Second, the *normative reeducative model* is based on the belief that norms from the basis of behavior and change come through reeducation in which old norms are discarded and supplanted by new ones. To quote Bennis, Benne, and Chin (1969) "Changes in normative orientation involve change in attitudes, values, skills, and significant relationships. It is not just change in knowledge and information or intellectual rationals" (p. 34). Emphasis is on experimental learning as an ingredient for all enduring changes in human systems (Bennis, et al., 1969). This system centers on the belief that "people technology is necessary in working out desirable changes in human affairs."

Third, *application of power* assumes the compliance of those with less power with those with greater power. When working within and without institutions, it is essential to understand the three models. At times, all three are factors in institutional decision making.

I believe, judging from my experience, that changing people's attitudes and values is the most important ingredient in the implementation of any new program. For this reason, I believe in a values-oriented approach to the training of people. Organizational change begins with people because people constitute the institution.

A normative reeducative model was used in developing a Comprehensive Rape Crisis Program at the Greater Lynn Community Mental Health Center (see Appendix C).

Taboo topics like rape usually bring out feelings of anxiety coupled with resistance. When dealing with any taboo topic, a values-oriented approach to training focusing on changing people's attitudes is essential to the success of the program. The mental health center staff and community advocates attended 100 hours of training over a 2-year period. The training dealt with the societal values, myths, and realities of rape; counseling victims; sexuality; "rap groups;" the legal system; and advocacy. The program is still functioning.

Because maintaining innovation is difficult, there is a built-in need for retraining annually. Goodwin Watson and Edward Glaser offer this warning:

Many an innovation brought in with great fanfare is superficially accepted, and months or years later things drifted back to the way they were before. Nobody may have openly resisted the change. Nobody revoked it. It just didn't last. (Cited in Havelock, 1973, p. 133)

Change Agents: Advantages and Disadvantages

Change agents is a term used to indicate people inside and/or outside a system who are planners and innovators. Over the last decade, I have functioned as both a change agent working in the community and as a change agent working inside institutions. There are advantages and disadvantages to both roles. The inside change agent has the advantage of knowing the system, speaking the language, identifying with the system's needs and aspirations, and being a familiar figure. Disadvantages facing the inside change agent include lacking perspective, not having adequate knowledge, having to live down past failures, not being able to move independently, and facing the difficult task of redefining ongoing relationships with other members of the system.

Advantages of functioning as an outside change agent include starting fresh, being in a position to be objective, being independent, and bringing in something which is genuinely new. The disadvantages faced by outside change agents are that they are strangers to the system, they may lack knowledge of the insiders, they may not care enough, and they may appear threatening to insiders.

Project PEOPLE, mentioned earlier, provides an example of a program developed by a group of outside change agents. The effect that PEOPLE's prepared childbirth class had on the local community hospital was to demonstrate a need for and to mobilize the institution to offer hospital-based and-controlled childbirth education classes. The PEOPLE's childbirth classes illustrated the effect that the national prepared childbirth movement had on hospitals throughout the country. Most hospitals now offer childbirth classes.

One solution for program planners is to develop a team approach involving inside and outside change agents. An example of this approach is the rape crisis program previously mentioned. In this program I served as an inside change agent representing the Greater Lynn Community Mental Health Center working with outside change agents, the Community Task Force, which is a volunteer group.

Freda Klein, who served as a consultant to the group, published an article on the experience entitled, "Developing New Model Rape Crisis Centers" (Klein, 1977). She described it this way:

Autonomy was a crucial question from the outset. Because the Community Mental Health Center funded the initial training and offered resources including meeting space, and typing and mailing costs, the Task Force's obligation became murky. After a long, sometimes tense process, we have developed a unique model: the Community Task Force, the Greater Lynn Community Mental Health Center and Union Hospital . . . three separate bodies working cooperatively to provide comprehensive services to rape victims and community education-preventive programs. This model is an outgrowth of the anti-rape movement, which won reforms from institutions. Since the Community Mental Health Center and the hospital must treat rape victims within a certain geographical area, there was no possibility for the community task force to become the only rape crisis center . . . .

We are without the burden of basic fundraising because the Community Mental Health Center provides a 24-hour hot line staffed by its Crisis Intervention Team members (calls are then referred to volunteer advocates screened and trained by the Task Force) . . . . Another trade-off concerns outreach. While the Community Mental Health Center has greater resources to conduct systematic outreach campaigns than do most volunteer centers, it is difficult to assess how many victims will avoid our advocacy services because of institutional ties.

The divergent practical conditions facing current anti-rape organizing and organizing of a few years ago are striking. But just as I'm longing for the good ol' days of political purism (and trying to ignore how steeped in privilege that model is), it becomes clear that our new predicaments can be turned into new bargaining positions of strength. (p. 10)

The new model did come with strings. It is incorporatd into a 4.5 million dollar mental health center. Its uniqueness and degree of community visability is married to a large diverse institution. However, in the 1980s many grass-roots women's health centers and rape crisis programs have been forced to close because of insufficient funding. The Greater Lynn Rape Crisis program with its institutional marriage is "alive and well." It has a life of its own, a 24-hour telephone hot line covered by professional counselors, and annual staff retraining programs.

Conclusion

In my 20s and 30s, I was involved in many causes including day care, antiwar, women rights, sex education, civil rights, education for parenthood, and affirmative action movements. My daughter used to play at writing agendas for meetings instead of playing house. It appeared that many battles had been won: fathers were allowed into the delivery rooms, a national daycare bill passed the House and Senate, the Vietnam War ended, *Our Bodies, Ourselves* was on the best-seller's list, abortion was legalized, and affirmative action was being taken seriously. Slowly, in my late 20s, things began to change. While teaching in a Massachusetts community college, I was struck by the apathy of students and the lack of social and political interest—there were no more protests. The aim of the students was to work hard, make money, and "play the game."

I am not yet 40, and I see the victories of my 20s erode. I see the National Human Service System which was assembled over the last decade being dismantled, I see race relations and affirmative action going "out of style." I saw the nation's daycare bill vetoed by former President Nixon and I am currently watching the Community Mental Health Systems Act being dismantled. The 1978 *President's Commission Report on Mental Health* cited primary prevention as one of the top priorities of the national community mental health system. Some ask the question, "Has primary prevention's time come and gone?"

Yes, many of us are fighting the same battle again, but this time we are no longer naive. In the words of Ellen Goodman, "It hits the generation that came into adulthood in the 1960s the hardest. They saw their piece of time as a straight line instead of a cycle. They saw progress as an arrow instead of a pendulum" (Goodman, 1981, p. 15).

I have learned that ground won in battle needs to be continually staked out and consciously held. The test before us lies in whether we can learn the lessons of the earlier activists who learned in lean times how to regroup, change, develop new strategies, and maintain their goals and energies over difficult times. We are fortunate that we have history to lean on and a new generation to join our ranks.

Today society faces a serious challenge. There are those who would wish to control the free dissemination of information concerning human sexuality. Special interest groups have begun to appear whose intention is to disrupt the advancement of study and sensitivity with regard to human sexuality. I feel strongly that we must protect our accomplishments as well as strive to improve the quality of our life goals in the future.

Powerful, knowledgeable people who have an understanding of the system must work together as change agents inside and outside and in coordination with systems to insure that all people receive quality human sexuality programs throughout their life-span. It is essential to work together toward this end to ensure freedom of privacy, freedom of religion, freedom of choice, and control of our sexuality and destiny. Perhaps it would do well to recollect the following passage written during the rise of Hitler by Pastor Martin Neimoller:

They came after the Jews,
    and I was not a Jew, so I did not object.
Then they came after the Catholics,
    and I was not a Catholic, so I did not object.
Then they came after the Trade Unionists,
    and I was not a Trade Unionist, so I did not object.
Then they came after me,
    and there was no one left to object. (cited in Gordon, 1981, p. 2)

As Edmund Burke once said, "All that is necessary for the triumph of evil is for good men (people) to do nothing."

References

Aborting deformed fetuses opposed by Reagan's top health advisor, would end pregnancy only to save woman. *Boston Globe,* May 28, 1981, p. 8.

American College of Obstetricians and Gynecologists, Committee on Maternal Health. *National study of maternity care and survey of obstetric practice and associated services in hospitals in the United States,* Chicago, Ill., 1971.

Bennis, W. G., Benne, K., and Chin, R. *The planning of change* (2nd ed.). New York: Holt, Rinehart and Winston, 1969.

Boston Women's Health Book Collective. *Our bodies, ourselves* (2nd ed.). New York: Simon and Schuster, 1971.

Bradford, L. E. Evangelism: The electronic church and conservative politics. *Big Mama Rag,* December 1980, p. 20.

Cramer, D. Birth without doctors. *Boston Globe Magazine,* April 12, 1981, pp. 12-13; 24, 29, 30.

Decade of legal abortions in New York proves benefits. *Nation's Health,* December 1980, p. 20.

The feds and the family. *Boston Globe,* Feb. 2, 1981, p. 10.

Feinstein, R., Goldman, J., Hatch, H., and Wolpent, E. It ain't necessarily so. In *Myths and facts about racism and the Klan in Boston.* Docudrama, 1980, p. 18.

Fishman, W. K. *The right-wing attack on women.* Paper presented at annual meeting of the American Sociological Association, Boston, Massachusetts, August 1979.

Goodman, E. The second battle is the tough one. *Boston Globe,* March 5, 1981, p.15.

Gordon, S. Sexual politics and the far right. *Impact '80: Journal of the Institute for Family Research and Education,* October 1980, p. 2.

Hamlin, N. Project PEOPLE proposal. Massachusetts Department of Children, 1972, pp.1-3.

Havelock, R. G. *The change agent's guide to innovations in education.* New Jersey: Educational Technology Publication, 1973.

Kirkendall, L. A. The assault of sex education. *The Humanist,* May/June 1973, 13-14.

Klein, F. Developing new models: Rape crisis centers. *FAAR News,* July/August 1977, pp.9-10.

National Foundation of March of Dimes, Committee on Perinatal Health. *Toward improving the outcome of pregnancy,* 1976, pp. 30-33.

Out of wedlock births doubled. *Nation's Health,* November 1980, p.15.

Schiller, P. *Creative approaches to sex education and counseling.* New York: Association Press 1973.

Sullivan, P. Newport Training Institute: Prevention programs, community education and professional development. *Consultation and Education Models that work.* Springfield, Mass., 1980, pp.1-4.

Wheeler, W. H. *Developing and administering mental health services to minorities*. Staff College, National Institute of Mental Health, January 1980, Module 1, 5.

Willis, E. Abortion rights: Overruling new fascists. *Village Voice*, February 4, 1980, pp.8-9.

Appendix A

On a Moral Majority letterhead, showing a logo depicting the U.S. Capitol and an address at 499 S. Capital Street, and with "Confidential" stamped across the top in block capitals, the follow letter was received (dated January 1, 1981).

DEAR MR.— — —
We have only begun to fight!
If the liberals and advocates of pornographic sex education think that, by smearing me, they can stop the Moral Majority's campaign to remove offensive sex education materials from our public classrooms . . . they have another guess coming! We cannot compromise our children's moral principles this nation was founded upon!

Mr.— — —I'm sure you've read in your local newspaper there in— — —about our campaign to alert the parents of America to the insidious efforts of secular humanists to destroy the moral convictions of our boys and girls in some public schools.

Sometimes, they call it sex education — at other times "values clarification,"etc.

Perhaps you even received my letter where I gave you actual excerpts from a textbook so that you could see for yourself how offensive some sex education material is.

But now, we have discovered another book that has been used a reference book in several public school libraries that makes *Life and Health* (the book I mentioned last November) seem almost acceptable.

And that's why I say, we have only begun to fight!

The book is entitled *Our Bodies, Ourselves* and it was published in 1973 by Simon and Schuster. It is possible that material like that which is being used in this book may be found in many school libraries. I want you to help us obtain information on this matter.

Here are just a few of the book's chapter titles:

Living with Ourselves and Others: Our Sexual Relationships

In Amerika They Call Us Dykes

Our Changing Sense of Self

The Anatomy and Physiology of Sexuality and Reproduction

Venereal Disease

Abortion

I tell you, my friend—the little bit of this book that we have read is not only disgusting, it is shocking!

"Most of us were taught sex belongs in marriage. The linking of virginity and marriage often forces us into marriage before we are ready, before we know whether it's something we want."

"Those of us who grew up in religious families may feel that to lose our virginity before marriage is to have sinned."

"If you have never masturbated, we invite you to try. You may feel awkward, self-conscious, even a bit scared at first. You may have to contend with voices within you that repeat, 'Nice girls don't . . .' or 'A happily married woman wouldn't want to . . . .' Most of us have had these feelings too, and they changed in time."

Do you want your children or the children of your loved ones reading this type of immoral trash? This is out and out humanistic garbage!

The parents in Renton, Washington, thought so when they pulled it out of the 9th grade health class in their high school, and the people in Ludlow, Massachusetts, felt the same way when they removed it from their high school after this book had been used for one entire year.

I don't know what this country is coming to when some of our schools openly teach that premarital sex is not sinful—that the moral values that you and I grew up with are outdated and backward.

This is all part of the humanists' attempt to change our society. They realize that we will not endorse free love, free sex, so they are brainwashing our children.

Here are some of the humanists' basic beliefs:

They believe that there are no absolutes (no right, no wrong)—that moral values are self-determined and situational. Do your own thing, "as long as it does not harm anyone else."

They believe in removal of the traditional and distinctive roles of male and female.

They believe in sexual freedom between consenting individuals, regardless of age, including premarital sex, homosexuality, lesbianism, and incest.

So, my friend, if you don't know what books are being used in your public school systems in the sex education classes, I strongly advise that you find out today!

Moral Majority is trying to learn where offensive sex education books like *Our Bodies, Ourselves* and *Life and Health* are being used.

Will you help us obtain that information?

Examine your public school' libraries and textbooks for immoral, anti-family, and anti-American content. Arrange to see the films shown in classrooms. If you find obscene books, films, or other such material being used by our young people in schools, please advise us right away.

We will then publish this information in our Moral Majority Report newspaper and inform the public on our daily radio commentary.

Then, you can politely, but firmly, take reasonable action where you live, Mr. — — —!

We do not oppose sex education when it is taught as a biological science. Reproduction, puberty, hygiene, and other such matters should be taught.

And, take into consideration, sometimes objectionable books and materials inadvertently find their way into good schools, where no one intentionally did this. Always be reasonable and gracious. Nothing is ever accomplished by being unkind, belligerent, or violent.

Across the top of this letter was "handwritten": "Please destroy this letter and the sheet I've enclosed immediately after reading them."

Another letter from the Moral Majority, to the same address, was sent in an envelope stamped CONFIDENTIAL - SEXUALLY EXPLICIT MATERIALS EN-CLOSED—DO NOT LET THIS LETTER FALL INTO THE HANDS OF SMALL CHILDREN.

It contained the following letter and enclosures:

Any objectionable material should be taken to the principal. If he is unresponsive, go to the school board, state legislators, the governor, and U.S. congressmen.

Do you want your child to choose his values free from your influence and free from any standard of right or wrong based on issues like premarital sex, extramarital sex, homosexuality, lesbianism, and bisexuality?

Do you want books like *Life and Health* and *Our Bodies, Ourselves* being used to influence your child's decisions?

I say "no" Mr. ———, and I will fight until my last breath to make sure that books like these two are removed from our public schools once and for all.

I'm not against sex education, when taught as a biological science, but I am against offensive sex education materials that distort and warp our children's minds and moral values.

But I need your help in this fight, and that's why I'm writing you today.

The Moral Majority is already working with several organizations to remove these harmful sex education materials that distort and warp our children's minds and moral values.

But I need your help in this fight, and that's why I'm writing you today.

The Moral Majority is already working with several organizations to remove these harmful sex education materials from classrooms. But all this takes money!

Your gift of $10, $15, or even $25 will help us fight to remove books from public schools like *Our Bodies Ourselves* and *Life and Health*.

In addition, Mr ———, your gift will be used to help us publish our Moral Majority Report newspaper, produce our daily radio commentary, underwrite our large national staff and, in general, to help return this nation to moral sanity.

Believe me, you and I are slowly losing control over what our children are being taught!

And parents are legally responsible for the actions of their children, so it is only proper that they have an interest and a VOICE in what their youngsters are taught in the public schools and the textbooks that are being used!

So won't you help us remove sex education books that are harmful to our children once and for all?

Your gift to the Moral Majority today could make the crucial difference in a child's life!

I hope you will take a moment to look over the special sheet I've enclosed for you today so that you can see for yourself why it is so important that we remove offensive materials from our classrooms and libraries immediately.

Then I encourage you to sit down right away and write me a check for the largest amount you can possibly sacrifice and send it back immediately.

Please let me hear from you soon. Each day counts when a small child's mind and morals are at stake. I will be anxiously awaiting your reply.

Working to Save Our Children,
Jerry Falwell

P.S. Remember—our children's moral values are at stake! Please rush your special gift to Moral Majority right away.

I ask that you destroy this letter and the special sheet I've enclosed immediately after reading it so that it will not fall into the hands of an innocent youngster.

SPECIAL REPLY FORM

Jerry,

   I promise I will do everything in my power to help you remove offensive sex education materials that are being used in our public school systems.

_____
(Please sign here)

☐ YES! I will inquire in our local public libraries and let you know if "Our Bodies/ Ourselves" and/or "Life and Health" is available to our young people.

   Mr. _____

   _____

   _____

Dear Jerry,

   ☐ YES! I want to help! Enclosed is my special gift to help the Moral Majority continue its fight against offensive sex education materials and to help its other national programs!

Appendix B

IMPORTANT   ADULTS ONLY!

The following are actual excerpts from the book, Our Bodies, Ourselves:

PAGE 26   Photograph of woman using mirror to examine self plus advocating the use of a plastic speculum.

PAGE 39   Chapter entitled SEXUALITY—"When I made love with Jack I felt like he was feeding me. I felt full with his — — — inside me. When I wasn't with him I would feel hungry again. Often I didn't have — — —. I kept coming back to him, though it was an impossible relationship, because I needed to be fed. Later I realized he was mothering me. I was asking him to be my mother. That was a revelation!" Page also has photograph of a nude woman.

PAGE 41   Section entitled SEXUAL LANGUAGE—"I was dancing with a man I liked a lot. We were feeling very sensual. As we moved our bodies to the music I could feel his — — — and — — — pressing on me. He whispered in my ear, 'I bet your — — — is warm and juicy!'"

PAGE 42   Section entitled SEX IN OUR IMAGINATION: OUR FANTA-SIES—"I've had fantasies of having to drink — — — from a man's — — — while he was — — —."

"I used to have a recurring fantasy that I was a gym teacher and had a classful of girls standing in front of me, nude. I went up and down the rows feeling all their — — — and getting a lot of pleasure out of it. When I first had this fantasy at thirteen I was ashamed. I thought something was wrong with me. Now I can enjoy it, because I feel it's okay to enjoy other women's bodies."
I fantasize making love with horses, because they are very sensuous animals, more so than cows or pigs. They are also very male animals—horse society is very chauvinist."

PAGE 43   Section entitled VIRGINITY—"I confined my sexual involvement to heavy petting, since the Catholic Church makes intercourse seem like such a sin. The day I left the Church was the day I had an argument in the confessional with the priest about whether having intercourse with my fiance was a sin. I maintained it wasn't; he said that I would never be a faithful wife if I had intercourse before marriage. He refused me absolution and I never came back."

PAGE 47   Section entitled SEX WITH OURSELVES: MASTURBATION—"It's exciting to make up sexual fantasies while masturbating or to masturbate when we feel those fantasies coming on. Some of us like to insert something while masturbating. Some of us find our— — — or other parts of our bodies erotically sensitive and rub them before or while — — —. Enjoying ourselves doesn't just mean our — — —. We are learning to enjoy all parts of our bodies."

"If you have never masturbated, we invite you to try."

"It's this letting go of control that enables us to have — — —. If you do not reach — — — when you first try masturbating, don't worry. Many of us didn't either. Simply enjoy the sensations you have. Try again some other time."

PAGE 49   "... sometimes I — — — to get away from the tightness and seriousness in myself."

PAGE 36   "Marijuana is rumored to be helpful. If your symptoms are relieved by the heaviest flow of your — — —, try to have an — — — or take a sauna or steam bath, all of which can speed up the flow considerably." Section entitled THE UTERINE CYCLE : MENSTRUATION.

PAGE 51   Section entitled THERE'S MORE THAN INTERCOURSE—"We can — — — and — — — our partner's — — — to — — — or as a part of lovemaking that later may include intercourse. This is called — — —. With our mouths and tongues we can experiment with ways to delight our partners and ourselves. The — — — can be stimulated with — — —. The — — — is highly sensitive to erotic stimulation. However, it is not as elastic as the — — —. Be gentle and careful and use a lubricant (saliva, — — — such as K-Y Jelly) if you have — — — the — — — within the — — —" Note: No medical warning regarding the danger of using foreign object (slender object)! ... "We can excite each other with *erotic pictures*, by sharing our fantasies, with the stimulation of a vibrator. Use your imagination. The possibilites are endless. For further suggestions see *The Joy of Sex* and *More Joy* edited by Alex Comfort." Editor's note: See *Washington Post* 9/10/77 - "Raymond Louis Urgo, a Georgetown hairdresser, convicted last June of involuntary manslaughter in the shooting death of his girlfriend at a sex and drug party at his apartment ... One psychiatrist testified yesterday Urgo possessed pornographic literature that gave him the idea of using his revolver—a 357 magnum—as a sexual stimulant by placing the gun's barrel in Miss Kisacky's mouth."

PAGE 113   "Not until we have an economic-social system that puts people before profit will everyone be able to participate."

PAGE 217   Section entitled HISTORY OF ABORTION LAWS AND PRAC-

TICE—"Last and perhaps more insidious, a highly moralistic group obsessed with banning 'sex for pleasure' struck up a campaign against both abortion and birth control."

PAGE 229 Photograph of girl having abortion in her street clothing and caption so notes the fact.

PAGE 233 Section discusses a COMPARISON OF SALINE AND PROSTA-GLANDIN ABORTIONS. Prostaglandin: "There is a likelihood that the fetus will be expelled with signs of life and not expire until shortly afterward—this is why the prostaglandin method is not often used beyond 20 weeks LMP"

PAGE 234 "With saline, the fetus is almost always dead. With prostaglandins the fetus often will show signs of life for a few minutes."

PAGE 243 Section entitled PARENTING IN A COMMUNE—"Communes are often attractive places for single or married parents to live in because child-rearing can be shared with others."

PAGE 353 Photograph—"The obstetrician-gynecologists' view of women."

Although this book is available at various places, we object to our tax dollars being used to provide this explicit, immoral information in our libraries and our schools. We are still "one nation under God."

Appendix C

COMMUNITY MENTAL HEALTH AND RAPE "THINGS TO THINK ABOUT"

1. Reassess your community.
2. What structure best suits your community?
   a. Feminist
   b. Hospital based
   c. Community based
   d. Combination of any of the above.
3. You can work with GLCMHC by coordination of:
   a. direct services
   b. consultation
   c. education
   d. training
   e. hot line
   f. space
   g. secretarial help
   h. information and referral
4. Why work with a mental health center
   a. longevity of service
   b. most # of victim served
   c. financial need
   d. coordination of services
5. Can you re-structure your Center without changing your philosophy?
6. If you don't integrate with a CMHC can you identify key consultants at the mental health center?
7. Why does a mental health center need grass-root groups?
   a. to fulfill their mandate to provide services to victims
   b. to fulfill their mandate of consultation and education

Preparing Young People for Responsible Sexual Parenting

Sol Gordon and Peter Scales

The dramatic changes that have occurred in American families during the past 25 years are accompanied by significant changes in how parents and children interact. "Increasingly, children in America are living and growing up in relative isolation from persons older or younger than themselves" (National Academy of Sciences, 1976, p. 39). Studies have indicated that children today are more dependent on their age-mates than children were a decade ago (Condry and Siman, 1974) and that "peer-oriented" children tend to be pessimistic about the future, measure lower in responsibility and leadership, and are more likely to commit illegal acts than "adult-oriented" children (Siman, 1973). Although there is a danger in the careless application of such labels, recent changes in the expressed values of American parents support the view that the pattern of decreased communication between parents and children is continuing. According to a national study of 1,230 families with children under 13, two-thirds of all parents agree that "parents should have lives of their own" even if this means spending less time with their children; and 46 percent of the "new breed" of parents (comprising 43 percent of the total sample) feel strongly that parents should not "sacrifice in order to give their children the best" (General Mills, 1977, p. 30).

In the midst of these value shifts, one of the key questions facing educators, researchers, and social planners is what kinds of families today's children will establish as adults. A parallel question is how society can best prepare young people today to successfully develop and maintain the family life they desire.

WHAT NEEDS TO BE DONE?

It does not suffice to blame the self-destructive behavior of youth on a "pathological" or "sick" society. Fixing blame in this way precludes a sense of individual responsibility for the kind of education provided for one generation by others. Lying, cheating, and stealing have almost become norms in the American culture of the 1970's. Perhaps these norms will be short-lived, but their pervasiveness in an economically ever-competitive world is undeniable. We need to recognize that adult Americans provide the models and the excuses for this kind of behavior. We create the need to cheat when we set up grades and teacher approval as the tickets to future success without providing the child with sufficient training and legitimate tools to achieve academic success. A 15-year study of one college's graduates suggests that "increasing scholastic aptitude in adolescence may be related to increasingly interpersonal immaturity in adulthood" (Fiske, 1977). For many young people, we create the need to steal not for profit but for sensation and attention. We create the need to lie when we ourselves are less than open about the issues that matter most.

What can be done to solve some of these problems? First, we need to redefine the values of the family. Despite the emergence of a new breed of parents whose personal lives may often be more important than spending time with their children, 68 percent of the new breed and 77 percent of the traditional parents in the General Mills study (1977) indicated that "strict, old-fashioned upbringing and discipline are still the best ways to raise children" (p. 80). It is precisely in this strict authoritarian family, however, that the likelihood of open communication is least likely to occur and, as a result, opportunities for parental caring, teaching, and involvement necessary to help children avoid some of the social problems discussed are also less likely to occur. We cannot have a return to the traditional family where the father alone was provider and the mother's lot was to bear and raise many children before she died: this would mean reverting to a scene which "often preoccupied itself with a grim struggle for survival [and] opposed the egalitarian strivings of both women and children, as well as those of men . . . [and where the father's] dominance more often than not created a wall between him and the rest of the family" (Gordon, 1975, p. 18).

Despite the professional talk about the death or demise of the family, and despite statistics showing an increase in both age at marriage and in the rate of divorce, Americans are the marrying kind. Over 90 percent will marry at some point, and most will have two children (Population Institute, 1977). Furthermore, four out of every five divorced adults remarry, half within four years (Everly, 1977). Therefore, the structure of the family as a basic social unit is not dead; but some of the values that ordered the traditional family are dying, lip service to the contrary notwithstanding. Gordon (1975) described the emergence of this more egalitarian family:

> For the first time in history, we are beginning to see glimmerings of the excitement, the joy, and the power of family life, based fundamentally on the fact that the husband and wife marry, not for political or economic reasons, but because they love each other. Women and men respect each other and if they decide to have children it is because they want them. They can spend time having fun together, and many are beginning to discover that religion is neither a burden nor a farce, but a faith, a ritual, and an affirmation of the spirit that brings joy, comfort, and relaxation to a hectic, complex life.
> Children are discussing their ideas with their parents, who no longer feel that the less their children know about sexuality and other "adult" pleasures, the safer they will be. Parents are communicating with their children, devoid of demands consisting entirely of "don'ts" with no rationale. (p. 19)

Unfortunately, this hopeful description is not yet typical of the communication between parents and children. In most families sex is the first communication block, the first evidence a child has that there are some things that cannot be discussed or can be talked about only under certain conditions. In their preoccupation with avoiding it, many adults have rendered sex vastly more important than most young people consider it to be. Seventy-seven percent of Sorensen's (1973) teenagers agreed that "some people I know are so much involved with sex that it's the most important thing in their lives"; but this should be considered along with the additional finding that, of 21 activities to be ranked in order of importance, sexual activities came near the bottom for both boys and girls. Most important for all adolescents were "having fun" and "learning about myself"; for 13- to 15-year-olds, "getting along with parents" was very important; for 16- to 19-year-olds, "becoming independent" and accomplishing "meaningful things" were primary goals.

PARENTS AND RESPONSIBLE SEXUALITY

Although Sorensen's study is marred by some methodological shortcomings, he did report provocative data. Nearly 40 percent of the 411 adolescents said they had not gotten to know their fathers, and one-fourth said they had not gotten to know their mothers. Is it any wonder that an estimated 577,500 youths between 10 and 17 ran away from home in 1975 (Opinion Research Corporation, 1976), or that children under 15 are the only age group that has recently shown an increase in admission rates to mental hospitals (Ford Foundation, 1977)? Sorensen (1973) found that many children only tell what they think parents want to hear, a finding supported by the General Mills (1977) study. Although young people who talk with their parents about sex and contraception tend to delay intercourse and to use contraception (Cahn, 1976; Furstenberg, 1971; Lewis, 1973; Miller and Simon, 1974; Shah, Zelnik, and Kantner, 1975), most young people do not talk with their parents about sex (see Scales, 1976) or about such other sensitive issues as death, money, family problems, and personal feelings (General Mills, 1977). When there is parent-child communication, it is likely to be moralistic and to stress prohibitions and behavioral restraints. It is a sad irony that studies consistently show that those who feel most guilty about their sexual feelings and behavior are also most likely to get pregnant (Hacker, 1976; Moore and Caldwell, 1976; Mosher, 1973).

The foundations for parent-child communication rests with communication between the parents themselves. How many children grow up believing that touching is only a prelude to sexual intercourse? That any demonstration of affection invariably leads to deep physical involvement? That their own parents rarely, if ever, are playfully affectionate with each other? How many children begin their own relationships thoroughly ignorant of how to communicate about sensitive issues because they have only caught furtive glimpses of how parents and other adults deal with important matters? How many have had their curiosity deflected with "words like 'when you're older' [that] must appease" them (Mitchell, 1974)?

Parents themselves need to be educated about sex before they can become more effective sex educators of their own children (Gordon, 1975). Although statistical change is just one measurement of a program's impact, we found in our own research that whereas mothers who took sex education programs did not increase their knowledge or become more liberal in their attitudes, they did benefit in several areas of reported communication about sex with their children. Fathers showed no such change—a predictable finding, since mothers in our society have traditionally taken the lead in caring for and responding to children. The extent to which these mothers reported change may have reflected a greater readiness to make practical use of what they learned (Institute for Family Research and Education, 1977a, 1977b; Scales and Everly, 1977).

HELPING PARENTS WITH SEX ROLES AND COMMUNICATION

We can help young people avoid destructive and irresponsible sexuality not only by becoming more approachable as parents, but also by helping them with difficult issues. How do young lovers communicate in the sexual situation and what are the different ways of communicating that lead to responsible and irresponsible sexual behavior? The discussion of such questions requires that adults accept young people as sexual beings. We cannot help youth make judgments about love and caring if they think our main intention is to keep them from having sex.

USING SCHOOLS AND OTHER COMMUNITY RESOURCES TO PROMOTE SOCIAL COMPETENCE

The schools can play a significant role in general education for life. Why should children who hate a particular subject and do poorly in it never be given the opportunity to take another course they have an interest in? It is a mistake to assume that all students need or want to learn the same skills at the same time, in the same order, and at the same pace. Schools might do well to rethink their notions of competence. Competence lies in the ability to approach life with a hopeful perspective, with an eye that has learned to see alternatives, a mind that can choose among options, to create visions of possibility. It is not necessary to abandon the goal of a literate and thoughtful society. With the freedom and cultivated ability to express visions may come the desire to learn the fundamental skills of information processing and expression, the same skills in which today's youth are becoming increasingly deficient.

For example, we need to help schools define their responsibilities in teaching about sex roles (Guttentag, 1977). Can the schools really afford to adopt a hands-off approach to the double standard and to other moral issues? Schools could take a moral stand by using texts and other nonsexist resources (cf. *Girls are Girls and Boys are Boys*, New York: John Day, 1974) to teach that women who define themselves only in terms of approval from men have little to contribute to any relationship. Schools also have a responsibility to teach that the principles of democratic freedom apply to choice of sexual life style as well as to work and family relations. The schools need to teach that even a majority vote cannot abrogate the fundamental rights of the handicapped and the retarded, or of sexual, ethnic, religious, and racial minorities. Democracy depends not on majority rule but on the preservation of the rights of those less numerous and powerful. What if the rights of blacks or, in earlier periods, those of Irish and Italian immigrants had been decided by the same process that resulted in Florida's 1977 disgraceful revoking of the rights of homosexuals to equal opportunity, including the opportunity to teach in the public schools?

❖   Sex education needs to be more broadly defined to reflect these principles. More important than how many schools teach sex education is the kind of education that is provided and the roles which schools, churches, and other community resources assume in preparing youth for a society based on choice. We as educators are often mocked because research has not demonstrated a correlation between sexual knowledge and responsible behavior. Other educators frequently and wrongly try to legitimize the view that sex education has no value. Without analyzing the reasons for their research results, they merely present the statistics that show sex education has a weak relationship to behavior. Yet, by neglecting to introduce broader concepts of the psychology of attraction, like and dislike, the meaning of different sex roles and the effect they have on communication, the place of women's liberation, the idea that readiness for parenting represents a total life outlook that needs to be re-examined and tested in relation to another person, we prevent young people from actively protecting their own and others' welfare. Comprehensive sex education which includes these elements is based on the beliefs articulated as part of our National Family Sex Education Week campaigns:* knowledge is not harmful, no one has a monopoly on morality, controversy is interesting and enhancing, not threatening.

Schools, however, are frequently oversensitive to extremist elements and are thus in too delicate a position to offer this degree of comprehensive sex education. Only six states and the District of Columbia mandate sex education of some type. Sixty percent of the districts in those states *exclude* the topic of birth control (Alan Guttmacher Institute, 1976). How can a school effectively help young people consider what it means to become a parent if it cannot teach them how to delay or avoid parenthood until such time as they freely choose it? Given the current restrictive climate of school sex education, it is doubtful that more thoughtful, eclectic approaches will soon characterize most public classrooms. A preparation for parenthood curriculum is, however, one suggested alternative (Gordon and Wollen, 1975).

MEDIA

One new approach to reducing sexism and ignorance has been to raise consciousness among media persons, including producers, performers, and the disc jockeys of rock music. The messages frequently contained in popular music communicate that having someone's baby is a great way to show your love, or that having sex with someone as soon as you meet is a great way to get to know each other. Efforts are being made, especially through the Population Institute's Rock Project, to promote the writing of responsible lyrics and to give less extensive airplay to records with sexist and irresponsible messages. Although this effort is greatly complicated by the enormous profits made by records promoting quick sex and pregnancy, it has generated interest and success throughout the country as a different way of reaching young people who "don't want to be preached at" (Population Institute,

*See Institute for Family Research and Education, *Impact Newsbriefs,* Syracuse, N.Y.: Ed-U Press, May 1977.

1977). Other new projects using the media have been developed by Chicago Planned Parenthood (a traveling theater group to reach youth on responsible sexuality), Oakland's Planned Parenthood (uses outreach to videotape teens talking about sex in their favorite hangouts and invite the teens to the clinic to see themselves on television and talk more about sex), and the Institute for Family Research and Education (a two-minute 16 mm film in which the boy gets pregnant and the girl tries to deny responsibility). (See Gordon and Scales, 1978, for more details on these and many other projects.)

GENERAL PRINCIPLES, TELEVISION, AND FREEDOM OF INFORMATION

In addition to using creative ways of communicating, we need to focus more on general psychological and social principles in educating youth. Drug abuse programs, for example, have often failed, not for want of money or professional input, but because responsible drinking is not the issue; boredom and loneliness are. We need to offer general guidance to people who are missing life's opportunities. This should include an understanding that all significant relationships and activities involve the risk of rejection or failure; if people like you only for sex, then they don't care for you very much.

Not only do we need to deal with crisis, we also need to provide techniques for the prevention of social ills. Runaway centers, alcohol treatment programs, and schools for pregnant girls are just a few examples of our orientation to crisis rather than prevention. We need to become more concerned about victims of crime and ignorance instead of glorifying what is criminal, irresponsible, and reckless. The decision of the Wisconsin judge that rape was a normal reaction to females' provocative clothing (*Chicago Tribune*, May 28, 1977) is as immoral as blaming child molestation on the seductiveness of a seven-year-old. Providing life competencies based on the general principles of choice and self-respect is the first step in reorienting our society to a concern with prevention of crime, ignorance, and social disillusionment. We need an atmosphere in which information and new ideas circulate freely without fear of censorship, so that old myths can be exposed and discarded.

For schools, this means encouraging new approaches to teaching basic skills. For parents, it means debunking the fancy interpretations of parent-child interaction. We have to teach parents that they do not have to be comfortable talking about everything related to sex in order to be good sex educators, that it is impossible to overstimulate a child with knowledge, that seeing parents have intercourse does not necessarily traumatize children or necessitate five years of psychoanalysis, that it is a myth girls who get pregnant "really wanted to" anyway. Girls get pregnant because they have had intercourse and/or they are stupid.

Most of all, we need to encourage and stimulate youthful curiosity. One way is to offer alternatives to television, the "plug-in drug" (Winn, 1977a). It is estimated that preschool children spend an average of 50 hours a week watching television and that, by the time children graduate from high school, they will have spent more time watching television than in any other activity except sleeping (Bronfenbrenner, 1976). Are the decreasing accomplishments of youth in scholastic activities really surprising when most of their formative years are spent in an experience that "permits so much intake while demanding so little outflow" (Winn, 1977b, p. 38)?

❖   People have the impression that young people today are well informed. They imagine that with all the sex education in the schools and all the sex on television and in other media the current generation of young people cannot help being informed. Critics of sex education imply that sex education in the schools encourages promiscuity. This is one of the great modern myths.

Many television programs commonly use themes of violence, sadomasochism, and rape. Advertisements are plainly designed to be sexually stimulating. But all of this is not responsible sex education. When is the last time you watched a mature, accurate program about sex education? The efforts of Norman Lear to present mature sexual themes in his situation comedies and programs like "My Mom's Having a Baby" (ABC) and "Guess Who's Pregnant" (PBS) are notable exceptions to an overwhelming onslaught of themes that demean sex.

A question of great concern to young people is whether or not they are "normal." Professionals have often encouraged a preoccupation with distinguishing normal from abnormal simply by reciting the often misleading statistics of research without explanation. To say that more and more teenagers are having sex at earlier ages is not enough. This is an accurate conclusion from the latest nationally representative study of teenage girls (Zelnik and Kantner, 1977), but it doesn't address the relationship between the partners, doesn't question whether they are enjoying and growing from the experience or whether it is a dreary and frightening initiation into adulthood. "By setting up familiarity with sex as an extremely important rite of passage without which one will forever remain a child, we tend to make it difficult for the average teenager to delay, to say no . . . (and so) encourage them to rush at an early age toward the image they have of the 'normal' teenager's sexual experience" (Gordon and Scales, 1977).

❖ CONCLUSIONS AND PRESCRIPTIONS FOR PREVENTION

Tomorrow's family will consist of a man and woman with comparable education, both of whom will work outside the home most of their adult lives and take turns staying home with their growing children. Right now, millions of women are working outside the home and returning to prepare meals, clean the house alone, and do all the other tasks implicit in the sexual double standard—and they are resenting it. We need to prepare youth for the new roles essential for tomorrow's family by eliminating this kind of prejudice and inequality.

Preparation is equally important for the liberation of men. Men would like to extend their life expectancies equal to those of their wives. They are tired of being diagnosed for having close relationships with other males, frustrated at watching their children grow up strangers. We need to prepare youth for the time when need, social compulsion, and sexual exclusivity will give way to the new words, to love, friendship, and priority.

We have overemphasized the importance of sex. In egalitarian relationships, the most important thing is not the pursuit of the ultimate, simultaneous, multiple orgasm. *The message we have for youth is that the real turn-on is getting to know and care about another person.* This, not sex, is the most important factor in a loving relationship. The second would be having a good sense of humor, followed by good conversations together. A satisfying sexual relationship would perhaps be ninth, and last would be cleaning the house together—cheerfully. For those who object that sex is so far down on the list, we say that of the 7,223 things important in relationships, sex is still in the top ten!

In developing a society of egalitarian families, we need to take the long view and teach young people that one's particular form of family life is precious only when it is freely chosen. When it is thrust upon people by others who have imposed their moral standards, it is utterly hateful:

At this time in the history of our earth there is no social need to press any individual into parenthood. We can free men and women alike to live as persons—to elect single blessedness, to choose companionship with a member of their own or the opposite sex, to decide to live a fully communal life, to bring up children of their own or to be actively solicitous of other people's children and the children of the future. In the process, those who elect marriage and parenthood as their own fullest expression of love and concern for human life also will be freed. For they will know that they have been free to choose, and have chosen each other and a way of life together. (Mead, 1976, p. 249)

NOTES

Note 1: Buder, J., Scales, P., and Sherman, L. "On becoming a non-virgin." Syracuse, N.Y., Institute for Family Research and Education. 1977, Unpublished data.

Note 2: Gordon, S., and Scales, P. Sexual communication among college undergraduates. Syracuse, N.Y., Institute for Family Research and Education. 1977, Unpublished data.

REFERENCES

Alan Guttmacher Institute. *11 million teenagers.* New York: Planned Parenthood, 1976.

Baldwin, W. H. Adolescent pregnancy and childbearing—growing concerns for Americans. *Population Bulletin*, 1976, *31*, entire issue.

Bane, M. J. Children, divorce, and welfare. *The Wilson Quarterly*, 1977, *1*, 89–94.

Bronfenbrenner, U. The disturbing changes in the American family. *Search*, 1976, *4*, 4-10.

Cahn, J. *Adolescents' needs regarding family planning services.* Paper presented at World Population Society Conference, Washington, D.C., November 19-21, 1975.

Clinch, T. A. The great comic book controversy. In S. Gordon and R. W. Libby (Eds.) *Sexuality today and tomorrow.* North Scituate, MA: Duxbury, 1976, 124-133.

Condry, J. C., and Siman, M. A. Characteristics of peer- and adult-oriented children. *Journal of Marriage and the Family*, 1974, *36*, 543-554.

Donovan, P. Student newspapers and the first amendment: Their right to publish sex-related articles. *Family Planning/Population Reporter*, 1977, *6*, 16-17, 23.

Everly, K. New directions in divorce research. *Journal of Clinical Child Psychology*, 1977, in press.

Fiske, E. B. High marks seen as no guarantee of later success. *The New York Times*, June 5, 1977, p. 19.

Ford Foundation. Growing up forgotten. *Ford Foundation Letter*, 1977, *8*, 1.

Furstenberg, F. F. *Unplanned parenthood: The social consequences of teenage childbearing.* New York: Free Press, 1976.

Furstenberg, F. F. Birth control experience among pregnant adolescents: The process of unplanned parenthood. *Social Problems*, 1971, *19*, 199-203.

General Mills Incorporated. *Raising children in a changing society.* Minneapolis: General Mills, Inc., 1977.

Glick, P. C. Some recent changes in American families. *Current Population Reports*, 1975, Series P-23, No. 52.

Gordon, S. *If you loved me, you would . . .* New York: Bantam, 1978.

Gordon, S. *Let's make sex a household word.* New York: John Day, 1975.

Gordon, S. The egalitarian family is alive and well. *The Humanist*, 1975, *35*, 18-19.

Gordon, S., and Conant, R. *You—A survival guide for youth.* New York: Quadrangle, 1975.

Gordon, S., and Scales, P. The myth of the normal outlet. *Journal of Pediatric Psychology*, 1977, *3*, 101-103.

Gordon, S., and Scales, P. *The sexual adolescent.* North Scituate, MA: Duxbury, 1978.

Gordon, S., and Wollen, M. *Parenting: A guide for young people.* New York: Oxford Book Co., 1975.

Guttentag, M. The prevention of sexism in primary prevention of psychopathology. In G. W. Albee and J. M. Joffe (Eds.), *Primary Prevention of Psychopathology.* Vol. 1. Hanover, N.H.: University Press of New England, 1977.

Hacker, S. *The effect of situational and interactional aspects of sexual encounters on premarital contraceptive behavior.* Ann Arbor, MI: University of Michigan, School of Public Health, Department of Population Planning, 1976.

Institute for Family Research and Education. *A training manual for organizers of sex education programs for parents.* Syracuse, NY: Ed-U Press, 1977. (a)

Institute for Family Research and Education. *Final report: A community family life education program for parents.* Syracuse, NY: 760 Ostrom Avenue, 1977. (b)

Institute for Juvenile Research. *Juvenile delinquency in Illinois, highlights oj the 1972 adolescent survey.* Chicago: Institute for Juvenile Research, 1972.

Judge blames rape on sexy clothes. *Chicago Tribune.* May 28, 1977, p. 6.

Lelyveld, J. Drive-in day care. *The New York Times Magazine,* June 5, 1977, p. 110.

Levinger, G. Where is the family going? *The Wilson Quarterly,* 1977, *1,* 95–102.

Lewis, R. A. Parents and peers: socialization agents in the coital behavior of young adults. *Journal of Sex Research,* 1973, *9,* 156–170.

Mathias, C. Senate bill no. 1–Jobs for youth. *Parade,* March 6, 1977, 6–7.

Mead, M. Bisexuality: What's it all about. In S. Gordon and R. W. Libby (Eds.), *Sexuality today–and tomorrow.* North Scituate, MA: Duxbury, 1976, 245–249.

Menken, J. *The health and demographic consequences of adolescent pregnancy and childbearing.* Paper presented at National Institute of Child and Human Development, Conference on the Consequences of Adolescent Pregnancy and Childbearing, Rockville, Maryland, October 1975.

Miller, P. Y., and Simon, W. Adolescent sexual behavior: context and change. *Social Problems,* 1974, *22,* 58–76.

Miner, M. Research firm identifies the new lost generation. *Chicago Suntimes,* May 9, 1977, p. 65.

Mitchell, J. *The circle game.* New York: Siquomb Publishing Co., 1974 Asylum Records.

Molinoff, D. D. Life with father. *The New York Times Magazine,* May 22, 1977, pp. 12–17.

Moore, K., and Caldwell, S. *Out of wedlock pregnancy and childbearing.* Washington, D.C.: The Urban Institute, 1976 (Working Paper 992-02).

Mosher, D. L. Sex differences, sex experience, sex guilt, and explicitly sexual films. *Journal of Social Issues,* 1973, *29,* 95–112.

National Academy of Sciences. *Toward a national policy for children and families.* Washington, D.C.: National Academy of Sciences, 1976.

National Alliance Concerned with School-Age Parents. Young parents: Special problems. *NACSAP Newsletter,* 1977, *5,* 12–13.

National Assessment of Educational Progress. *Education for citizenship: A bicentennial survey.* Denver: National Assessment, 1976 (Report No. 17-CS-01).

National Center for Health Statistics. Advance report, final natality statistics 1975. *Monthly Vital Statistics Report,* 1976, *25,* (Supp., HRA 77-1120).

Opinion Research Corporation. Runaway incidence ascertained. *University Newsletter,* July 1976 (Princeton, New Jersey).

Pike, A. R. Turning the menace into magic. *Parents' Magazine*, 1977, *52*, 39ff.

Population Institute. Focus: All in the family. *Population Issues*, March/April 1977, p. 1.

Population Institute. *Pregnant pause*. March 1977, Issue No. 3.

Prescott, J. W. Abortion or the unwanted child. *The Humanist*, March 1975, pp. 11-15.

Ross, H. L., and Sawhill, I. V. The family as economic unit. *The Wilson Quarterly*, 1977, *1*, 84-88.

Scales, P. *A quasi-experimental evaluation of sex education programs for parents*. Unpublished doctoral dissertation, Syracuse University, 1976.

Scales, P. Males and morals: Teenage contraceptive behavior amid the double standard. *Family Coordinator*, 1977, *26*, 211-222.

Scales, P., and Everly, K. A community sex education program for parents. *Family Coordinator*, 1977, *26*, 37-45.

Scales, P., and Gordon, S. The effects of sex education. In S. Gordon and P. Scales, *The sexual adolescent*. North Scituate, MA: Duxbury, 1978.

Shah, F., Zelnik, M., and Kantner, J. F. Unprotected intercourse among unwed teenagers. *Family Planning Perspectives*, 1975, *7*, 39-44.

Shellenberger, J. A. Today's teenagers have no heroes; are not against marriage, college or family influence. New York: Anna M. Rosenberg Associates, 444 Madison Avenue. *Press Release*, 1975.

Siman, M. A. *Peer group influence during adolescence: A study of 41 naturally existing friendship groups*. Unpublished doctoral dissertation, Cornell University, 1973.

Sorenson, R. C. *Adolescent sexuality in contemporary America*. New York: World, 1973.

Study finds drinking—often to excess—now starts at earlier age. *The New York Times*, March 27, 1977, p. 38.

Syntex Laboratories. An in-depth look at the male role in family planning. *The Family Planner*, 1977, *8*, 4.

Teevan, J. J. Reference groups and premarital sexual behavior. *Journal of Marriage and the Family*, 1972, *34*, 283-291.

United States Bureau of the Census. *Status: A monthly chartbook of social and economic trends*. Washington, D.C.: Bureau of the Census, October 1976.

United States Commission on Population Growth and the American Future. *Population growth and the American future*. New York: New American Library, 1972.

What the statistics show. *The Wilson Quarterly*, 1977, *1*, 76-83.

Winfrey, C. Week without television tunes several families into different channels. *The New York Times*, June 5, 1977, pp. 37, 42.

Winn, M. *The plug-in drug*. New York: Viking Press, 1977. (a)

Winn, M. The hazards of the plug-in drug. *Parents' Magazine*, 1977, *52*, 38ff. (b)

Zelnik, M., and Kantner, J. F. Sexual and contraceptive experience of young unmarried women in the United States, 1976 and 1971. *Family Planning Perspectives*, 1977, *9*, 55-73.

Prevention of Psychopathology of Blacks

Thomas O. Hilliard

Those who profess to favor freedom and yet deprecate agitation are men who want crops without plowing up the ground, they want rain without thunder and lightning. They want the ocean without the awful roar of its waters.

—*Frederick Douglass*

An effort should be made to attenuate the viciousness of a system of which the doctrinal foundations are a daily defiance of an authentically human outlook. . . . The function of a social structure is to set up institutions to serve man's needs. A society that drives its members to desperate solutions is a non-viable society, a society to be replaced.

—*Franz Fanon*

The colonial condition cannot be adjusted to: like an iron collar, it can only be broken.

—*Albert Memmi*

❖   The subject matter of the present paper—the role of political and social action in preventive mental health and the discipline of Black psychology—reflects an interface of two fields, in each of which the ignorance would seem to far exceed the understanding of the phenomenon in American psychology. Nevertheless, the present paper is focused on a beginning or preliminary formulation of prevention theory and intervention with Blacks and, by implication, other oppressed people. However, in my opinion, it is not feasible to formulate effective social or political intervention strategies without an implicit or explicit conception of the dynamics and development or etiology of the dysfunction. The relationship between a theory of psychopathology and the corresponding intervention is crucial. For instance, if you conceptualize the cause of psychological disorder in Blacks as resulting from the lack of congruence between ideal/self perceptions, then techniques such as clarification and reflection of feelings are appropriate therapeutic responses; or if you adopt a more psychoanalytic notion involving neurotic defenses organized around the repression of sex and aggression impulses stemming from unresolved oedipal conflicts, then therapeutic strategies such as the interpretation of defenses and conflicts, and the manipulation of transference relationships are logical sequelae.

❖   In striking contrast to the void in most prevailing theories of personality, psychopathology, or psychotherapy, clinicians who work with personal problems of Blacks, particularly low-income clients, are acutely aware of the failings of the social system and its contribution to the stress and psychopathology of Black people. Similarly, another important source of contemporary work on mental health relevant to Blacks and other oppressed people is the cross-cultural work of Franz Fanon (1963, 1967), Albert Memmi (1965), and Joseph Howard III (1972), who have written poignantly about the "social psychology of colonialism." Each has described the social processes of colonialism as a form of oppression and the impact of its social processes on colonized or oppressed people.

Thus my attention will focus on problems or impediments to an appropriate frame of reference for Black psychology, my conception of a preliminary conceptual framework for Black psychology, and an identification of the political and social action implications that flow from such a "world view."

The overriding point of view of this paper, based on my clinical experiences and personal observations, is that the nature and cause of severe Black dysfunctions, particularly with low-income people, stem less from psychogenic factors and more from political and social oppression, although psychogenic explanations and political/economic analyses need not operate independently of each other. Despite the considerable controversy over the role and potency of political/economic and psychogenic explanations, the issue seems not to be a choice between psychogenic and political/economic variables, since in many cases, both classes of variables operate, and in fact, interact. The critical issue, from the point of view of mental health strategy, may be at what point or level should the intervention be directed. Nevertheless, the focus of the present social analysis is on the properties of the social order or social system and its relationship to human suffering, pain, and dysfunction. This social analysis need not discount the role of the family in child development, nor does it assume that all faulty child-rearing practices or other deleterious experiences can be attributed to the sociopolitical conditions. Rather, in my opinion, it demonstrates the substantial explanatory potency of a sociopolitical perspective that operates in conjunction with an analysis of individuals. The importance of a sociopolitical perspective is reflected in the recurrence of studies, based on an ecological model, which consistently demonstrate socioeconomic correlates of the incidence and prevalence of severe psychopathology (Faris and Dunham, 1939; Hollingshead and Redlich, 1958; Langer and Michael, 1963; Srole, Langer, Michael and Rennie, 1962), rates of chronic alcoholism (Faris and Dunham, 1939; Harper, 1976), and drug addiction (Drug Abuse Survey Project, 1972). In addition, there are countless other works that describe the role of racism, poverty, and other forms of sociopolitical oppression on the quality of life of Blacks in this country (Willie, Kramer, and Brown, 1973; Jones, 1972).

Nevertheless, despite the obvious association between poverty and racism and the psychological functioning of Blacks, there has been only a limited amount of work on oppression and its role in the development, precipitation, and maintenance of psychopathology. In fact, when discussions of the role of political and economic phenomena are approached, they are disguised by the use of euphemistic and more palatable terminology that refers to "disadvantaged populations," "inner city problems," and "cultural deprivation." The prominence of such terminology as a replacement for a more appropriate delineation of the details of the oppressive experiences is more than semantic. Rather, such confused terminology avoids depicting the core causes of social problems and in fact distorts the reality of Black life. This jargon or terminology shifts the cause of the problem from societal conditions to properties or traits of the "casualties" or "victims."

The "scholarly" treatment of the Black family by behavioral scientists represents a prime example of how victims and their institutions and milieus are viewed as the causes of their own problems. Scientific studies, from this vantage point, provide an endless recitation of data and statistics to describe the deteriorating family structure, high crime rates, number of welfare recipients, problems of illegitimacy, and so forth. This proclivity to focus almost exclusively on social pathology of Blacks caused Benjamin Quarles (1967), a Black historian, to note:

When we pick up a social science book, we look in the index under "Negro," it will read "see slavery," "see crime," "see juvenile delinquency," perhaps "see Commission on Civil Disorders"; perhaps see anything except the Negro. So when we try to get a perspective on the Negro, we get a distorted perspective. (p. 29)

The classic example of this social orientation is the so-called "tangle of pathology" thesis by Moynihan (1965), which utilizes correlational data to infer that there are causal relationships between the instability of the Black family and the social conditions of Blacks. Although paying "lip service" to the relationship of oppression to the social pathology in Black communities, this view implies that a kind of "culture of poverty" occurs in which certain destructive aspects of poverty become self-perpetuating and, in a sense, are functionally autonomous of external forces that spawned them and have a momentum of their own. Similarly, Albert Memmi (1965), in his study of colonialism in North Africa, describes the "mythical portrait of the colonized" which distorts the characteristics of the colonized and thereby provides rationalizations for the continued existence of colonialism as a system of oppression. More recently, William Ryan's *Blaming the Victim* (1971) provides a systematic explication of the nature and role of "victim analysis" in American thought. He concludes that "the logical outcome of an analysis of social problems in terms of the deficiencies of the victims is the development of programs aimed at correcting these deficiencies" (p. 4). For instance, the present emphasis on child abuse and neglect has been criticized for its almost exclusive emphasis on parental abuse without a corresponding concern with eliminating institutional or other forms of child abuse (Gil, 1971; Hilliard, 1978a). Thus, this myopic view of social problems causes a critical defect in the philosophy, content, and objectives of intervention programs.

Impediments to an Appropriate Conceptual Framework for Black Behavior

Assuming the appropriateness of a theoretical perspective that includes political and economic phenomena for Black psychology, some of the major impediments to such a view are the following:

1. AN OVEREMPHASIS ON PSYCHOGENIC/PSYCHODYNAMIC EXPLANATIONS OF BEHAVIOR

Consistent with the nature of education and training in mental health, and the attendant compartmentalization of the study of human behavior, prevailing mental health theory and practice have maintained a narrow psychogenic orientation, which excludes political phenomena. Thus mental health professionals have relied almost exclusively on variables such as self-concept, ego strength, impulse control, locus of control, passivity, the nature and adequacy of defense mechanisms as explanations for Black behavior. Joseph Howard (1972), for instance, in criticizing the apolitical orientation of mental health, noted the failure of traditional theories of dreams, dream symbolism, and dream interpretation, with their overemphasis on latent libidinal impulses, to account for the political content of dreams of oppressed people, particularly activists. As an example, he reports a dream of a Black college student in psychotherapy, at a large midwestern university during the campus protests and student rebellions in the 1960s, who was grappling with identity issues as a Black in a predominantly White university. The following scenario unfolds in her dream. In therapy the student recalled being enclosed in an all white mass or tent, of trying vainly to escape from the tent and, yet, of being afraid of breaking out. Finally, after considerable vacillation and anxiety, she burst her way out of the white mass that surrounded and engulfed her. As she burst out of the white mass, she recalls that the first things that she saw were the colors red, black, and green. She then woke up. Obviously, these colors must be interpreted as representing the liberation colors of Marcus Garvey and symbolizing her assertiveness and personal liberation as a Black.

Another political limitation in clinical theory is reflected in the psychodynamic treatment of "superego" issues focusing narrowly on morality associated with sexual and aggressive impulses. However, few theorists describe the "political superego" or morality issues that are associated with group identification and system challenging or other political behavior presented by young Black and other minority clients.

More broadly, there is a paucity of work that systematically assesses the relationship between the sociopolitical system, situational stresses, and the resulting personality issues. An exception is *The Politics of Therapy* by Seymour Halleck (1971), which outlines how political phenomena impact on personality and the consequences for psychotherapeutic intervention.

2. LIMITATIONS OF THE CLINICAL ROLE

Psychiatry and the other traditional mental health fields that followed and emulated its tradition started as service oriented approaches with the responsibility for ministering to the problems of individuals. Thus, the focus of the therapy has been the intrapsychological deficiencies of "sick" individuals. This model, largely for practical reasons, has implicitly discounted or minimized other variables that are perceived as inessential to the treatment process. In its most traditional form, it has been widely criticized as an adjustment model, designed to preserve the status quo. In fact, some accounts have suggested that the community mental health system is designed to reduce social conflict (Kenniston, 1968), a role similar to that of the social welfare system in relation to unemployment (Piven and Cloward, 1971). Thus, as an ancillary and supportive service model dealing only peripherally with core issues such as the structure of society, the nature and role of economic resources, the relationship of political power on human relationships, etc., its perspective on human development has been quite limited.

The limitations of the clinical role and its perspective are reflected in the following statements espoused by a former president of the American

Psychiatric Association regarding the social role of organized mental health.

It is my opinion that psychiatric services should not be the tool for restructuring society or solving economic problems or for determining new human values. Psychiatric services should be continued as patient oriented activities designed to reduce pain and discomfort and to increase the capacity of the individual to adjust satisfactorily. . . . The purpose of community mental health centers was originally directed toward the prevention of psychiatric disorders and treatment in the community familiar to the patient. Any attempt to dilute or divert the activity of the community mental health center into a non-medical social agency or a political instrument is extremely detrimental to achieving the primary objective of providing adequate psychiatric services for all citizens. (Halleck, 1971, p. 11)

Similarly, Halleck (1971) stated, in response to political activism at a national professional conference:

I would be remiss in my convictions if I did not raise a strong protest to this sort of thing. We are psychiatrists and as such are physicians whose entire level of competency has to do with emotional and mental disorders. . . . Nor do we by virtue of being psychiatrists have any more basis for opinions in the area of politics than would a garbage collector, policeman, lawyer or secretary. Again, it seems to me that our only area of competency is in the framework of medical practice, not social work or social theorizing. (p. 12)

Although these views may be dismissed as representing an extreme position on the social role of the mental health professional, they reflect, in my opinion, a widespread point of view among mental health professionals.

3. PERSONAL FEARS ASSOCIATED WITH CHALLENGING THE POLITICAL AND ECONOMIC SYSTEM

In addition to the influence of intellectual or cognitive determinants on the conceptual frameworks and intervention strategies in mental health, there are, in my opinion, powerful psychological or motivational factors that impede a proper analysis of the basic political and economic issues that underlie mental health issues. In fact, at times the limited perspective of mental health professionals that fails to acknowledge the role of social and political oppression is merely a device or "security operation" to avoid the confrontations and personal dilemmas associated with a social change role. The proclivity to focus almost exclusively on intrapsychic phenomena results, at times, from what I term a "flight into psychogenics." Essentially, this mechanism is interpreted as avoidance behavior designed to reduce anxiety and minimize the impending personal and moral dilemmas. Another mechanism utilized to cope with the fears and insecurities and, in fact, the existential dilemmas associated with confrontations with societal institutions has been referred to by the Reverend Jessie Jackson as "the paralysis of analysis," an obsessive compulsive defense. The essential feature of this mechanism is the incessant need to collect more data in order to achieve "scientific certainty" about causes before any actions or interventions can be initiated. Again the purpose of this security maneuver is to immobilize and to prevent any action.

Toward a Frame of Reference for Black Psychology

In an attempt not merely to criticize the prevailing efforts at conceptualizing the behaviors of Blacks, I will outline what are some of the core principles that may serve as the foundation of a conceptual framework for Black psychology. Although this frame of reference was designed to understand Black behavior, it would seem to be especially applicable to preventive mental health issues with Black people (Butler et al., 1979). Black psychology, according to this view, may be characterized by the following principles or guidelines.

1. A set of philosophical assumptions that provide a basis for defining a value system that is consistent with the essential nature of Black people and, as such, is consistent with the goal of "liberating" the Black mind.
2. A historical perspective that encompasses both the African heritage of Blacks and our unique experiences in this country.
3. A political/economic perspective that permits considerations of the relationship between the modal behavior of contemporary Blacks and the economic and power dynamics of White society.
4. A broad social/psychological view that facilitates the examination of the role of social institutions in determining Black behavior patterns.

Philosophical/Theoretical Assumptions

During the reexamination of formulations and approaches regarding Blacks, substantial attention is being directed to questions about the validity and appropriateness of the philosophy and the assumptions inherent in the psychological theories and approaches (Butler et al., 1979; King, 1975). At the center of these concerns is the belief that psychological theories reflect the value orientations, cultural perspective, and "world view" of the theorist and that these are responsible for the development of the theories. As an example, recent revelations about the major proponents of the IQ testing movement suggest that political ideologies may greatly influence ideas and theories that may have the trappings of scientifically based conclusions. Yet, these theoretical assumptions and philosophical premises may have far-reaching implications. As Butler et al.

(1979) state, in reference to assumptions underlying a discipline:

The nature of these assumptions is critical, for the fundamental premises in which a discipline is grounded determine both the goals and methodologies that the discipline will embrace. . . . Moreover, these premises also delimit the legitimate area of study, the kind of data that will be accepted as valid, and the kinds of principles that will be invoked to explain phenomena of interest. (p. 4)

Although systematic scrutiny of the assumptions and value orientation inherent in American psychology and, indeed, in Western science has only recently begun, there are several concepts that might appropriately serve as good starting points for review. For instance, a major thrust of American psychology has been guided by the notion of "the psychology of individual differences." From this point of view, the superordinate objective of psychological inquiry has been to detect the underlying differences between people or to identify their distinguishing or unique attributes in domains such as intellectual functioning, personality, interests, etc. (that are presumed to exist). But, it would seem that assumptions and related procedures of American psychology are set up to manufacture the expected differences between people. The technology of testing represents perhaps one of the best examples of how "the presumption of individual differences" dictates the approaches that provide data to further support it. For instance, in item analysis related to test development, items are deliberately selected to differentiate between people (confirming preexisting beliefs). Test items that do not differentiate are rejected. This practice and the underlying theory place, in fact, a value on human diversity and differences, and at the same time devalue human commonality.

A corollary concept that seems to provide support for the psychology of individual differences is the normal distribution curve. In fact, although the normal distribution curve is presented as a neutral or value-free concept, it has major political and economic implications. Essentially implicit in the theoretical bell-shaped curve in which the majority of people cluster in the center, with a small percentage at each end of the curve, is a hierarchical social arrangement that influences the distribution of resources and opportunities. One of the most blatant examples of its use to order society is in the use of the normal distribution curve as the basis for distributing grades in educational settings (that is, grading on the curves). In other situations, the "curve" determines the relative place of individuals in terms of a given attribute. For instance, often the "intellectually gifted" in public education are determined not by qualitative features of intellectual performance, but by their relative position on the theoretical normal distribution curve (that is, the top 5 percent on IQ).

Nobles (1972) has similarly criticized the theoretical limitation inherent in western definitions of "self" for the emphasis on the "i" rather than the "we" as reflective of a more individualistic orientation. In contrast, he describes the extended self-concept—or the "we"—as reflecting a more collective orientation, which he sees as more compatible with the ethos of African people.

In summary, the view expressed is that in order to develop a psychology appropriate for the study of Blacks, the underlying philosophical and theoretical premises must be compatible with the nature and social condition of Black people. The assumption and approaches of scientific inquiry must likewise be reexamined in order to insure their appropriateness.

HISTORICAL ANALYSIS

An axiomatic principle of psychology is the notion that in addition to the role of contemporary forces, human behavior is shaped by prior experiences and events. In fact, a historical perspective is as essential to an understanding of a people as a longitudinal developmental analysis is to the understanding of individual Blacks. Yet psychologists have traditionally ignored the historical context within which Black behavior is situated, which would provide critical information and data relative to Blacks and Whites. A proper historical analysis, while outlining the critical and potent role of slavery in determining contemporary Black behavior, must involve a treatment of African history prior to slavery in the United States. Clark (1972) criticizes others' objections to the study of Black historical events as having happened "too long ago" to have contemporary relevance. Nevertheless, a number of accounts have identified, for instance, African retentions in the language patterns of Blacks in the United States (Turner, 1949; Smith, 1978), while others have described the philosophical and religious orientation and patterns of family life as African in origin (Nobles, 1972, 1974).

Numerous other historical accounts have described in great detail the brutalizing nature of slavery and racism and its impact on individual Blacks and institutions. In fact, Nobles (1977), in *A Formative and Empirical Study of Black Families: Final Report,* found that the second most prevalent theme of stories that the Black families reported being told by their parents as children was the impact of slavery on the ancestors of Black people. This empirical study, then, provides quantitative documentation of the saliency of memories of slavery in the present.

A companion clinical study that similarly points out the force of historical experiences in influencing contemporary Black behaviors examined the military trials of the Black Marines involved in confrontations with the White Marines who were self-avowed Ku Klux Klansmen (Hilliard, 1978b). Using extensive clinical data from examinations of the Black defendants, 10 of the 14 of whom were from the deep South, a "collective consciousness" of Blacks was identified, which was amplified by the Black Marines' own personal experiences of racism and bigotry in growing up and in the military. These unique historical and cultural factors that Blacks share as a group combined with situational and personal factors to determine their response. Again, these studies suggest the need to examine historical factors systematically in order to understand the behavior of Blacks.

POLITICAL/ECONOMIC PERSPECTIVE

As stated previously, there is a particular need to delineate the relationship between Black psychology and political/economic variables. Perhaps, the clearest example of the relationship between political and economic factors and the psychology of Black people is reflected in the history of slavery. That is, slavery in America provides one of the best examples of how an entire society and its institutional practices, including religious, educational, and legal institutions, worked conjointly to support the subjugation of Black people for economic gain. Winthrop Jordan (1968) traces in elaborate detail the changes in attitudes, and the development of well articulated anti-Negro attitudes, as the need for slave labor increased. Similarly, Higgenbotham (1978) describes the process of developing legal doctrine to justify and ensure an effective subjugation of Blacks. These and other studies of slavery in the United States provide a political/economic basis to the development of racism, rather than basing it on primarily psychological motivation. At times, the misreading of the history of slavery has caused the misconception that slavery was as Rhodes and Montrero (1968) state, a relationship "between individual slaves and slaveowners rather than essentially social relations between metropolitan White society and colonial Black society in which the rapid development of the former society occasioned the veritable destruction of the other." Franz Fanon, in his study of colonialism and oppression, has warned that racism should not be considered as an individual trait or "quirk," but rather as the most visible sign of a more systemized oppression. In describing the psychological consequences of this "organized domination," Fanon (1967) states:

The social group, militarily and economically subjugated, is dehumanized in accordance with a polydimensional method. Exploitations, tortures, raids, racism, collective liquidation, rational oppression take turns at different levels to make of the native an object. . . . Because no other solution is left, the racialized group tries to imitate the oppressor and thereby tries to deracialize itself. (p. 35)

Although the writings of Franz Fanon and Albert Memmi draw on their experiences in more well-defined colonial situations in Africa, both writers were well aware of the parallels between the colonial situations and the social conditions of Blacks in the United States.

A more recent body of studies suggests a continuation of direct relationships between political and economic variables and Black psychology, and indeed, Black psychopathology. For instance, Brenner in his book, *Mental Illness and the Economy* (1973), provides empirical data to demonstrate the relationship between the economy and the rate of mental illness. Using admission rates to mental hospitals in New York State as the measure of mental illness, he examines the effect of periods of economic instability, such as the Great Depression in the 1930s and recessions on the incidence of major mental illness. Brenner concludes, in contradiction to previous studies of the relationship of the Great Depression to mental illness by Komora and Clark (1935) and Pollocks (1935), that there is an inverse relationship between the state of the economy and mental illness, which has been stable over the past 127 years.

Brenner's analysis is in agreement with the research of Dohrenwend (1973) on the relationship of social status—or more appropriately, socioeconomic positions—to exposure to stressful life events. Not surprisingly, her research, which indicates that low social status groups experience more stressful life events such as death in the family, marital breakdown, job loss, etc., is consistent with the research of Brown and Birley (1968) on the relationship of stressful events to the presence of schizophrenia, and severe depression, respectively. This study by Dohrenwend (1973) further suggests that Blacks have more exposure to stressful life events than ethnic groups with higher social status.

The foregoing studies strongly suggest the relationship between economic, political and social stresses, and psychopathology, particularly among poor people. The impact of these stresses may be experienced directly by individuals or more directly through undermining or destroying basic social institutions that are responsible for Black development, survival, or support. For instance, variables such as limited economic resources, underemployment, or unemployment, poor housing conditions, meager health and nutritional resources may have a direct impact on the mental health of individuals or groups. However, in addition, political and economic stresses that have an indirect but deleterious influence on primary social institutions such as the family, education, and mass media may be more insidious. Frequently, in fact, social policies are espoused, such as the "best interests of children" or "the least detrimental alternative," which profess commitment to the quality of life of children, without a corresponding emphasis on strengthening the basic social institutions responsible for their nurture and development.

SOCIAL-PSYCHOLOGICAL PERSPECTIVE

A critical aspect of a broad social-psychological perspective in conceptualizing Black psychology is the role of the major social institutions or
agents of socialization. Traditionally, the responsibility for socialization
of the young has been delegated to institutions such as the family, religion, and education. These institutions have provided permanence and
continuity for cultural traditions, mores, norms, and values. At an individual level these institutions have been major determinants of identity,
morality, beliefs, attitudes, political awareness, and so forth, and thus, in
a real sense, influence personal and personality development. However,
although these institutions retain a major responsibility for Black child
development, in recent years there has been an apparent rearrangement
of the role and potency of the various social institutions in relationship to
Blacks. These major changes in social institutions, which have had the
net effect of reducing the control of the Black community, particularly
the Black family, over the socialization process of children, include the
following:

1. The reduction in the role and influence of religion
2. The diminished role of the Black community in policy decisions in
   public schools largely due to the nature of implementation of desegregation in public education
3. The ascendance of the mass media, particularly television, as a major
   social institution

Although recognizing the role of the Black family in socialization, and
to a lesser extent religion, the focus of this section is primarily on providing a very brief overview of the role of education and the mass media.
The rationale underlying this emphasis reflects the belief that in a mechanistic and technologically oriented society, these institutions, over which
the Black community has minimal influence, have usurped much of the
traditional role of the family in socialization.

The role of education as a social institution is critical at every level for
its role is far greater than merely providing technical skills, it also has a
major role in transmitting a cultural perspective. As Maulana Ron Karenga (1969) stated: "Education . . . is basically a political thing and it
provides identity, purpose, and direction within an American context"
(p. 39). This cultural perspective is reflected in curriculum content, books
and materials, formal and informal communications by staff, and the role
modeling that occurs in relationship to the major personnel that staff the
schools. The educational literature contains voluminous evidence of the
deleterious consequences of American education for Black children. In

commenting on the widespread devaluation of Blacks that occurs in public schools, Butler et al. (1979) warn:

Public schools have traditionally made use of content and practices that rob children of self-esteem and encourage an identification with White mainstream culture and a rejection of Black culture. For example, until recently, primary education programs generally exposed children to readers and fictional literature that contained exclusively White characters acting in predominantly middle-class milieus. Moreover, children's books . . . such as "The Hardy Boys," "The Bobbsey Twins" and "Tom Sawyer" consistently depicted Blacks as lazy, ignorant, and subservient to Whites, and consistently referred to Blacks . . . as "niggers," "darkies" and "coons." (p. 16)

The devaluation of Black children that is experienced in educational institutions ranges from a general contempt toward Black culture and experiences, abuses of standardized testing that culminate in the disproportionate and inappropriate assignments of Blacks to lower tracks, to overt racism. Obviously, the negative impact of these experiences, which have increased with the widespread removal and demotion of Black administrators under current desegregation practices, have major implications for the mental health of Black children.

During the post-1950s period, the mass media—particularly television—have demonstrated a substantial increase in potency as a social institution. The powerful role that television has in the shaping of the informational base and world view, as well as attitudes, beliefs, and identity, particularly of Black children, has been supported by research data. Several studies have concluded that:

1. Black children spend a disproportionate amount of time watching television, in comparison to their White counterparts (Bogart, 1962; Greenberg and Dominick, 1969).
2. In general, the total time spent by Black children watching television is greater than time spent in classrooms (Greenberg and Atkin, 1978).
3. There is a substantial belief by children that what they view on television is real (Greenberg and Reeves, 1976).

These data on the television viewing habits of Black and other minority children must be read in conjunction with other data that indicate the overall exclusion of Black characters, the racism inherent in the images, the low status of Black characters, and so forth (Bay Area Association of Black Psychologists, 1973; Black Efforts for Soul in Television, 1972; Butler et al., 1979; Greenberg and Atkin, 1978). These research studies suggest the potential of television, particularly in the formative years of children, for molding self-concept or identity, level of aspirations, values, and coping styles.

Although limitations of time and space have precluded an overview of the socializing role of other forms of the mass media, such as movies, newspapers, or magazines, suffice it to say that they might be reasonably inferred to present the same problems.

IMPLICATIONS FOR SOCIAL AND POLITICAL ACTION

The point of view expressed throughout the paper is merely that the mental health of Blacks is inextricably tied to the overall economic, political, and social status of Black people. Simply stated: Unless there is a substantial reduction in the political and economically based oppression, there will not be an overall improvement in mental health. From this vantage point, mental illness as a large scale social problem is inherently a political and economic problem requiring political and economic solutions. Thus the present one-to-one model of patient care has no potential for a substantial reduction in the incidence and prevalence of mental illness or human suffering. Societal conditions are manufacturing psychiatric casualties more quickly and in greater numbers than we have the capacity to treat effectively now or in the foreseeable future. Thus, any substantial mental health strategy for Blacks must align itself with the total liberation struggle of Black people.

The starkness or bleakness of this assessment of the one-to-one clinical model should not be interpreted as an evaluation of its social utility, for if it can truly demonstrate that it is a viable modality for bolstering the human spirit, stimulating maximum utilization of psychic resources or relieving psychic pain and suffering, these are not achievements that are easily dismissed. Yet mental health strategy must also be evaluated in terms of its potential for the reduction of mental dysfunction as a social problem rather than merely individual dysfunction.

The purpose of this paper was not to attempt to define the specific political actions or tactics to be utilized in eradicating the social conditions generating mental illness and minimizing growth or mental health. Suffice it to say that the full range of political and social actions utilized for social change are appropriate. The objective of this paper, then, was to provide a theoretical context within which to place mental health theory and practice with Blacks.

References

Albee, G. W. The relation of conceptual models to manpower needs. In E. L. Cowen, E. A. Gardener, and M. Zax (Eds.), *Emergent approaches to mental health problems.* New York: Appleton-Century-Crofts, 1967.

Bay Area Association of Black Psychologists. *The effects of children's television programming in Black children*. Position paper presented by Dr. Carolyn Block to Federal Communications Commission, January 1973, Washington, D.C.

Black efforts for soul in television, Content analysis of Black and minority treatment on children's television. Best, Action for Children's Television, 1972.

Bogart, L. American television: A brief survey of research findings. *Journal of Social Issues*, 1962, *18*(2), 36–42.

Brenner, M. H. *Mental illness and the economy*. Cambridge: Harvard University Press, 1973.

Brown, G., and Birley, I. Crises and life changes and the onset of schizophrenia. *Journal of Health and Social Behavior*, 1968, *9*, 203–214.

Butler, P., Khatib, S., Hilliard, T., Howard, J., Reid, J., Wesson, K., Wage, G., and Williams, O. In R. L. Jones (Ed.), *Sourcebook on teaching in Black psychology: Perspectives and course outlines*, Vol. 1, 1–29. Washington, D.C.: Association of Black Psychologists, 1979.

Clark, C. Black studies or the study of Black people? In R. L. Jones (Ed.), *Black psychology*. New York: Harper & Row, 1972.

Dohrenwend, B. S. Social status and stressful life events. *Journal of Personality and Social Psychology*, 1973, *28*, 225–235.

Douglass, F. West India emancipation speech, August, 1857. In P. S. Foner (Ed.), *Frederick Douglass*. New York: Citadel Press, 1969.

Drug Abuse Survey Project. *Dealing with drug abuse*. New York: Praeger Publishers, 1972.

Fanon, F. *The wretched of the earth*. New York: Grove Press, 1963.

Fanon, F. *Toward the African revolution*. New York: Grove Press, 1967.

Faris, R., and Dunham, H. *Mental disorders in urban areas*. Chicago: University of Chicago Press, 1939.

Gil, D. G. A socio-cultural perspective on physical child abuse. *Child Welfare*, 1971, *50*(7), 389–395.

Greenberg, B. S., and Atkin, C. *Learning about minorities from television: The research agenda*. (Paper prepared for conference.) Television and the Socialization of the Minority Child, Center for Afro-American Studies, University of California, Los Angeles, April 1978.

Greenberg, B., and Dervin, B., with the assistance of J. Dominick and J. Bower. *Use of mass media by the urban poor*. New York: Praeger Publishers, 1972.

Greenberg, B., and Dominick, J. Racial and social class differences in teenagers' use of television. *Journal of Broadcasting*, 1969, *13*, 3331–3344.

Greenberg, B., and Reeves, B. Children and the perceived reality of television. *Journal of Social Issues*, 1976, *32*, 86–97.

Griffin, M. The influence of race on the psychotherapeutic relationship. *Psychiatry*, 1977, *40*, 27–40.

Halleck, S. *The politics of therapy*. New York: Science House, Inc., 1971.

Harper, F. *Alcohol abuse and Black America*. Alexandria, Va.: Douglas Publishers, 1976.

Higgenbotham, L. *In the matter of color*. New York: Oxford University Press, 1978.

Hilliard, T. Psychology, law and the Black community. *Law and Human Behavior*, 1978, *2*, 10–131. (a)

Hilliard, T. *The Ku Klux Klan and the Black Marines*. Unpublished paper, 1978. (b)

Hollingshead, A. B., and Redlich, R. C. *Social class and mental illness*. New York: Wiley & Sons, 1958.

Howard, J. Toward a social psychology of colonialism. In R. L. Jones (Ed.), *Black psychology*. New York: Harper & Row, 1972.

Howard, J. H. *The political socialization of the black community*. (Unpublished paper) Annual Convention of Association of Black Psychologists, San Francisco, Calif., 1972.

Joint Commission on Mental Illness and Mental Health. *Action for mental health*. New York: Basic Books, 1961.

Jones, E. Social class and psychotherapy: A critical review of research. *Psychiatry*, 1974, *37*, 307–320.

Jones, R. L. *Black psychology*. New York: Harper & Row, 1972.

Jones, R. L. *Sourcebook on teaching in Black psychology*. Washington, D.C.: Association of Black Psychologists, 1979.

Jordan, W. *White over Black*. Chapel Hill: University of North Carolina Press, 1968.

Karenga, M. R. The black community and the university: A community organizer's perspective. In A. Robinson, C. Foster, and D. Ogilvie (Eds.), *Black studies in the university*. New Haven: Yale University Press, 1969.

Kenniston, K. How community mental health centers stamped out the riots. *Transactions*, 1968, *5*, 21–29.

Kessler, M., and Albee, G. Primary prevention. *Annual Review of Psychology*, 1975, *26*, 557–591.

King, L. (Ed.). *African philosophy: Assumptions and paradigms for research on Black people*. Proceedings for the First Annual J. Alfred Cannon Research Series Conference, April 1975.

Komora, P., and Clark, M. Mental disease in the crisis. *Mental Hygiene*, 1935, *19*, 289–301.

Langer, T. S., and Michael, S. T. *Life stress and mental health: The midtown Manhattan study*, Vol. 2. New York: Free Press, 1963.

Memmi, A. *The colonizer and the colonized*. Boston: Beacon Press, 1965.

Moynihan, D. *The Negro family: The case for national action*. Office of Policy Planning and Research, United States Department of Labor. U.S. Government Printing Office, March 1965.

Nobles, W. African philosophy: Foundations for Black psychology. In R. L. Jones, *Black psychology*. New York: Harper & Row, 1972.

Nobles, W. African roots and American fruit: The Black family. *The Journal of Social and Behavioral Sciences*, 1974, *20*, 66–77.

Nobles, W. *A formative and empirical study of black families: Final report*. Washington, D.C.: Office of Child Development, 1977.

Piven, F., and Cloward, R. *Regulating the poor*. New York: Vintage, 1971.

Pollocks, H. The depression and mental disease in New York state. *American Journal of Psychiatry*, 1935, *91*, 736–771.

Quarles, B. Quoted in R. Staples, *The Black Family*. Belmont, Calif.: Wadsworth Publishing Co., 1971.

Rhodes, R., and Montrero, A. Papers on colonialism, 1968–69. Unpublished.

Roth, R., Berenbaum, H. L., and Hershenson, D. *The developmental theory of psychotherapy: A systematic eclecticism*. Unpublished paper, Illinois Institute of Technology, 1967.

Ryan, W. *Blaming the victim.* New York: Vintage, 1971.

Smith, E. A. *The retention of the phonological, phonemic, and morphophonemic features of Africa in Afro-American ebonics.* Seminar series paper, Department of Linguistics at California State University (Fullerton), 1978.

Srole, L., Langer, T., Michael, S., and Rennie, T. A. *Mental health in the metropolis: Midtown Manhattan study*, Vol. 1. New York: McGraw-Hill, 1962.

Turner, L. *Africanisms in the Gullah dialect.* Chicago: University of Chicago Press, 1949.

Willie, C., Kramer, B., and Brown, B. *Racism and mental illness.* Pittsburgh: University of Pittsburgh Press, 1973.

Overcoming Self-Hate in Gays

Brian R. McNaught

When the American Psychiatric Association's board of directors voted unanimously in December 1973 to remove homosexuality from its *Diagnostic and Statistical Manual of Psychiatric Disorders*, it did not "cure" the nation's 22 million gay men and women overnight.

When Ford and Beach demonstrated in 1951 that homosexual behavior is evidenced in every species of mammal, gay people did not suddenly think of their sexual activity as "natural."

When the Catholic Theological Society of America's Committee on Sexuality insisted (Kosnick, Carroll, Cunningham, Modras, and Schulte, 1971) that scriptural passages traditionally used to condemn homosexuality had been taken out of context and misinterpreted, gay men and women did not suddenly feel loved and accepted by God.

Despite all of the advances in the last 60 years in our understanding of human sexual response; despite the studies and subsequent statements by social scientists which underscore the appropriateness of homosexual behavior for some persons; despite evidence of an increased tolerance of gay people in many segments of society, including some quarters of the Catholic Church, I believe self-hate continues to be the biggest hurdle for many gay people. Ignorance, I believe, is the creator of this hurdle and therefore the enemy of gay men and women and of all those persons who are dedicated to serving the needs of gay people, such as counselors, clergy, therapists, educators, and social workers.

Despite all the public emphasis on civil rights, I suggest that the greatest goal of gay men and women today is to love and to be loved maturely. In conquering self-hate through education, the gay person begins the important process of growth toward love of self and of others, and learns to

From Brian R. McNaught, "Overcoming Self-Hate through Education: Achieving Self-Love among Gay People," in George W. Albee, Sol Gordon, and Harold Leitenberg (eds.) *Promoting Sexual Responsibility and Preventing Sexual Problems.* Copyright © 1983 by the Vermont Conference on the Primary Prevention of Psychopathology. Reprinted by permission.

overcome the obstacles which currently discourage meaningful relationships.

These conclusions are drawn from the observations of personal experiences and through written and verbal communication with a large cross-section of gay men and women throughout the United States and Canada. The communication with the gay people resulted from articles I have written, speeches I have given, or media interviews with me on the subject of homosexuality, conducted since 1974.

Seven years ago, on a nondescript Saturday morning, I grabbed a bottle of paint thinner and drank it. At the time, I seemingly had everything for which to live. I was 26 years old, attractive and intelligent. I was an award-winning columnist on the staff of a Catholic newspaper, a frequent host of a church-sponsored television talk show, and a popular speaker at parish functions. My family celebrated my presence, even when I was accompanied by my handsome and articulate lover, a minister.

My goal in life was to be God's best friend, or a "saint" as we would say in the Catholic Church. I desperately wanted to be loved and associated love with approval. The approval of others, I reasoned, was the only sign we had that it was appropriate to like yourself. In my attempt to experience self-love, I eagerly sought the approval of everyone I encountered, from aunts and uncles to grocery store clerks. If I could make them smile, I must be a person worthy of love, I insisted. I was good at getting smiles, but they were never enough. People who find their worth in the approval of others, I learned, have an insatiable appetite.

Of particular concern to me was the approval of my church, the institution around which nearly all our family social life revolved; the institution which had educated me for 16 years and nurtured in me the idea I was special. Considered a "prince of a boy" by the nuns in grade school, the brothers in high school, the Catholic readers of my weekly column, I was polite, creative, sensitive, and likeable. Nevertheless, I lacked an important sense of self-worth.

I am convinced that my lack of self-esteem resulted from my lifelong awareness of homosexual feelings. To be sexual at all in an Irish Catholic environment in the 1950s was discouraged. Sex was an inappropriate topic for discussion. Because no one ever spoke of homosexuality (boys loving boys and girls loving girls) except in the crudest jokes, I kept my feelings a secret from the time I developed my first crush on a male lifeguard at age 9 and dreamed at night about sleeping with Tarzan.

Like every gay person with whom I have talked, I did not think of myself as a "queer" when I was a youngster; at least I would not accept the term as an accurate description of my feelings. Queers were "sissies" and I was no sissy; I excelled in a variety of sports. Queer boys were supposed to hate girls and at the same time want to be a girl. I liked being a boy and had lots of girl friends. "But if I'm not a queer, what am I?" I wondered.

The myths surrounding homosexuality were presented as truths when I was in grade school and, in many places in this country, they continue to be. Children with a homosexual orientation grow up thinking there is something "queer" about their feelings; something sick and immoral; something which when revealed will eliminate the love and respect of their parents, siblings, and friends.

By the time I entered high school, I figured out that my feelings for other men—my attraction to the male aura—made me a homosexual. Still, I did not see the contradiction between liking the bodies of other boys and eventually getting married. Like millions of other gay people throughout history, I reasoned that I must be the exception.

I do not remember reading anything in popular literature about homosexuality. There was no available book or copy of the *Saturday Evening Post* to which I could turn. Outside the office of the guidance counselor there was a rack of pamphlets on a variety of subjects like drinking, dating, and drugs but nothing on homosexuality; nothing that could answer my questions.

"If you come into my office and tell me that you've screwed a chick, I'll talk to you," declared the guidance counselor in a talk to my all-male senior class, "But if you tell me you're queer, I'll kick you out of the office." Until he made that announcement, I had seriously considered telling the counselor my long-held secret. He frightened me into maintaining silence, which I was as good at as I was in securing his approval of me in other areas. When I graduated, the guidance counselor was one of the faculty members who voted unanimously to honor me with the Christian Leadership Award.

The process of learning to hate myself was well underway. I knew, for instance, that I would never win the high school award if I revealed my sexual feelings. Even though I felt I was a good person, insofar as I kept the Ten Commandments, discouraged "impure thoughts," and enthusiastically performed various "acts of charity," I began to believe that homosexuals, as a group, were bad people and that I shared somehow in that sin.

I lived two lives—a public one which drew positive attention and a private one which was tormented with fear and anxiety. When I drank the paint thinner, I did so to escape the contradiction between my public and private self. I feared losing the affirmation of others and at the same time could no longer bear lying about my sexual orientation. As far as I was concerned, I was going home to God to whom I would explain myself and from whom I would seek an answer to my pain. How could a father who loved his child allow him or her to be a homosexual?

As I had my stomach pumped, I decided that my secret was literally killing me and that if I cared to live, I had to learn to be myself, accept myself, and love myself regardless of the consequences. It was while sitting on the table in the emergency room of the Catholic hospital that I decided never again to live my life based on other people's expectations. Shortly thereafter, I broke up my relationship because it was beyond repair; I started reading about homosexuality and I joined an organization of gay Catholics called Dignity. After attending a conference on Christian ministry to the homosexual, I wrote a column for the Catholic newspaper on the beauty of gay love. I formed a chapter of Dignity in the city and told the editor and each of the staff people about my homosexuality.

Within a month of opening my new inner-city apartment as a center for gay people, I agreed to be interviewed in a daily newspaper. The next working day, my column was dropped from the Catholic newspaper. In the following weeks, I began legal proceedings against the Church, organized pickets of the newspaper, and began speaking publicly about homosexuality. Three weeks after my column was dropped, I undertook a hunger strike in protest of the sins of the Church against gay people. The fast ended after 24 days when the bishops of Detroit wrote me a letter in which they pledged to work to educate the clergy about homosexuality. The following day I was fired from the remainder of my responsibilities at the newspaper.

In the process of this public ordeal, I alienated my family, most of my readers, and my television viewers. All of the signs of my sainthood, my acceptance, were stripped away. I lost my job, my friendships with many gay and nongay people, the approval of my Church, and my high school Christian Leadership Award (for a period of time). Yet, for the first time in 26 years, I felt authentic, adult, and worthy of admiration and love.

Today, I am in a relationship with another man which is honest, open, sensitive, and supportive. I have many friends who love and support me as a whole person. While I may lack many of life's traditional signs of success, like write-ups in the alumni newsletter and a healthy salary for my work, I have never contemplated suicide again, and I feel fully alive.

My understanding of my homosexuality today is that it is a natural variation; that the genital expression of same-sex feelings ought to be responsible; that gay people are beloved children of God and, like heterosexuals, are called to reach our full potential. My position on the Catholic Church's official teaching is that they are in error when they suggest homosexuality is an "abomination," and that they will one day change their stand.

For me, the process of emerging from an image to a reality, from a secret to a song, from self-hate to self-love is ongoing. Frequently there are temptations to be inauthentic, to return to the closet, or to an image for the sake of approval. The tools I use to continue that growth process remain the same. The most important step I took was educating myself to the truths about homosexuality, truths which tore down the myths of the past and helped me rebuild a positive self-image.

❖ The negative self-image frequently manifests itself in alcohol and drug abuse, irresponsible contact with sexual partners by individuals who know they have a venereal disease and, certainly the most tragic, the physical abuse of one homosexual by another. Humphreys and Miller (1980) found evidence to suggest that homosexual victims of violent crimes are most often those most fearful of being identified as gay. For this reason, gay men and women who seek my help receive homework reading assignments. There are a variety of worthwhile books on the market which I can enthusiastically recommend.

Young people who are confused by their sexual feelings are encouraged to read *A Way of Love, A Way of Life* by Frances Hanckel and John Cunningham (1979). I also encourage teachers of high school and college students to show the filmstrip *The Hidden Minority: Homosexuality in Our Society* (Guidance Associates, 1979).

As general resource books I suggest Tripp's (1975) *The Homosexual Matrix*; *Society and the Healthy Homosexual* by George Weinberg (1972); *Loving Someone Gay* and *Living Gay* by Don Clark (1977, 1979); and *Positively Gay*, edited by Robert Leighton and Betty Berzon (1979).

Women who are interested in reading more about the lesbian experience are encouraged to read *Our Right to Love: A Lesbian Resource Guide*, edited by Ginny Vida (1978); *The Joy of Lesbian Sex* by Emily Sisley and Bertha Harris (1977); and Rita Mae Brown's (1973) *Rubyfruit Jungle*.

Materials recommended for men include *The Joy of Gay Sex* by Charles Silverstein and Edmund White (1977); *Men Loving Men* by Mitch Walker (1977); *The Best Little Boy in the World* by John Reid (1976); and *The Front Runner* by Patricia Nell Warren (1974).

Religion, I have found, is a critical area for many gay people. Too many educators and therapists who are not interested in religion overlook the tremendous influence a religious background can have upon an individual's sense of self-worth. Today, especially, with the so-called Moral Majority and other reactionary groups using the Bible as a weapon in their war against gay civil rights, it is important that gay people and their families have accurate information about the Scriptures and their approach to homosexuality.

Most of the books I recommend are by Catholics but, because of their treatment of both the Old and New Testament, I feel they are helpful to persons of both Christian and Jewish backgrounds. By far, the most important book on the subject is *Christianity, Social Tolerance and Homosexuality* by John Boswell (1980). Also quite helpful are *The Church and the Homosexual* by John McNeill, S.J. (1976); *Embodiment* by James Nelson (1978); and *Human Sexuality: New Directions in American Catholic Thought*, a study commissioned by the Catholic Theological Society of America (Kosnick et al., 1977).

Another critical area of concern for gay people which often influences their ability to love themselves is the response of their families to homosexuality. My parents had many questions, which I attempted to answer, but they seemed to be especially helped by reading books by "impartial" observers whom they could trust. Of particular help at the time was Laura Hobson's (1976) book, *Consenting Adult*. Since then, Betty Fairchild and Nancy Hayward (1979) have written *Now That You Know: What Every Parent Should Know about Homosexuality*, a book which has been successful in moving many parents from a position of fear to one of understanding.

It is not uncommon to hear skepticism from a gay person who has read his or her first book on homosexuality. The opinions of one author who affirms homosexuality are welcomed but distrusted by readers who have spent 18, 30, or 50 years learning to approach their sexuality negatively.

However, learning positive new things about one's sexual orientation is not unlike eating peanuts: it is not easy to stop. The people with whom I have worked generally ask for a more extensive book list, with fiction, poetry, history, and biographies included.

A second step which I took and which I recommend to people seeking to build positive self-images is associating with other gay people. I met my minister lover in a bar to which I vowed I would never return once I had "roped" him into a relationship. I viewed the people in the bar as the pathetic "queers" who had been described to me throughout my life and with whom I could not relate. Had I attempted to talk with them, I would have made new friends and therefore probably would not have felt so trapped in my relationship. However, I saw my lover as "not like those others," and I did my best to keep us both away from their influence.

When I broke up my relationship, I soon began meeting a variety of gay people. Some of them I liked very much and some of them I did not, but I came to a growing awareness that "gay" is an adjective and not a noun; that I was a gay man who was part of a community. I met other gay Catholics and gay atheists. I talked with gay Republicans, Democrats, and also gay anarchists. I listened to people defend monogamy and defend open relationships. In this process I felt liberated to choose my own path, to say "I am doing this because it is 'Brian's way' and not because it is the 'gay way.' "

The knowledge which I accumulated by reading enabled me to feel more secure when I encountered other gay people and nongay people. It enabled me to begin taking *responsibility* for my life, to see the need to *care* for my uniqueness, and to *respect* myself. The gay men and women I encourage to join local gay organizations, attend religious services for gay people, and participate in gay social functions return with similar stories. Some people begin dressing in clothing they prefer as opposed to the clothing they wore because they thought it was "gay." Those who find the gay bars to be compromising situations or places in which they are prone to drink too much begin to avoid them and feel better about themselves for doing so. Other people report that while they used to use terms like "queen," "faggot," "fruit," and "fairy" to describe themselves and their friends, they no longer see these terms as humorous or appropriate.

In order to find the gay organizations, the gay religious services, or the social functions sponsored by the community, I suggest that people purchase a copy of the *Gayellow Pages*. This national directory lists all the organizations, publications, and services for gay people in each city in the United States and Canada. It is an invaluable resource for gay men and women and for professionals seeking to meet their needs.

Although I would avoid at all costs "pushing" someone out of the closet, I do believe that "coming out" is an important part of the self-affirmation process. Individuals who are constantly forced to lie to parents, peers, and fellow workers about their social life are denying the joy and beauty of their same-sex feelings and undermining the positive attitudes they might have developed through private reading. While some persons find leading a double life a small price to pay for a successful career or similar goal, most persons with whom I have talked seem unwilling to play the games. Those persons who have "come out of the closet"—who have affirmed their sexual orientation to themselves and to significant others—frequently pay an initial price of rejection by some people, but at the same time they report a unique sense of self-determination, worth, and honesty.

In addition to coming out, I believe participating in your own liberation is important to the notion of care, respect, and responsibility. For many years, I had worked with other disadvantaged minorities in their struggles for civil rights. I did so as a white, presumed-to-be-heterosexual male. As such, my privileged status was maintained, and I was limited in my ability to feel the sense of growth experienced by those more intimately involved. When I lost my column, and then my job, however, I had to begin fighting for my own rights and, in so doing, experienced the same pride which I had seen in the faces of the black people, the Hispanics, and the women with whom I had marched.

There are two national gay organizations which I encourage gay people and their supporters to join. The first is the Gay Rights National Lobby (GRNL), located at 930 F Street, N.W., Washington, D.C., 20004. GRNL is the organization which lobbies Congress to pass legislation favorable to the civil rights of gay people. The National Gay Task Force (NGTF), located at 80 Fifth Ave., New York, N.Y., 10011, is the organization which monitors the media's presentation of homosexuality, works to educate the general public, solicits nondiscrimination clauses from major corporations, and acts as a liaison with the White House and others on issues of concern to the gay community. Persons interested in working for changes in their respective churches are also encouraged to join the gay caucuses which exist in nearly every denomination. Their names and addresses are available in *Gayellow Pages.*

From my discussions with various gay men and women, I suggest that the primary concern today for gay people is being enabled to love and be loved maturely. I have read that one-third of the population (gay and straight) wants a long-lasting relationship with another person, one-third says they want one but are unable to maintain a committed relationship, and one-third has no interest in being involved with the expectations and demands of a one-on-one marriage.

Perhaps because of my reputation as a gay man who supports relationships, the majority of the people with whom I have talked want to be in a committed relationship and dream of it lasting the rest of their lives. Although the men tend to be more flexible than the women on the subject of genital exclusivity, members of both genders talk enthusiastically about having one special person whom they would love and by whom they would be loved. The two questions most frequently asked are: "How do I meet a potential mate?" and "How do I maintain the relationship when there are no role models and no support systems?"

Professionals who would like to assist gay people in this process need to remember that most gay people have been denied the important period of dating and have missed the many lessons such a period teaches. Because most gay people were confused and closeted in high school and college, they generally faked the dating ritual and frequently selected a safe companion for the sake of appearances. When an individual comes out at age 21, he or she has probably never had the experience of kissing, holding the hand of, or even dancing with a person of his or her choosing. The male or female walking into their first gay bar has never had the intimate opportunity to learn that the most sexually attractive person does not necessarily possess the best personality, that race, religion, sense of humor, intelligence, and economic background frequently influence whether or not one person will be compatible with another. Furthermore, many gay people do not have a sexual experience with another homosexual until they have come out of the closet. When they do finally emerge into a gay social scene, they frequently conduct themselves like children in a candy shop, or, as I did, rush into a relationship merely for the sake of affirmation and security. Both the gay person and the professional should be aware that individuals who have only recently come out of the closet will need a period of time for social and sexual adjustment; to expect otherwise is to invite disappointment and more negative self-images.

Because of social attitudes toward homosexuals, the number of healthy social settings available to gay people are limited, though they have increased tremendously since 1969, the birth year of the modern Gay Pride Movement. Gay bars continue to be the most popular meeting places but are not always conducive atmospheres for getting to know another person. In fact, some gay people complain they have never had an intelligent conversation in a gay bar, due in no small part to the loud music, dim lighting, and sexually tense aura of most gay bars.

Gay newspapers (also listed in *Gayellow Pages*) generally record weekly or monthly social activities, such as picnics, sporting events, parties, and so forth, which are designed to meet the needs of the community. They also list organizations such as the gay mountain climbing group, the lesbian mothers' group, and the gay college athletes' association. These different organizations enable gay people to come into contact with people of similar interests. Each year, new social and professional groups are formed, offering that many more opportunities for gay people to find someone with whom they might establish a relationship.

Maintaining a relationship in a society which discourages permanence is difficult enough for heterosexuals, but for gay people who generally receive no support for their efforts from family, employers, the church, or the state, the task can seem impossible. They are forced to make choices. With whom should they spend the holiday—unsuspecting parents or a lover? With whom do they attend office social functions—lover or friend? How do they make sacred their commitment, when their church discourages their union? How do they share a home when some communities will not sell to two unrelated persons of the same gender and many apartment owners prohibit rentals to the same? Is it any wonder that many gay people find it difficult to maintain a committed relationship?

On the other hand, because there are no preconceived notions or role models for gay relationships, they are free to grow into their own unique shapes. Gay couples most successful at maintaining a committed relationship discourage roles and insist on open, honest communication. With increasing frequency, gay couples and liberated heterosexual couples are seeing that their relationships are virtually the same. They share the same goals, many of the same problems and frustrations, and the same joys.

Successful gay relationships are those in which the individuals are sensitive to each other's needs, share tasks equally, leave space for growth, and encourage each other's creativity. If sexual activity is to be engaged in outside of the relationship, it is done with mutual consent.

In this paper I have concerned myself mainly with encouraging gay people to love themselves by eliminating negative self-images through education. My approach has been to destroy the myths of the past through the reading of current literature and contact with other gay people and to encourage in the gay person respect, care, and responsibility. A person who has learned to love himself or herself is able to love another person maturely.

But what about our efforts in behalf of those boys and girls who are aware of homosexual feelings but have not yet had those feelings polluted by ever present myths? While it is important that we meet the needs of yesterday's and today's victims of hatred, fear, and ignorance, it is essential that we not merely try to repair their wounds, but also get about the business of primary prevention.

Young people need to learn at an early age that it is OK to be different from the majority; they need to know that there is no such thing as an unnatural thought. From their school texts, the attitudes of their teachers, sex education courses, television programs, magazine and newspaper articles, popular songs and church sermons, youngsters need to learn that it is all right to be homosexual. Although some parents seem concerned that presenting homosexuality in a positive light will encourage their children to become homosexual, no study supports such fears. On the contrary, healthy, broad-based sex education tends to create healthy, confident people, regardless of their sexual inclinations. Sexually mature people are not intimidated by the sexuality of others.

Educators and others with access to the public need to include "gay people" in sentences where appropriate, have books and other resources available for interested persons, and discourage the telling of antigay jokes. Persons interested in helping homosexual men and women develop positive attitudes toward sexuality and self should diligently watchdog the media, praising the networks and commercial sponsors when the gay subject matter is handled well and criticizing them when it is not, or when there is no attention given to gay people. Letters to the editor in local and national publications which comment on a gay news event or feature are another means of raising public consciousness, eliminating ignorance, and guaranteeing that more people will grow up with a healthy attitude toward themselves and others.

Finally, I applaud the courage of heterosexual men and women who publicly support the healthiness of homosexuality and who champion gay civil rights at the risk of being identified and scourged as homosexual. Although whites can march with blacks, and men can march with women without losing their "privileged status," nothing separates the heterosexual from the homosexual in the front page photo of a gay pride march.

In the same breath, I suggest that professionals, such as my high school guidance counselor, who ought to be comfortable with gay men and women but are not, should examine other career options.

References

Boswell, J. *Christianity, social tolerance and homosexuality.* Chicago: University of Chicago Press, 1980.

Brown, R. M. *Rubyfruit jungle.* New York: Daughters, 1973.

Clark, D. *Loving someone gay.* New York: Signet, 1977.

Clark, D. *Living gay.* Millbrae, Calif.: Celestial Arts, 1979.

Fairchild, B., and Hayward, N. *Now that you know: What every parent should know about homosexuality.* New York: Harcourt Brace Jovanovich, 1979.

Ford, C. S., and Beach, S. A. *Patterns of sexual behavior.* New York: Harper and Bros., 1951.

Fromm, E. *The art of loving.* New York: Bantam Books, 1967.

Gayellow Pages. (Obtainable from Renaissance House, Box 292, Village Station, New York, N.Y. 10014. Published annually.)

Guidance Associates. *The hidden minority: Homosexuality in our society.* White Plains, N.Y.: Guidance Associates, 1979.

Gutiérrez, G. In Sr. C. Inda and J. Eagleson (Eds. and trans.), *A theology of liberation.* Mary Knoll, N.Y.: Orbis, 1973.

Hanckel, F., and Cunningham, J. *A way of love, a way of life.* New York: Lothrop, 1979.

Hobson, L. *Consenting adult.* New York: Warner Books, 1976.

Humphreys, L., and Miller, B. Lifestyles and violence: Homosexual victims of assault and murder. *Qualitative Sociology,* 1980, *3,* 169-185.

Kosnick, A., Carroll, W., Cunningham, A., Modras, R., and Schulte, J. *Human sexuality: New directions in American Catholic thought.* New York: Paulist Press, 1971.

Leighton, R., and Berzon, B. (Eds.). *Positively gay.* Millbrae, Calif.: Celestial Arts, 1979.

McNeill, J., S.J. *The church and the homosexual.* Mission, Kans.: Sheed, Andrews and McMeel, 1976.

Nelson, J. *Embodiment.* Minneapolis: Augsburg, 1978.

Reid, J. *The best little boy in the world.* New York: Ballantine, 1976.

Silverstein, C., and White, E. *The joy of gay sex.* New York: Crown, 1977.

Sisley, E., and Harris, B. *The joy of lesbian sex.* New York: Crown, 1977.

Tripp, C. A. *The homosexual matrix*. New York: McGraw-Hill, 1975.

Vida, G. (Ed.). *Our right to love: A lesbian resource guide*. Englewood Cliffs, N.J.: Prentice-Hall, 1978.

Walker, M. *Men loving men*. San Francisco: Gay Sunshine Press, 1977.

Warren, P. N. *The front runner*. New York: William Morrow, 1974.

Weinberg, G. *Society and the healthy homosexual*. New York: St. Martin's Press, 1972.

IV. Programs Involving Social and Political Change

This section presents some examples of programs involving efforts to bring about social change. Our consumer-oriented society fosters the further disintegration of the family and contributes to the growing numbers of single parents, particularly women, who must shoulder the burden of child rearing without adequate financial resources and often without support groups. Other at-risk powerless groups include the growing number of elderly people, particularly elderly women, who are at high risk for being poor as well as powerless, and the growing number of persons crowded into our prisons and dumped from mental institutions onto the streets of the cities. Further social pathology results from the deterioration of our schools, our neighborhoods, our communities—here are reports of action programs aimed at major social change in these areas. Over and over, the same themes are repeated: It is the children, particularly the children of the poor, and women, particularly single parents and elderly women, it is the minorities and the handicapped, who suffer most from oppression. The lack of adequate day care, the impoverishment and meaninglessness of our school system, and the urgent necessity for restructuring our schools, our neighborhoods, our communities—all these are considered in this section.

A Vision of Child Care in the Future

Edward Zigler and Matia Finn

❖ A Time for Action

Over the course of the International Year of the Child many of the short-falls outlined above became worse. In large measure, this was due to in-flation and inaction, but perhaps our lack of commitment was really the primary cause. Evaluated in these terms, the International Year of the Child can be viewed as a failure.

But let us take another viewpoint. We have come a long way in the process of assessing what we are doing and not doing to optimize the development of our nation's children. In 1979 we were forced to educate each other on the problems facing children and families, and this has re-sulted in consciousness raising about the unmet needs of children in America. We have garnered vital information. Now is the time for ac-tion. The International Year of the Child can serve as our launching pad for greater activity in behalf of children, and, as such, the year may in-deed be considered a success. To this end, we want to share with you our vision for child care in the 1980s.

Recommendations

We order our agenda for the 1980s around the social institutions that are most critical in determining the quality of the lives of the children in this country. These institutions, in order of their importance in influencing the lives of children, are, the family, the school, and child care outside the home.

Before we address ourselves to changes that need to be made, we raise a very basic question. That is, will the action be at the federal, state, or local level? While we have come to be dependent on federal initiatives for the many programs begun on behalf of children since the 1960s, it is our belief that the role of the federal government will diminish during this decade. We are in the midst of an era of uncontrollable inflation and

Proposition 13 mentality. We cannot afford to wait for federal action. As will become clear in the course of our discussion, any changes to the benefit of children and families will come about through state and local initiatives and through greater involvement in matters pertaining to family life by the private sector.

The Family

The family will remain the first and foremost institution in determining what is going to happen to children. It is imperative, however, that we acknowledge the multiple forms that now constitute a family. Whereas our national policies and rhetoric are directed to the traditional nuclear family where the husband is the breadwinner and the mother the housewife and where there are two or more children living at home, the fact is that fewer the 7 percent of Americans now live in this kind of family arrangement (U.S. Bureau of the Census, 1979). Other arrangements include both parents who are wage earners, with one or more children living at home; married couples with no children, or none living at home; single parent families; unrelated persons living together; and one person living alone.

Families, then, are significantly different today than they were a quarter of a century ago or even a decade ago. There have been deep and far-reaching changes in American society in recent years that have contributed to the changes in family structure. These are significant in that they influence not only the way children are being raised and educated but our attitudes toward young people as well.

These attitudinal changes are reflected in shifting demographics. Because of recent trends, ours has become an aging society, with relatively few children and with mounting numbers of elderly. Twenty-nine percent of today's population is under age 18, in contrast with 34 percent in 1970. Since that year the 25- to 34-year-old group increased by 32 percent, and the number of those over 65 increased by 17 percent. There is an overwhelming trend toward late marriage and childbearing, and an increasing number of couples are choosing to have no children at all (U.S. Bureau of the Census, 1979). During the past decade, the number of children under 15 has decreased by 6.4 million. It is important for us to consider what will be the role of children and youth in an aging society and in an increasingly childless one. Will taxpayers be more caring toward children or will the needs of the young be seen to conflict with adult goals?

The past decade has also been a period of great change in the economic realm. Rampant inflation, sluggish growth, increased energy costs, and balance of payments problems have contributed to pressures on families as well as to people's loss of confidence in the economy. A survey by

Yankelovich, Skelly, and White in 1974–1975 found that Americans had less faith in the economy than they previously had and were more fearful of the future. The sluggish economy has also contributed to cutbacks in spending, especially in social services.

Accompanying these changes has been the increase in working mothers. As indicated in an earlier section of this chapter, working mothers now constitute a substantial portion of the labor force and there are indications that the trend will continue, especially in the case of mothers of infants and young children. Women not only constitute a greater proportion of the labor force than ever before, but more and more women have more than one job. Latest statistics reveal that while in 1969 16 percent of the women who worked held more than one job, by 1979 30 percent of the women working held at least two jobs. Eleven percent of these women held two part-time jobs but the remaining 19 percent held two full-time jobs (Brozan, 1980). While changing roles for women contributed to the initial reasons for women joining the labor force, today mothers are working not so much because they want to but because they have to. This has been noted in a recent article by feminist writer Betty Friedan, who contends that women no longer have a choice between staying at home and working, "because it isn't really a free choice when their paycheck is needed to cover the family bills each month; [and] when women must look to their jobs and professions for the security and status their mothers sought in marriage alone" (Friedan, 1979, p. 94).

Another trend reflected in the statistics cited in the beginning of this section is the increase in single parent families. Single parents grew by about 1 million (or 40 percent) between 1960 and 1970 and by nearly 2 million between 1970 and 1978 (Norton, 1979). The majority of single parent families are headed by low-income women, although a small portion is headed by men. One reason cited for the increase in single parent families is the escalating divorce rate. After divorce, the most rapidly growing category of single parenthood, especially since 1970, involves unmarried women (Advisory Committee on Child Development, 1976).

Preceding these recent social changes is the demise of the extended family. With transition from an agrarian to an industrial civilization, the family's role as an economic unit was gradually eroded. Work roles for men and women became more sharply differentiated and children, once an asset in terms of their productivity, came to be regarded as liabilities. At the same time, industry required a mobile labor force. As a result, and in the process of multiple moves, the extended family was lost as a resource in time of trouble and as a natural teaching and socializing agent. Families no longer had immediate access to the experience and wisdom of their elders, nor the support systems for child care and education which they could once count on.

Not only are families separated from their kin but they also face increased isolation and alienation within their own communities. Friendly neighborhood stores have given way to interstate highways, impersonal supermarkets, and shopping malls. With the advent of desegregation and busing, schools no longer serve children from the same community. Having very little in common, families rarely interact with their neighbors. According to a recent survey (Yankelovich et al., 1975), these changes have resulted in serious psychological and emotional problems among people of all socioeconomic levels.

For the family to remain viable during these times of transition and in the face of changing demographic and socioeconomic conditions, we must commit ourselves to supporting and strengthening family life. An important element missing in families today is support, which is perhaps why grass roots help groups proliferated during the 1970s. In numerous communities people joined groups for feminists, single parents, divorced parents, abusive parents, battered spouses, and so on. Some groups depended on their membership for support; others sought the advice of "experts" who ran such programs as reality therapy, sensitivity training, parent effectiveness training, and so on.

With this in mind, every single one of our recommendations for the 1980s is consistent with the notion of family support systems (Zigler and Seitz, in press, a; Caplan, 1978). For the remainder of the chapter, we will focus on several concrete and inexpensive ways to achieve this. It is imperative that we realize, however, that these are but suggestions. Some may work out well, and some may not. It is important that as a nation we begin what Campbell refers to as an "experimental approach to social reform" (Campbell, 1969). With such an approach we try out new programs and learn from the experience whether or not they are effective. If they are, we retain them. If not, we modify or discard them and try new programs.

Referral Centers

One of our suggestions in support of family life involves developing referral information centers in each community. There are several options available—for example, day care centers, food stamps, community legal and health services—which families are often not aware of. Information referral centers would provide the links between families and community services. A network of such services would also provide us with statistics—how many people inquire about day care? What are some of the concerns parents have? With people all over the country showing up at these referral centers inquiring about day care facilities, we doubt that any administration would again proclaim that there is no need for increased day care services in this country.

Home Visitor Programs

Another suggestion is the home visitor program. We are not referring here to a home visitor program for the poor but rather a program for all families regardless of their socioeconomic status. Families today function in isolation. They experience a sense of aloneness, alienation, and helplessness. We know that this isolation and sense of helplessness are contributing factors in many cases of child abuse (Helfer and Kempe, 1972; Maden and Wrench, 1977). With the home visitor program, families who wished to could have someone visit them occasionally to discuss how they were doing, what they might need, and so forth, and could provide them with emotional support and information. For the home visitor program we could utilize an important resource—this nation's senior citizens. Such home visitor programs could prove to be useful not only to families but also to many older retired people who are themselves isolated and lonely. There are several examples of successful home visitor programs. One is Henry Kempe's program in Denver (Kempe and Helfer, 1972); the other is the Home Start program which was started at the instigation of the senior author during his tenure as director of the Office of Child Development (Scott, 1974; Zigler and Valentine, 1979). The Child and Family Resource Program, referred to in greater detail in a later section of this chapter, also includes several home visitors or "family advocates." These individuals work to establish a close, trusting relationship with each family and to serve as resource persons who can advise families of services available in the community (Zigler and Seitz, 1980).[3]

Foster Care

Next to support of the family we recommend that changes be instituted in our present foster care system. Our recommendations are that as many children as possible be kept at home and preventive services to families at risk, as adoption subsidies, be made in order to ensure a permanent home for children. Preventive services and adoption subsidies are cost-effective. Out-of-home care for a child between the ages of 2 and 19 years is $100,000. The alternative we recommend is cheaper. The Children's Bureau, for example, has developed several models for preventive services that have been instituted in several communities (e.g., Burt, 1976). These models show conclusively that minimal financial support to families in times of need as well as other services, coupled with counseling

3. For more information on the early childhood and family education programs in Minnesota, refer to "A Policy Study of Issues Related to Early Childhood and Family Education. A Report to the Minnesota Legislature. January 15, 1979." Available from the Minnesota Council on Quality Education, 722 Capitol Square Building, St. Paul, MN 55101.

and follow-up support, can substantially reduce the number of children placed in foster care. The money now spent on foster care and institutional placement of children should be channeled to these types of family support services.

Subsidizing adoption is also important if we are to achieve permanent homes for children, especially older children, black children, or retarded or otherwise handicapped children. There are many fine families who would adopt such children if only they could afford to. Instead of spending money on foster care or institutionalization of these children, why not subsidize their adoption? Senator Cranston, among others, proposed this idea in legislation to provide for increased adoption assistance (Cranston, 1979).

The School

The second most important socializing institution is the American school. Consistent with the notion of family support systems, we envision that the school of the future will serve children before they are born. Research studies are indicative of the importance of early intervention and our ability to prevent some handicapping conditions. If parents enroll in the school during pregnancy, they could receive support and education relevant to prenatal care that would prevent unnecessary disabilities in children. After birth, parents and children would continue to receive educational services that would further enhance adult–infant interaction and promote optimal development of the child. Should there be anything wrong with a child—speech impediment, or hearing difficulty, for example—these would be identified during the preschool years and help provided before the problem compounded itself to the detriment of both the child and the family. We have available to us screening and other identification devices, as well as programs for handicapped infants and young children. Yet children with disabilities often go undiagnosed until they reach school age simply because their families do not come into contact with an institution such as the school until then.

The types of school services we are referring to are already in existence. The Brookline Early Education Project in Massachusetts is one example (Pearson and Nicol, 1977). Also, many states are cognizant of the school's failure to help preschool and younger children and are developing new programs to combat the problem. The Minnesota Legislature, through the Minnesota Council on Quality Education, has been funding pilot early childhood and family education (ECFE) programs in Minnesota elementary schools. By law, the programs have geographic boundaries to their service area. *All* families and expectant parents of children o through kindergarten within a program's service area are eligible to participate.

Services offered by the programs include parent/family education, concurrent child development activities, family resource libraries, early health screening and referral, parenting education for adolescents and expectant parents, and coordination of community services for families.

Through these types of services, there occurs a natural situation wherein parents and schools act in partnership. As it stands now, parents do not have to send children to school until the child reaches the age of 5 or 6. By that time, school is viewed as an alien and often hostile environment. Teachers and parents are often at odds or, at best, parents are unaware of what schools are trying to achieve. An important outcome of Headstart and other early childhood education programs of the 1960s has been the realization that the parent is the child's primary teacher. Any help schools try to give children must be in conjunction with the parent if it is to be at all effective (Bronfenbrenner, 1975; Valentine and Stark, 1979).

Education for Parenthood

Besides reaching out to would-be parents and parents of young children, schools should also offer education for parenthood classes to students of all ages. With the demise of the extended family and the increase in two-paycheck families, children no longer benefit from learning about child-rearing and development. To compensate, we should include in school curricula courses relevant to the role and responsibility of parents. Such courses should also offer options of internship in child care. For example, high school students could be sent out to work at Head Start programs and day care centers. There are Education for Parenthood model programs instituted in 2,000 school districts that include internship experiences in child care. These were developed by the U.S. Office of Child Development in 1972.

Corporal Punishment

As we mentioned earlier in the chapter, corporal punishment in schools is not only a barbaric form of discipline, it also serves to further child abuse in the home. We recommend that the practice be abolished. There is absolutely nothing in favor of corporal punishment. Studies are conclusive in indicating that corporal punishment is the least effective way of shaping human behavior (National Education Association Task Force on Corporal Punishment, 1972). Furthermore, it escalates aggression in children and promotes violent tendencies, factors which may contribute to the already rampant crime among our nation's youth. Many states require teachers to report parents suspected of child abuse. Yet very few states have statutes that make schools accountable to the parents by banning corporal punishment and requiring school personnel to use other forms of discipline.

Child Care Outside the Home

The institution which overlaps the school (for the purposes of the discussion we refer to it as a separate institution) is child care outside the home. As we have seen, more and more women are entering the work world and childrearing, once the responsibility of the family, is increasingly delegated to babysitters and other nonrelatives in publicly supported or private child care facilities, day care centers, and family day care homes.

While the need for more day care facilities remains acute, there are other problems associated with child care outside the home. We shall offer suggestions to the solution of some of these problems in two separate, albeit overlapping sections, one dealing with publicly supported programs for low-income families, and the other dealing with the child care needs of all families, regardless of income or structure. The latter section will be discussed under the heading of work and family life.

Publicly Supported Child Care and Early Intervention Programs

Federal spending on child care amounts to more than $2 billion a year. This includes expenditures for Head Start and other related early childhood programs (e.g., Home Start) and subsidizing day care facilities for low-income families through Title XX of the Social Security Act. Intervention programs during the preschool years may prevent unnecessary retardation and/or other complications to development later in the life of children. While some of the programs, Head Start in particular, have been shown to work well (Palmer and Anderson, 1979; Zigler and Seitz, in press, a,b) and are cost-effective, only a small percentage of those families eligible for services actually send their children. One of the problems associated with publicly supported programs is, then, the need for more services to accommodate the numbers of low-income families requiring such services. It may not be realistic to expect that all those eligible receive some sort of preschool experience or day care placement, but priority should be given to those who are most in need, including children of bilingual background, children of single parents, and handicapped children. These children are at a high risk for developmental delays and associated learning and other disabilities, so services should be offered to them regardless of income.

Child and Family Resource Programs

The family support system of the future may be exemplified by the Child and Family Resource Program (CFRP), which has been experimentally implemented in 11 locales across the nation. This model approach to early intervention has been praised by the Comptroller General in a report (1979) as comprehensive and cost-effective. Briefly described, CFRPs are designed to offer a variety of services tailored to the unique developmental needs of children. The services are provided from the prenatal period through the child's eighth year and include health, nutrition, and education components. What is unique about CFRPs is that not only do they offer comprehensive support services for the entire family as well as the child, but that they utilize existing community services and act as a referral system and linkage between families and public agencies. According to the Comptroller General's report (1979), the benefits of CFRPs include better preventive health care and nutrition for young children; rapid assistance to families during crises, correction of problems such as inadequate housing, and general improvement in overall quality of life.

Child Care Professionals

Another important change, already in the offing, is the professionalization of child care workers. This applies not only to federally subsidized centers but to all child care centers. The most important aspect in determining how a child is going to develop rests in the nature of that child's interaction with adults (Abt Associates, 1979). Providing optimal care to a group of 15 or 20 children is not as simple as caring for 1 or 2 children in a home setting. Those who work with children in group situations should be trained in the principles of child development and should be cognizant of their impact on the children's growth and socialization. It is imperative, if we are to have quality child care, that we spend additional funds on training child care workers.

In the same vein, parents must be assured that their children are taken care of by competent adults. To this end, the senior author in 1972 was supported by several national organizations concerned with child development and welfare who sought the establishment of a consortium whose sole focus was to upgrade the quality of care children receive. Known as the Child Development Associate Consortium (CDAC), this nonprofit organization, with the help of the nation's leading psychologists and early childhood educators, developed an assessment and credentialing system for child care workers (Ward, 1976). Those child care workers who receive the CDAC credential are regarded as competent to take care of preschool children in group situations. Since 1972 close to 7,000 child care workers have received the CDAC credential. While significant, the number is low given our needs today. We not only need a greater number of CDACs, but the concept itself should be expanded to meet the needs of our changing society. We need, for example, to develop a similar assessment and credentialing system for infant day care workers, school-age day care workers, and family day care "mothers."

The organizational structure of the CDAC should also reflect social changes over the years. In order to mobilize efforts toward professionalizing child care, HEW, as the department was then known, funded the Consortium. Although it is a nonprofit organization and thus able to develop other means of fund raising, the consortium remains operative at the mercy, so to speak, of federal grants (Zigler and Kagan, 1980). The Consortium should be financially independent. We suggest that it reorganize as a mandated corporation, much on the same lines as public television. Although this change would still entail developing an aggressive fund-raising program, the Consortium would nonetheless have a financial security granted to it by Congress and it would operate independently of any government agency.

Regulating Day Care Centers

Regulating responsibility that falls within the realm of the federal government is the regulation of day care centers and the establishment of national day care standards that would be adhered to by all child care facilities. Despite an increase in federal involvement in day care in the last decade and the $2 billion plus price tag that it entails, the principle of federal responsibility for day care has not yet been established. The history of moratoriums and revisions of Federal Interagency Day Care Requirements are explained in other publications (Beck, 1979; Cohen and Zigler, 1977; Zigler and Heller, 1980). Suffice it to add here that child care advocates have been fighting for very basic standards that would do no more than ensure compliance with health and safety codes and a reasonable staff:child ratio. These have not been forthcoming for over 10 years. As mentioned earlier in this chapter, a victory was scored recently with the announcement by Health and Human Services Secretary Patricia Harris that implementation of the revised standards would take effect in October 1980 (Federal Register, March 19, 1980). Several weeks after the Secretary's announcement, a congressional finance committee delayed FIDCR implementation for yet another year, this time due to budgetary reasons. There is considerable dispute as to how much, if anything, will actually be saved by this delay. In the meantime, children and families suffer the consequences. It is imperative that the press and the public impress upon this nation's leaders that day care is not an issue to be treated lightly. Day care should be tailored to the needs of the many children it serves. (Zigler and Goodman, 1980).

Work and Family Life

With the two-paycheck family the norm rather than the exception, and the increase in single parenthood, the impact of the workplace on family life becomes an issue of concern. The relationship between the two institutions has been the subject of several recent studies which emphasize an important point: work and family life are not separate worlds as has been assumed but are, rather, interdependent and overlapping, with functions and behavioral rules within each system influencing processes within the other (Brim and Abeles, 1975; Kanter, 1977).

When there are children present, life for the dual-career family is stressful. Day care arrangements must be made for the infant and pre-school child; before and after school facilities have to be found for the older child; school vacations and days when the child is sick bring with them the need for yet other solutions. Since worker satisfaction and productivity have been found to be a function of family stability and other processes within the family system (cf. Kanter, 1977), it behooves industry to offer relevant services and benefits that would facilitate family life.

The role of industry in facilitating family life has been slow to develop. However, some of our suggestions with regard to work and family life have been tried by several of the major corporations. These include changes in the work structure to accommodate flexible working arrangements, part-time work opportunities, and job sharing. Companies are required by law to offer maternity leaves (Bureau of Business Practice, 1979). At best, these constitute 3 months, although school teachers, for example are able to take up to a year's leave of absence without pay in order to stay with their newborn infants. Some school systems offer maternity and paternity leave so as not to exclude the father from childrearing. However, as a nation we lag far behind other countries. According to Kamerman and Kahn (1976), European nations' pronatal policies include 6 to 12 months maternity or paternity leave with pay in order to facilitate childbearing, and provisions for child care are made when both parents work.

Several major corporations have instituted a variety of day care programs in support of their employees. Stride Rite Corporation, in Boston, has a company-based day care center as one of its employee benefits packages. Employees pay at the rate of 10 percent of their salary for the day care to a maximum of $25 a week (McIntyre, 1978). Levi Strauss and Company, in San Francisco, after 7 years of research and experimentation, concluded that day care services should be close to where people live rather than where they work (McIntyre, 1978). As a result of these findings Levi Strauss's policy is to "advocate the concept" of home day care. However, the company, while it is supporting research on the issue, does not have a reimbursement program for employees who use family day care homes.

Since company-based day care centers may not be entirely satisfactory and subsidizing such centers is expensive, several businesses could together support programs central to where their employees work. This would prove convenient to the employees as well as inexpensive because several business would contribute to the cost of one center. Part of the cost for child care might be paid by employees with the rest subsidized either by companies or unions. Children from low-income families who attend the facility could be subsidized by the state or federal government.

Industry could also support other activities that would promote interdependence among families within neighborhoods. For example, a PTA block-mother type arrangement (Mead, 1970) wherein parents take turns looking after children could be instituted. Such an arrangement would only work in conjunction with flexitime or other types of restructuring of the traditional work week. This service would be important not only in alleviating the stresses families currently face but also in promoting neighborhood stability.

Another option might be supporting a referral center or a network of senior citizens who could serve, for pay, as housekeepers or child care workers. This could be done in a center-based location or through referring families in need to those older citizens who wish to work in such capacities. This service might prove especially useful in alleviating the school-age day care problem, since it involves fewer hours per day of care, except at times when children are sick or vacationing. With grandparents usually not in the same locality, the use of senior citizens could also add another important dimension to the lives of children.

Support from Philanthropy

Much of the literature calling for business support of family life is related to industry's involvement through restructuring of working arrangements and including other relevant services as part of employee benefits. Industries could also channel support dollars through their corporate funding program (Zigler and Anderson, 1979). By law, corporations can generally donate as much as 5 percent of their net profits for charitable causes. They choose, however, to contribute less than 1 percent (Cmiel and Levy, 1980), despite the fact that these contributions are tax deductible. Furthermore, money that is donated by industry is channeled to sources that have little to do with family life. According to a recent analysis on corporate philanthropy (Cmiel and Levy, 1980), 49.1 percent of corporations changed their policies to reflect the impact of inflation and the retrenchment of government programs. Of those listing some changes, the most commonly cited changes were increased aid to higher education followed by cultural organizations. This means not so much a change as a reaffirmation of traditional priorities of corporate philanthropy (Finn, 1978). In terms of urban programs and community groups (these include children's programs) that might lose government programs, Cmiel and Levy note that "expressed corporate interest has not yet been translated into action." This is unfortunate considering the investment, in terms of employee satisfaction and productivity, corporations would be making if they provided financial aid in support of family life.

Conclusion

We have outlined in this chapter several ideas that could be tried out in response to problems facing children and families. It would be unrealistic to expect at these times of financial restraints revolutionary changes that involve eliminating societal stresses through the provision of jobs and adequate housing for everyone or the restructuring of our entire economy, as has been suggested by some writers (e.g., Keniston, 1977). We must acknowledge, however, that new patterns of family life that affect all people, but especially our children, are just now beginning to emerge. The social transition we are experiencing is difficult: a simple response is not the solution. Rather, a broad spectrum of options is needed, options that may be tried out without vast organizational expenditures.

Our nation cannot be transformed into a child-oriented society overnight. Progress and changes are gradual processes, and the first steps are undoubtedly the most difficult. The International Year of the Child has brought us to the threshold of our first steps toward becoming a nation that is concerned with and responsible for the optimal development of children. Parents, communities, and industry must now work together to ensure that our most valuable resource, our children, receive the care they deserve.

References

Abt. Associates. *Final report of the national day care study: Children at the center.* Executive Summary. Cambridge, MA: March 1979. (Contract No. HEW 105-74-1100).

Advisory Committee on Child Development. *Toward a national policy for children and families.* Washington, D.C.: National Academy of Sciences, 1976.

Albert, N., and Beck, A. T. Incidence of depression in early adolescence: A preliminary study. *Journal of Youth and Adolescence,* 1975, *4,* 301–307.

Anderson, R., and Henry, D. *A literature review and analysis on the use of corporal punishment in the care of children.* Austin, TX: Center for Social Work Research, University of Texas, 1976.

Beck, R. Child care: Story of neglect. *American Federationist,* 1979, *86,* 9–13.

Blatt, B. The pariah industry: A diary from purgatory and other places. In G. Gerbner, C. J. Ross, and E. Zigler (Eds.), *Child abuse: An agenda for action.* New York: Oxford University Press, in press.

Blatt, B., and Kaplan, F. *Christmas in purgatory.* Boston: Allyn and Bacon, 1966.

Boocock, S. S. A cross-cultural analysis of the child care system. In L. G. Katz (Ed.), *Current topics in early childhood.* Vol. 1. New Jersey: Ablex, 1977.

Brimm, O. G., Jr., and Abeles, R. P. Work and personality in the middle years. *Social Science Research Council Items.* 1975, *29,* 29–33.

Bronfenbrenner, U. Is early intervention effective? In H. J. Leichter (Ed.), *The family as educator.* New York: Teacher's College Press, Columbia University, 1975.

Brozan, N. Women now hold 30 percent of 2nd jobs. *New York Times,* June 24, 1980, B6.

Bureau of Business Practice. *Fair employment practice guidelines,* 1979, 170(9).

Burt, M. R. The comprehensive emergency services system: Expanding services to children and families. *Children Today,* 1976, 5(2), 2–5.

Campbell, D. T. Reforms as experiments. *American Psychologist,* 1969, *24,* 409–429.

Caplan, G. Family support systems in a changing world. In E. J. Antony and C. Chiland (Eds.), *The child in his family.* Vol. 5: *Children in a changing world.* New York: Wiley, 1978.

Cmiel, K., and Levy, S. *Corporate giving in Chicago: 1980.* Chicago: Donors Forum Library, 1980.

Cohen, D. J., and Zigler, E. Federal day care standards: Rationale and recommendations. *American Journal of Orthopsychiatry,* 1977, 47, 456–465.

Comptroller General of the United States. *Report to the Congress: Early childhood and family development programs improve the quality of life for low-income families.* Washington, D.C.: U.S. Government Accounting Office, February 6, 1979. (Document No. (HRD) 79–40).

Condry, J. C., and Siman, M. A. Characteristics of peer and adult-oriented children. *Journal of Marriage and the Family,* 1974, *36,* 543–544.

Condry, J. C., and Siman, M. A. *An experimental study of adult versus peer orientation.* Unpublished manuscript, Cornell University, 1976.

Congressional Record. January 15, 1979, S76–77.

Cranston, A. (Testimony). U.S. Congress. Senate Committee on Finance, Subcommittee on Public Assistance. *Proposals related to social and child welfare services, adoption assistance and foster care,* Ninety-Sixth Congress, September 24, 1979.

Edelman, M. W. Children instead of ships. *New York Times,* May 14, 1979.

Edelman, M. W. Newsletter distributted by Children's Defense Fund. June 1980.

Finn, M. Focus on foundation giving: Education. *The Philanthropy Monthly,* 1978, *11,* 20.

Friedan, B. Feminism takes a new turn. *The New York Times Magazine,* November 18, 1979, pp. 40, 92–106.

Furrow, D., Gruendel, J., and Zigler, E. *Protecting America's children from accidental injury and death. An overview of the problem and an agenda for action.* Unpublished manuscript, Yale University, 1979.

Gil, D. G. *Violence against children: Physical child abuse in the United States.* Cambridge, MA: Harvard University Press, 1970.

Harmon, C., Furrow, D., and Zigler, E. Childhood accidents: An overview of the problem and a call for action, *SRCD Newsletter,* Spring 1980.

Helfer, R. E. and Kempe, C. H. (Eds.). *Helping the battered child and his family.* Philadelphia: Lippincott, 1972.

Hofferth, S. L. Day care in the next decade: 1980–1990. *Journal of Marriage and the Family,* 1979, *41,* 649–657.

Kamerman, S. B., and Kahn, A. J. *European family policy currents: The question of families with very young children.* Unpublished manuscript, Columbia University, School of Social Work, 1976.

Kanter, R. M. *Work and family in the United States: A critical review and agenda for research and policy.* New York: Russell Sage Foundation, 1977.

Kashani, J., and Simonds, J. F. The incidence of depression in children. *Amrican Journal of Psychiatry,* 1979, *136,* 1203–1205.

Kempe, C. H., and Helfer, R. E. Innovative therapeutic approaches. In R. E. Helfer and C.H. Kempe (Eds.), *Helping the battered child and his family.* Philadelphia: Lippincott, 1972.

Keniston, K. *All our children.* New York: Harcourt, Brace, Jovanovich, 1977.

Keyserling, M. D. *Windows on day care.* New York: National Council of Jewish Women, 1972.

Knowles, J. H. (Ed.). *Doing better and feeling worse. Health in the United States.* New York: W. W. Norton, 1977.

Lash, T. W., Sigal, H., and Dudzinski, D. *State of the child: New York City (11).* New York: Foundation for Child Development, 1980.

Light, R. Abused and neglected children in America: A study of alternative policies. *Harvard Educational Review,* 1973, *43,* 556–598.

Maden, M. F., and Wrench, D. F. Significant findings in child abuse research. *Victimology,* 1977, *2,* 196–224.

Martinez, A. (Testimony). U.S. Congress. House Committee on Education and Labor, Subcommittee on Select Education. *Proposed extension of the Child Abuse Prevention and Treatment Act,* Ninety-Fifth Congress, March 11, 1977.

Martinez, A. (Testimony). U.S. Congress. Senate Committee on Labor and Human Resources, Subcommittee on Child and Human Development. *Child Care Act of 1979,* Ninety-Sixty Congress, February 21, 1979.

McIntyre, K. J. Day Care: An employer benefit, too. *Business Insurance,* December 11, 1978, pp. 11–36.

Mead, M. Working mothers and their children. *Childhood Education,* 1970, *47,* 66–71.

Mednick, B. R., Baker, R.L., and Sutton-Smith, B. *Teenage pregnancy and perinatal mortality.* Unpublished manuscript, study supported by the National Institute of Child Health and Human Development, Grant No. 75-7-060, 1979.

National Education Association Task Force on Corporal Punishment. *Report of the task force on corporal punishment.* Washington, D.C.: National Education Association, 1972.

Norton, A. Portrait of the one-parent family. *The National Elementary Principal,* 1979, *59,* 32–35.

Palmer, F.H., and Andersen, L.W. Long-term gains from early intervention: Findings from longitudinal studies. In E. Zigler and J. Valentine (Eds.), *Project Head Start: A legacy of the war on poverty.* New York: The Free Press, 1979.

Pearson, D. E. , and Nicol, E.H. *The fourth year of the Brookline Early Education Project: A report of progress and plans.* Unpublished report, 1977, Brookline Early Education Project, 987 Kent Street, Brookline, MA 02146.

Scott, R. Research and early childhood: The Home Start Project. *Child Welfare,* 1974, *53,* 112–119.

Siman, M. A. *Peer group influence during adolescence: A study of 41 naturally existing friendship groups.* Doctoral Dissertation, Cornell University, 1973.

Smith, R. E. (Ed.). *The subtle revolution: Women at work.* Washington, D.C.: The Urban Institute, 1979.

Smock, S. M. *The children: The shapes of child care in Detroit.* Detroit: Wayne State University Press, 1977.

U.S. Bureau of the Census. *Current Population Reports.* Series P-23, No. 84. Washington, D.C.: U.S. Department of Commerce, 1979.

U.S. Department of Health, Education and Welfare. *Monthly Vital Statistics Report.* Provisional Statistics, June 30, 1976, *24,* 13.

U.S. Department of Health and Human Services. *Monthly Vital Statistics Report.* Advanced Report, Final Natality Statistics 1978, April 28, 1980, *29,* 1 (supp.).

Valentine, J., and Stark, E. The social context of parent involvement in Head Start. In E. Zigler and J. Valentine (Eds.), *Project Head Start: A legacy of the war on poverty.* New York: The Free Press, 1979.

Ward, E. H. CDA: Credentialing for day care. *Voice for Children,* 1976, *9,* 15.

White House Conference on Children. *Report to the President.* Washington, D.C.: U.S. Government Printing Office, 1970.

Wooden, K. *Weeping in the playtime of others.* New York: McGraw-Hill, 1976.

Wynne, E. A. Behind the discipline problem: Youth suicide as a measure of alienation. *Phi Delta Kappan,* 1978, *54,* 307–315.

Yankelovich, Skelly, White, Inc. *The General Mills American family report 1974– 1975.* Minneapolis: General Mills, 1975.

Zelnick, M., and Kantner, J. First pregnancies to women aged 15 to 19: 1971 and 1976. *Family Planning Perspectives,* 1978, *10,* 11–20.

Zigler, E., and Anderson, K. Foundation support in the child and family life field. *The Philanthropy Monthly,* 1979, *12,* 12–14.

Zigler, E., and Goodman, J. On day care standards—again. *The Networker: Newsletter of the Bush Programs in Child Development and Social Policy.* New Haven, CT: 1980, *2*(1).

Zigler, E., and Heller, K. A. Day care standards approach critical juncture. *Day Care and Early Education,* 1980, *7,* 7–8; 47.

Zigler, E., and Kagan, S. L. *The Child Development Association: Has the 1970 challenge been met?* Unpublished manuscript, Yale University, 1980.

Zigler, E., and Seitz, V. Social policy implications of research on intelligence. In R. J. Sternberg (Ed.), *Handbook of human intelligence.* New York: Cambridge University Press, in press. (a)

Zigler, E., and Seitz, V. *Early Childhood Intervention Programs: A re-analysis.* Submitted for publication. (b)

Zigler, E., and Valentine, J. (Eds.). *Project Head Start: A legacy of the war on poverty.* New York: The Free Press, 1979.

Early Childhood Development as a Policy Goal

Richard H. de Lone

To speak of facilitating early childhood development is often to imply an agenda for public policy. The implication is that left to their own devices, some or all children do not develop optimally (whatever that means) in our society. Something must be marshalled—information, programs, transfer payments, professionals—through allocation of public resources.

That said, any policy approach to facilitating development must be based on good theory—a sound understanding of what development is and how it occurs—and it must be a theory that can be translated into action: that is, a set of resource allocations and decisions which will reliably lead to the desired outcomes predicted by the theory. In the world of public policy, a theory is no better than its application, and vice versa. So, for instance, Kohlberg's stage theory of moral development may strike one as beautiful and "true," but it has no more relevance for public policy than Keats's "Ode on a Grecian Urn" unless it can be put into operation as programs or strategies that promote moral improvement. Although these comments verge on truism, even a cursory acquaintance with the annals of public policy makes it clear that such policy is often based on interesting theories which cannot be effectively applied, or (more commonly, perhaps) on no theory at all. In the press of politics, any handle may be grabbed, whether it opens the right door or not.

Because developmental theory and public policy concerning family and children have been more closely allied than is true for most other issues in the social and behaviorial sciences, as I have argued elsewhere (de Lone, 1979), it may be worth pursuing this truism in more detail. An understanding of the requirements of public policy may help in deciding which policy alternatives (if any) are most likely to be effective in facilitating infant and child development.

There can, of course, be no public policy worth mentioning unless there is some shared understanding of goals and a consensus that these goals are sufficiently important to merit the allocation of scarce public resources. For present purposes, however, I will assume, perhaps foolishly, that a rough consensus exists that it is in the public interest to allocate resources toward making children smarter, healthier, emotionally better rounded and socially more competent, and that there is a general understanding, as well, of what these things mean. Accepting these givens, adequate public policy—in this or any field—must fulfill four criteria:

- It must be based on sound theory.
- That theory must be translated into an adequate policy framework through the legislative and administrative functions of government.
- There must be a "delivery system" capable of carrying out the policy.
- There must be a practicable and reasonably well-defined set of techniques (applications of theory) at the ultimate point of delivery.

One can be more or less rigorous in deciding what constitutes a sound theory for public policy. In matters of foreign policy, for instance, informed judgment has to serve in lieu of any theory that one might call "scientific," for inaction is not a permissable policy choice. But in matters of human development, as in matters like thalidomide, it is certainly desirable to have a theory that goes beyond mere descriptive plausibility or clinical hunches (valuable as those hunches may be in some settings). A sound theory for public policy aimed at facilitating child development should have predictive value, it should be dynamic, it should facilitate child development, and it should be empirically validated or scientific (in Popper's sense that it is disprovable). I would argue that, in addition, it should have a firm philosophical base, an epistemological self-consciousness. Since most empirical work in social science uses proxies to measure the thing, not the thing itself, it is entirely possible to sustain the illusion of empirical (and even of predictive, dynamic) validity by guileless confusion of epiphenomena with the phenomena. As Kessen (1966) has warned, if we ignore epistemological issues, we face the clear and present danger that "our conclusions about the development of human knowledge may derive in large measure from the preconceptions of the nature of man and the nature of reality that we have stuffed—or, worse, let slip—into our initial conception of the psychological task" (p. 61). Those words could serve as an epitaph for volumes of worthless controversy on the subject of IQ.

A further hazard for the social and behavioral sciences lies in the fact that so much theory is basically taxonomic, not dynamic: we break the phenomenon into pieces; give each piece a label (e.g., IQ; self-concept, demographic characteristic); express the label in quantitative terms; find mathematical relationships between quantities; and—forgetting that the thing itself is something more than, indeed different from, the sum of its labels—yield too often to the temptation to believe that the phenomenon has been explained. Thus, taxonomies masquerade as dynamic theories of causation. This error is particularly likely to occur as one moves from the academic literature to the lay interpretation of that literature for policy-making purposes, and it has a glorious history in the social sciences, too. One can consider, for instance, the history of the so-called Phillip's curve, which led economists to believe that there was an inevitable trade-off between inflation and unemployment (i.e., that high inflation would result from low unemployment and vice versa), a notion that OPEC and "stagflation" recently washed down the drain when it became apparent that the implicit model relating these two factors dynamically was too simple (see, for instance, Lekachman, 1976). Closer to home, the famous assertion of Bloom (1964)—that "in terms of intelligence measured at age 17, about 50 percent of the development takes place between conception and age 4," (p. 88)—was based not only on a questionable definition of intelligence but partly on erroneous reasoning which confused explained variance in test scores (at different times on different tests) with an explanation of development itself.

The second criterion, development of an adequate policy framework, also implies several subcriteria. One is that sound theory will inform legislative and administration policy planning. This, of course, is not always true because of political constraints, or because of the time lag required for research to enter the policy stream, or because of the insouciant ignorance of policy makers. But there is more to an adequate policy framework than good theory. Adequate policy also requires that the goals and objectives of the policy are logically connected to the theory, that resources and timelines are adequate for attainment of those objectives, and that what I will call the "sphere of agency" is properly conceptualized and inherently capable of performing what the theory and objectives of a policy would have it perform.

The well-known story of Head Start provides an illustration of the requirement that goals be logically related to theory. Let us assume for the sake of argument that Head Start was grounded in sound developmental theory about the importance of the early years for cognitive development. Alas, this does not mean that, even if the early cognitive gains experienced by many children in Head Start had been maintained that Head Start would have helped achieve the objectives of the legislation, which were ultimately to improve the economic status of blacks and other low-income children. For in fact, as numerous studies, most of which were thoroughly assessed by Jencks, Bartletts, Corcoran, Crouse, Eaglesfield, Jackson, McLelland, Mueser, Olneck, Schwartz, Ward, and Williams (1979) have shown individual differences in cognitive skills explain at best a minor part of variation in economic achievement.

Examples of policies that are inadequately funded or given impossible time constraints are legion, and the point needs no clarification. The notion of a proper sphere of agency is a bit subtler. At its simplest, it merely means that the delivery system—usually some set of bureaucracies—has the capacity and mandate to implement the policy. This condition is sometimes violated when agencies are asked to take on assignments for which they in fact have little or no experience, capacity, or incentive to perform. There may be subtler problems, however, with the sphere of agency. One major class of problems results from unintended consequences of social programs (consequences which are sometimes serendipitous but more often not). For example, when resources are scarce, policy must generally attempt to define the target population with the "problem" that the policy is supposed to resolve. But the act of definition can easily turn into an act of stigmatization which is counterproductive. Programs for slow learners, the mentally retarded, the emotionally disturbed, the socially maladjusted, and so on are examples. A second major class of problems can occur when the tacit functions of a system are in conflict with the explicit goals of a policy. For example, some have argued that the educational enterprise services the tacit function of social control and perpetuation of the status quo, in direct conflict with the explicit goals of many programs that have tried to use the schools to promote the development and social mobility of disadvantaged groups (e.g., Bowles and Gintis, 1976; Leacock, 1969). A third type of sphere of agency problem results from systemic contraditions. For example, in our cyclic economy, policies and programs intended to alleviate economic hardships are hardest to fund when needed most (i.e., when the economy is in a low). Similarly, many human service programs, because they more nearly resemble an art form than an engineering exercise, depend on the judgment and discretion of local service providers. But a counterforce, the pressure for accountability from remote funding sources (such as the federal government) may generate regulations and stipulations that severely limit the domain of judgement.

The next step in this continuum of policy criteria concerns the adequacy of delivery systems. Assuming the chosen delivery system is the proper sphere of agency, a host of everyday problems results which are no easier to solve because of their familiarity. Here we are largely concerned with intergovernmental relations, effective management, coordination of services, adequate planning, staff training, clinical practice, evaluation, and the like—the entire apparatus of public administration. Suffice it to say that it is always theoretically possible to do things well, but Murphy's law constantly asserts itself. The safest assumption is that large-scale efforts will be implemented with variable quality, and the modal performance will be, by qualitative standards, mediocre. Where excellence is required, public programs will always disappoint. De Lone's law says: if the thing is not worth doing in a mediocre fashion, it is not worth doing at all!

The final criterion is the availability of adequate technique (applied theory) to implement a policy which survives the above tests. To illustrate from another field, economists have a pretty good idea of what makes a small business viable or what makes a good investment. But the ability of economists (or anyone else) to translate that theory into concrete steps which would cut down the rather high failure rate of small businesses, or which would result in an investment portfolio that consistently outperformed the market norm, simply does not exist.[1] Similarly, one may conclude that Piaget has developed a valid model of cognitive growth and be completely unable to tell a teacher what kinds of interventions will hasten the process: perhaps this is just the state of the art, or perhaps it is that growth cannot be nudged; it just happens.

Linked to the criterion of technique is the question of evaluation. How do we know when something has worked? Problems of methodology and instrumentation aside, evaluating programs or policies that aim at fostering *development* is terribly hard to do. Even with adequate controls and pre-post measures, short-term studies are almost invariably subject to the suspicion that they measure learned (and hence forgettable) responses, not development which is, in the absence of extraordinary circumstances, irreversible. But longitudinal studies that are methodologically sufficient are few and far between, slow by definition, time-bound (as are all studies of social phenomena), and rarely capable of providing firm conclusions on more than a few points. Indeed, social science is generally better at telling us what has not worked than what will. But the problems are only in part methodological and logistical. They are also epistemological. Interpreting measurements requires that we reexamine the proxies used in evaluating effectiveness, the assumptions implicit in our theories, and the exogenous factors (for instance, flaws in the delivery system) which may have influenced results. Hence, the question of technique, which requires evaluation, leads to a closing of the loop and a return to the questions and issues posed in the first three criteria.

Table 1 summarizes the criteria listed here. In the balance of this paper,

---

1. To be sure, the market itself is the mediator of risk.

Table 1: Criteria for Effective Public Policy

Criterion	Tests
Sound theory	Descriptive plausibility
	Predictive value
	Dynamic properties (causal relations)
	Empirical validity
Adequate policy framework	Embodies sound theory
	Goals and objectives congruent with theory
	Resource and logistical adequacy
	Proper sphere of agency not unintended outcomes harmony of tacit and explicit functions absence of systemic contradictions
Effective delivery system	Management
	Planning
	Personnel
	Fiscal systems
	Evaluation systems
Viable technique	"clinical" lore
	"Evaluatability"

these criteria will be used to test some major choices which present themselves to anyone interested in selecting a public policy approach that will in fact facilitate infant and child development.

Traditionally, the children whose development has been of primary concern to public policy are children from low-income families, many of whom are members of minority groups. And while public policy has placed a particular emphasis on cognitive development (through early childhood education programs and other vehicles), the view of development implicit in much policy discussion is a rather broad (perhaps even loose) one. It includes health promotion, emotional growth, and social competence. Its aim is nothing less than facilitating the growth of capable, fully competent, and functional adults who can make their way in society and contribute something to it.

These broad goals are hard to fault. While developmental liabilities know no bounds of class or race, any review of the state of children in the United States leads to the conclusion that the children of low-income families face systematically more severe developmental hazards as a re-

sult of their social and economic status (e.g., Keniston, 1977). Yet there
has been a persistent tendency to confuse policies that aim at promoting
individual development with strategies for changing the social conditions
that produce developmental risk. This is an old tendency in our society,
as evident in early 19th century school reform (Katz, 1969) as in subsequent waves of social reform up to and through the Great Society (de
Lone, 1979). The reasons for this confusion lie deeply rooted in the heritage of classic liberalism which was and is our dominant social, political,
and economic heritage. For liberalism, as embodied in American culture,
views the individual as the *alpha* and *omega* of society. Not only is the
promotion of individual liberty and happiness viewed as the end of society, but the society is viewed as the sum and product of so many individual actors and actions—just as in the classic view of the free market, the
economy is the result of myriad individual choices and preferences,
guided by the invisible hand of the market.

Our pernicious cultural habit of equating virtue with economic success, and immorality with poverty (evident in 18th century legacies of
the British "poor laws" and in 20th century attitudes toward welfare recipients); our Horatio Alger mythology, as alive today as ever; and the
reams of regressions run by sociologists studying social mobility with
equations in which social status is the dependent variable and a host of
individual characteristics serve as the right-hand variables, are but a few
examples of the intellectual consequences of "explaining" society by studying individuals. But the apotheosis of this tendency, and a central
framework for public policy, has been the doctrine of equal opportunity.
This doctrine contains an admirable social goal but, as it becomes confused with a social fact and transmuted into a social theory, is also a dangerous sophistry.

In what I take to be the mainstream version of this cultural ideal/myth/
theory, the notion is that once "artificial" constraints such as discrimination, bad diets, and poor schooling are eliminated, individuals can,
should, and will make their way in the world more or less as their merits
dictate. The result will be a society in equilibrium, with each rewarded in
proportion to his or her contribution to the whole (e.g., Bell, 1973;
Plattner, 1979). To be sure, individual talents, propensities, and preferences are important and have an important bearing on social outcomes,
but it is apparent that this somewhat more sophisticated restatement of
the notion that every person is master of his or her fate ignores substantially the effect that social and economic structures may have not only on
social outcomes but even on individual development, as will be discussed
subsequently. Consider, for instance, the variety of studies which have
concluded that social origins (race and class at birth) have more influence

than any other factor on the likely status of adults, even when controlling for individual ability (cf. Sewell, 1971, regarding educational attainment; Bowles and Gintis, 1974, 1976; Brittain, 1977; and the comprehensive review and reanalysis of numerous studies by Jencks, 1979).

The relevance of all this to public policy for facilitating child development is simply this: historically, there has been a strange brew of developmental theory and social theory in our public policy. Developmental theory—and programs based on it—have played the role of the alchemical agent dropped in the pot of equal opportunity to turn the lives of the disadvantaged into gold. What the philosopher's stone has yielded is something else: an almost metaphysical confusion of developmental theory and social theory which has served neither policy—nor children—well.

I do not mean to suggest that the problem has been caused by mixing apples and oranges, developmental theory and social theory, or that development should be left to the psychologists and social change to others. Development occurs in society, and no one would seriously argue for long that it makes any sense to think about development out of social context. Conversely, a social theory which does not incorporate an understanding of the ways in which individuals develop will be a pale theory. Public policy based on either will risk failure. The question, in other words, is how to develop a developmental theory in proper relation to social theory (and vice versa) as the basis for policy.

That we need do so is apparent from the abundant literature which suggests the interplay between individual and socioeconomic factors. Virtually all studies which try to identify developmental risk end up listing socioeconomic indicators. For a typical example, there is the paper presented at the Vermont Conference last year by Rutter (1979), who cited the following risk factors associated with child psychiatric disorder: severe marital discord, low social status, overcrowding or large family size, paternal criminality, maternal psychiatric disorder, admission to the care of the local authority (e.g., the child welfare system), and possibly "scope of opportunity." What these have to do with Freud is problematic, but it is striking that almost all are associated, in greater or lesser strength, with parental poverty and its sibling, unemployment. Conversely, a copious literature illustrates the pathogenic effects of unemployment and poverty on adults (and through them, on children in a variety of ways). So Brenner (1976) has found that a rise of 1 percentage point in unemployment is associated with an 8.7 percent increase in narcotics use, a 5.7 percent increase in robberies, a 3.8 percent increase in homicides, and a higher incidence of mental illness; Eisenberg (1979), reviewing a large body of studies, concluded that any major breakthrough in the health status of low-income children in this country is likely to come from employment and income increases; Ross and Sawhill (1975) found that unemployment explains most of the difference between black and white rates of family dissolution. One could go on to cite ad nauseam studies linking poverty and poor nutrition, poverty and low school achievement, poverty and family breakup, and so forth. The ubiquity of these findings pushes us to conclude that there is some relationship between socioeconomic status and development, but the questions remain. Just what is that relationship? How should theory account for it? What are the dynamics of the relationship? What is the proper policy framework for addressing it, and what are the implications for delivery and technique?

To simplify the matter, I would suggest that there are two broad policy options which flow from an effort to accommodate this relationship. Implicitly or explicitly, these options reflect two divergent theories or models, to use a somewhat more apt term, of the relationship between development and socioeconomic conditions.

One approach can be called the micro model, and it has typified most efforts at social reform in the United States. The other I will call the macro model. To so distinguish is somewhat to caricature both, but for purposes of this short discussion, it may also help clarify some basic considerations.

The micro approach is based on essentially normative criteria of development. Although it may draw on a diversity of disciplines for its theories and models of development (biogenetics, epigenetics, behaviorism, neo-Freudianism, etc.), its overarching model of development has three basic parameters: (1) it views the early years as the plastic years, the critical period and even determinative period in human development; (2) it treats development as the result of a series of inputs (genes, nutrients, environmental stimulae) and interactions (between genes and stimulae, parent and child, etc), and (3) it treats environment as the child's immediate surrounding—family, neighborhood, school and, in more studies than not, simply "mom."[2] As a basis for policy, this model of development leads to an emphasis on funding programs which aim at identifying "at risk" individuals—that is, those whose development by normative standards is likely to be deficient—and providing them with targeted interventions which may run the gamut from early childhood education programs, to parent education, to maternal and infant health care, to genetic engineering, and more. These are interventions applied with more

2. Urie Bronfenbrenner and others, using a taxonomy somewhat similar to that used here, have referred to such institutions (family, school, neighborhood) as the mezzo-structure.

or less professional assistance, in a "helper/helpee" clinical framework. Publicly funded programs and hence public bureaucracies, including the education system, the health system, and the welfare system, are assigned the responsibility for implementing these programs, and to a considerable measure, the colleges and universities are involved both in training practitioners in the techniques used in these approaches and in evaluating their effectiveness.

The second broad approach, the macro approach, exists more in literature and argument than it does in fact, for it is by and large the road not taken by public policy. It views the criteria for development as essentially relativistic, not normative. And, while acknowledging the sensitivity and importance of the early childhood years, the macro model (at least in this writer's version) views development as a continuous process of the organism seeking equilibrium with its spatial and temporal environment, not only in early years but into adulthood. It defines the operative developmental environment as including not simply the immediate surround, but also the class, race, sex, and cultural group to which the individual belongs, and the social situation in which that membership finds itself at any moment in historical time (with a past, present, and prospective future). In this perspective, the immediate surround is viewed as a mediator, a filter, not a "causal" agent. The simplest way to make this rather abstract and complex generalization palpable is to consider a cross-cultural example. Michael Cole and his associates have made the point strikingly in their study of the reasoning and performance of American and Kpelle (Liberian) children (and adults). Although Kpelles fail to solve "riddles" which we consider ridiculously simple, Americans perform less well than Kpelles in certain tasks, such as sorting leaves into categories, that are intrinsic to the later group's culture. Yet no one would infer from such evidence that either group is developmentally deficient or incapable of problem solving. Rather, the more plausible conclusion is that "cultural differences in cognition reside more in the situations to which particular cognitive processes are applied than in the existence of a process in one cultural group and its absence in another" (Cole, Gay, Glick, and Sharp, 1971, p. 233). By the same token, children within one society who come from different racial, ethnic, class, and perhaps sex background, insofar as they depart from the norm *as a group* in developmental patterns, may be reflecting differences "in the situations" defined by their group membership.

Finally, this alternative model places an emphasis on the individual as theory builder or "map maker" whose personal contruction of reality, comes from the processing of information derived from his or her "situation", information which, in the early years in particular, is filtered through the immediate surround. The process implied is akin to developing, testing, and refining hypotheses about social reality and the child's likely future in it. These hypotheses guide development (both as internal structure and conscious behavior) of the kinds of skills, behaviors, and attitudes (tacit and conscious) which will be rewarded in it. This map or theory, in turn, structures each new encounter with experience and in some rather obscure sense guides subsequent development. (For a fuller treatment of this concept, and its progenitors, which trace back at least to Kelly, 1955, see Laosa, 1979 and de Lone, 1979.)

With this view of development uppermost, it becomes almost meaningless to argue that one child (or one group of children) develops less "well" than another. Rather, the judicious presumption should be made that all develop equally well in response to their circumstances, unless proven otherwise. Accordingly, if there are developmental differences which seem socially undesirable in their results, one should look to change the circumstances rather than attempt to change the individuals. For instance, if minority youth achieve poorly in school, drop out, cannot find work, and are more frequently convicted of crimes than majority youth, as they do, one should look to changing the circumstantial meaning of being black (or brown, or red) in the United States not only because such changes may be good things in themselves but also because they have developmental implications![3]

From this perspective, a relevant framework for a social policy which facilitates child development must encompass basic structural principles: the skills required by the occupational technostructure; the system of caste and class differentiation; the structure of opportunity (not simply educational pathways but, even more centrally, the distribution and control of capital investments which generate jobs and ration opportunities); and the distribution of income and wealth. The leading programmatic elements of such policy consist of full employment policies, economic development if beneficial to members of low-income groups and communities, affirmative action programs, minimum income supports, and similar efforts aimed at greater equality in the political economy. In current rhetoric, the foundation of a "family policy" is viewed as economic support. Again, one must turn to public bureaucracies to deliver such an approach, but the emphasis goes to the system of taxa-

3. This argument, it should be observed, is not equivalent to arguing that subcultural values should be altered, nor is it equivalent to romanticizing cultural differences. As Ogbu (1978) has argued, cultural heritages are not in themselves either an asset or a liability in terms of social outcomes. They may prove to be a strength, a weakness, or entirely neutral only with respect to the way in which they constitute a reactive adaption to the dominant groups' terms or in respect to the way the dominant group reacts to them.

tion and regulatory agencies, as opposed to human service bureaucracies. At the level of "technique," the issue is less one of "helping" or of clinical skill than it is one of creating incentives and opportunities for empowerment of the disenfranchised.

Before applying to these broad alternatives the policy tests suggested in the first part of this paper (which both will flunk in some aspects), it is important to indicate that the choices are not quite as polar as implied. For one thing, the notion of the child as theory builder, constructing reality and a way of processing it through interaction with the environment, has close analogies both in Piagetian and Skinnerian versions of reciprocal action between organism and environment.

For another, there will be individual variance in development even when sociocultural situations are similar, for reasons that are likely to be a problematic mix of genetic, micro environmental, and idiosyncratic "theory building" differences.

For another, to say that the family or other structure in the immediate surround is a mediating, not a primary influence on development does not gainsay the usefulness of studying those micro interactions (although it does alter their interpretation or meaning for policy purposes). Nor does it mean that all developmental liabilities are associated with class or racial status. Nor does the "macro" alternative imply the "micro" interventions can never affect the class- or race-related course of development. What it does suggest, however, is that the intervention, to have impact, must be sharp, major, and sustained. For example, when Kpelle children are placed in Western-type schools for a number of years (a sharp and sustained break with traditional, that is, nonschool, education in the village), they exhibit cognitive processes similar to those of Western children (Cole et al. 1971). By contrast, parent education programs, early childhood education, or other micro interventions are typically marginal and sporadic interventions which do not fundamentally alter the situation of the child. If they have much impact on development, the studies which demonstrate such impact have been carefully hidden.

But what, one may ask, about genes? This paper will not enter the heredity-environment controversy except to make a couple of points: one, there is no doubt a genetic component to intelligence and other aspects of development; two, insofar as genetic endowment places absolute limits on development, this fact is of little use for policy unless one resurrects eugenicism or dreams of a future of clones, for that which can be influenced by policy is the environmental side of the equation; and three, there is no reason to suspect that genes have much to do with determining the class structure or the inequality of social and economic conditions which characterizes this or any other society since individual characteristics explain only a small portion of the variance in social outcomes. Indeed, such specific factors as IQ are only mildly associated with adult success. McLelland (1973), for instance, found correlations of .2 between childhood IQ and adult success as measured by a variety of indicators; this would lead one to conclude that even with a robust claim for the influence of genetic endowment on intelligence, no more than 2 or 3 percent of the variance in social status can be explained by genetic contributions to intelligence!

Let us then consider the claims of these two approaches as the basis for public policy aimed at facilitating infant and early childhood development.

Adequacy as Theory

Current knowledge of the hows and whyfores of child development is, of course, imperfect. Yet, developmentalists can paint a fairly plausible picture of critical events, sequences, and factors (biological and environmental) in human development. However, such plausibility is not in itself sufficient for public policy if one assumes that the goal of policy should be, as suggested above, nothing less than facilitating the growth of capable, fully competent, and functional adults who can make their way in and contribute to society. To support this goal, a theory must not only tell us how children develop, it must include a description of how to intervene in a way that enhances development, and it must include a social theory which is able to identify systemmatically the childhood interventions which will lead with some predictability to adult outcomes. One result of the flurry of interest that occurred in the late 1960s and early 1970s in early childhood development programs was that many leading developmentalists were forced into an agonizing reappraisal of the limits of their knowledge. The effectiveness of interventions—especially in the area of cognitive development—is generally in doubt; the notion that the early years are "critical" to (or determinative of) adult development has been modified to the more modest and supportable claim that the early years are a "sensitive" developmental period, and, indeed, the ability to predict adult characteristics from childhood ones is quite limited (White, Day, Freeman, Hartman, and Messenger, 1973). It is not, in fact, until children reach the age of 8 or 9 (approximately the third grade) that one can begin to construct a plausible future scenario, based on such factors as correlations in year-to-year performance in school achievement, probabilities linking school achievement to school attainment, and the relationship of school attainment to occupational status. But even here, the predictions are very rough and based on crude variables. There remains a tremendous amount of individual variability, and it is by no means clear whether one's scenario is based on developmental stabilities or rigidities in social and institutional process, that is, predictable continuities of socially determined experience, not developmental stabilities (de Lone, 1979).

In short, the theoretical basis for the micro approach to developmental policy is shaky. The more ambitious the goals of that policy, the shakier it becomes. For instance, there is considerable theory and knowledge to support certain targeted services which aim at identifying and correcting individually specific developmental disabilities, from nutritional deficits to learning disabilities, in the sensitive period of childhood. There are important and proper, if modest, goals for public policy. But there is not adequate theory to support the micro approach if the effort is to facilitate the development of that class of children most "at risk" as a class—children of low income and minority groups. As suggested above, it has been the strange conjunction of liberal social theory and developmentalism which have made it easy for policy makers to commit the fundamental error of assuming that microdeterminants of individual development can be manipulated through program interventions to alter social outcomes. Our preconceptions of reality—of social reality, in particular—have been let slip or stuffed into our conception of the psychological task in this regard, and they must be unpacked.

Is the macro approach a theoretically superior alternative? It would be stretching things to attempt a definitive positive answer to this question. But there are reasons to believe it may be superior. It is a perspective which begins by attempting to imbed development in social context. On a priori grounds such an effort appears necessary if one is to take any but a very narrow view of what developmental policy should be. As such, it offers possibilities of yielding a dynamic conceptual framework which systematically relates individual development to social and economic structures and the contexts they produce. Further, it does not negate or disregard the main body of developmental theory so much as it places it in a different perspective and dynamic framework for policy purposes. In particular, its primary policy strategy involves supporting the economic status and security of the family, the agency which, for most of the children most of the time, serves as the source of nurture and the filter of experience. Common sense suggests that publicly funded, professionally delivered interventions are likely to be second-best substitutes for a secure family (however one defines that increasingly nebulous concept), and a body of evidence overwhelming in scale makes it clear that employment, and the economic security which goes with it, is *the* most important *single* determinant of family well-being. Further, such limited evidence as is available suggests that even *without changes in* employment status, simply increasing family income leads to benefits which most of us would conclude enhance the developmental milieu of families. Consider, for instance, this summary of findings from the income maintenance experiments:

The findings on family well-being are not uniformly positive or consistent, and they include some negative as well as numerous beneficial effects. But, taken together, they suggest the potential effects of a more adequate system of income support. These findings indicate that welfare reform that results in the kinds of programs tested in the experiments would contribute to less welfare dependency in the long run, which would (at least partially) offset the disincentive effects on work effort. Many families would use the payments to increase their long-run well-being and their earnings capacity, increase their savings, reduce their debt, obtain additional education and training, and migrate to areas with better opportunities. There would be improvement in nutrition and in the health of children at birth. Drop-out rates among teenagers would diminish, and perhaps there would be improvements in school performance. Finally, there would be less reliance on public housing. (Kehrer, 1979, p. 17)

On the other hand, much of the argument of the developmental payoff of a macro strategy relies on theory that is more intuitive than empirical. Cross-cultural studies are the best empirical source, and they do more to establish the broad fact that developmental patterns differ in distinctly different cultures than they do to illuminate the mechanics of development or the developmental importance of different socioeconomic contexts, social class settings, and subcultures within a society. The notion of the child as an actor in his or her own development through "map making" or the construction of a theory of social reality has a rather mysterious concept at its core, and it gains plausibility more from anecdotal data and analogies to cybernetics than from psychological research. Insofar as one demands a theory that meets all the tests sketched out above, then none is available. Insofar as one is forced to choose among these competing alternatives, however, a modest conclusion on the merits would seem to be that the macro alternative is as worthy of consideration as the prevailing micro choice. A more heroic assumption is that it is preferable. In any event, researchers can rest happy in the knowledge that more research is called for!

Sphere of Agency, Delivery Systems, and Technique

Beyond matters of theory, an effort to test systematically these two broad policy approaches against the criteria suggested above for adequate policy framework, effective delivery systems, and viable technique would require specification of policy strategies and lengthy discussion of implementational issues. It lies well beyond the scope of this paper, and, if theory is wrong, implementational issues are moot. A few overall points are worth making, however, beginning with an examination of micro approaches.

First, if an aim of public policy is to reduce the developmental penalties paid by children guilty of being born to low-income parents, it should be remembered that what is good for the goose is usually good for the gander. Thus, micro approaches which "improve" the development of poor children will also benefit affluent children (and are likely to benefit them more). While this may raise the developmental mean for the society as a whole, it will do nothing to eliminate the relative disadvantage of low-income children, who will remain relatively at risk by standards which are, finally, relative to any given society! Inequality can absorb individual interventions.

Second, when human service programs address the poor, sphere-of-agency problems do arise, as indicated briefly in the examples (stigma, systemic contradictions, etc.) given earlier. It is hard to be sure whether these problems outweigh the benefits, but it is entirely possible that they do, if the kinds of perverse effects frequently found in human service programs for older age groups apply in early childhood. Consider just one example: that recent studies show that vocational education programs not only fail to enhance the earnings and employment records of some (mostly male) recipients, but they also result in lowered aspirations, and in some groups lower rates of school attainment—a fact which probably damages future earnings prospects (Grasso and Shea, 1979).

Third, given the failure of evaluation research to find significant or lasting benefits of early childhood education programs, parent education programs, or similar developmental programs, one must conclude that if clinicians exist whose efforts have consistently positive results for reasons other than chance, they are few and far between. Occasional successes may be the result of exceptionally skilled clinicians, but it seems doubtful that public bureaucracies can replicate this scarce factor.

Again the question arises, do the macro alternatives meet these largely implementational tests any better? Again the answer is equivocal. Little in the past history of welfare programs, employment and training programs, or economic development programs gives one much to cheer about. Full employment, the prerequisite for an effective economic support program, is no easy thing to achieve and has been surprisingly unpopular as a political goal in this country (Nixon, 1973). Bureaucratic as well as technical obstacles exist. Yet, as economist Lester Thurow and others have argued, the basic issues are less those of economic theory, policy framework, or delivery than they are of political will (Thurow,

1973). It is not technically difficult to design or administer a credit income tax that would place a minimum income under every family and that would help to redistribute income (e.g., Keniston, 1977). Despite the bad public relations of the CETA system, evaluations have consistently found that the bureaucratic capacity to create publicly subsidized employment of reasonable (if variable) quality exists. And there is ample theoretical justification for the use of wage and capital subsidy programs which, without fueling inflation, can increase the employment opportunities for the so-called structurally unemployed (Eisner, 1978).

Child developmentalists cannot alone create the political will to drive this country toward an egalitarian family support policy. But in their professional lives, they can raise through research the kinds of macro issues that are important to the development of children, and in their personal lives they can be advocates. Things will not change easily or instantly, but if no one bothers to make the effort, they will not change at all.

References

Bell, D. Equality and merit. *The Public Interest,* 1973, *29,* 20–68.

Bloom, B. *Stability and change in human characteristics.* New York: Wiley, 1964.

Bowles, S., and Gintis, H. I.Q. in the United States class structure. In A. Gartner, C. Greer, and F. Reissman (Eds.), *The new assault on equality.* New York: Social Policy Books, 1964.

Bowles, S., and Gintis, H. *Schooling in capitalist America: Educational reform and the contradictions of economic life.* New York: Basic Books, 1976.

Brenner, H. *Estimating the social costs of national economic policy: Implications for mental and physical health and criminal aggression.* Joint Economic Committee, Congress of the United States. Washington, D.C.: U.S. Government Printing Office, 1976.

Brittain, J.A. *The inheritance of economic status.* Washington, D.C.: The Brookings Institute, 1977.

Cole, M., Gay, J., Glick, J.A., and Sharp, D.W. *The cultural context of learning and thinking.* New York: Basic Books, 1971.

de Lone, R.H. *Small futures: children, inequality and the limits of liberal reform.* New York: Harcourt, Brace, Jovanovich, 1979.

Eisenberg, L. *A research framework for evaluating health promotion and disease prevention.* Paper presented at the First Annual Alcohol, Drug Abuse and Mental Health Administration Conference on Prevention, Silver Springs, MD, 1979.

Eisner, R. A direct attack on unemployment and inflation. *Challenge,* 1978, *21,* 49–51.

Grasso, J., and Shea, J. *Vocational education and training: Impact on youth.* Berkeley, CA.: Carnegie Council on Policy Studies in Higher Education, 1979.

Jencks, C., Bartlett, S., Corcoran, M., Crouse, J., Eaglesfield, D., Jackson, G., McClelland, K., Mueser, P., Olneck, M., Schwartz, J., Ward, S. and Williams, J. *Who gets ahead?* New York: Basic Books, 1979.

Katz, M.B. *The irony of early school reform: Education innovation in mid-nineteenth century Massachusetts.* Cambridge, MA: Harvard University Press, 1969.

Kehrer, K.C. More on the income maintenance and welfare reform debate. *The MPR Policy Newsletter,* Mathematica Policy Research, 1979, *1,* 17.

Kelly, G. *The psychology of personal constructs.* New York: Norton, 1955.

Keniston, K. *All our children: The American family under pressure.* New York: Harcourt, Brace, Jovanovich, 1977.

Kessen, W. Questions for a theory of cognitive development. *Monographs of the Society for Research in Child Development,* 1966, *31* (5, Serial No. 107).

Laosa, L.M. Social competence in childhood: Towards a developmental, socio-culturally relativistic paradigm. In M.W. Kent and J.E. Rolf (Eds.), *Social competence in children,* Vol. 3: *Primary prevention of psychopathology.* Hanover, N.H.: University Press of New England, 1979.

Leacock, E. *Teaching and learning in city schools.* New York: Basic Books, 1969.

Lekachman, R. *Economists at bay.* New York: McGraw Hill, 1976.

McLelland, D.C. Testing for competence rather than for "intelligence." *American Psychologist,* 1973, *28,* 1–14.

Nixon, R.A. The historical development of the concept and implementation of full employment as economic policy. In A. Gartner, R.A. Nixon, and F. Reissman (Eds.), *Public service employment: An analysis of the history, problems and prospects.* New York: Praeger, 1973.

Ogbu, J.U. *Minority education and caste: The American system in cross-cultural perspective.* New York: Academic Press, 1978.

Plattner, M. The welfare state vs. the redistributive state. *The Public Interest,* 1979, *55,* 28–48.

Rutter, M. Protective factors in children's response in stress and disadvantage. In M.W. Kent and J.E. Rolf (Eds.), *Social competence in children,* Vol.3: *Primary prevention of psychopathology.* Hanover, N.H.: University Press of New England, 1979.

Ross, H., and Sawhill, I. *Time of transition: The growth of families headed by women.* Washington, DC: The Urban Institute, 1975.

Sewell, W.H. Inequality of opportunity for higher education. *American Sociological Review,* 1971, *36,* 793–809.

Thurow, L. Toward a definition of economic justice. *The Public Interest,* 1973, *31,* 56–80.

White, S., Day, M.C., Freeman, P.K., Hartman, S.A., and Messenger, K.P. *Federal programs for young children: Review and recommendations,* Vol.I. Dept. of Health, Education and Welfare. Washington, DC: U.S. Government Printing Office, 1973.

The Politics of Aging

Robert H. Binstock

The contemporary politics of aging do, indeed, present many dilemmas and opportunities. My basic message with respect to the opportunities is that they lie, ironically, in discarding the notion that the aging are a monolithic constituency. We thereby enable ourselves to focus on policy issues and political actions dealing with those subgroups within the aging population that are most seriously disadvantaged. I will consider the opportunities that can be presented through such a focus, shortly, after outlining some of the major dilemmas in American policies toward the elderly and then briefly reviewing the politics of aging which shapes them.

The Dilemmas of Our Policies on Aging

The contemporary dilemmas of American public policy toward aging have been shaped by four major factors.

The first, which has been termed "the graying of the budget" (Hudson, 1978), is that our national government's existing policy commitments toward the elderly currently lead it to spend one-fourth of the annual federal budget on programs for the aging. This is slightly less than the proportion spent on defense programs. The estimated total for federal expenditures in Fiscal Year (FY) 1980 is $531.6 billion; of that, $132.2 billion will go for programs on aging.

Second, the present policies do not substantially alleviate the severest problems—poverty, ill health, and inadequate services—experienced by millions of the most disadvantaged elderly.

Third, if present policies are maintained, the mere demographic increase in the number of older persons in America would lead federal expenditures on aging to more than triple in real dollars early in the next century and thus comprise 40 percent of total federal outlays (Califano, 1978, p. 1576). Today we have 24.4 million persons who are 65 and older; in the year 2000 we will have 30.6 million (Siegel, 1976, p. 3).

And fourth, there are no foreseeable elements in the future of the

American economy or in the characteristics of the emerging elderly population that will eradicate the severest problems of old age. Today's policies will cost even more in the future, but millions of older persons will still experience severe deprivation.

The central dilemma posed by these factors would seem to be whether to retrench collective responsibility for alleviating some of the dire hardships experienced by older persons or to carry forward, even increase, our responsibilities to the aging at the cost of other national goals. Before considering how the politics of aging may bear on the resolution of this issue, let us examine how this broad dilemma of policy toward the aging is expressed in more specific forms for several sectors of social policy concern.

ECONOMIC SECURITY

The need for adequate income is perhaps the most critical problem confronting the aging population of the United States. To be sure, the federal government is spending a great deal on income programs for the elderly; in FY 1980 it will provide more than $96 billion in direct cash benefits and $33 billion in health care benefits to older persons. Additional tens of billions will be paid out through state and local governments and private pension plans. But the fact remains that a substantial percentage of older persons experience severe poverty.

❖ HEALTH

Receiving less attention than economic security in the past few years, and probably far more difficult to deal with in the long run, are issues concerning the improvement of older persons' health. Older persons are subject to more disability than younger persons, see physicians 50 percent more often, have about twice as many hospital stays and, once hospitalized, will stay there twice as long (Brotman, 1978, p. 1624).

The Medicare and Medicaid programs enacted in 1965 have helped to defray the costs of seeing doctors, staying in hospitals, and obtaining several additional specific health services and goods. But these programs do not seem to have had much impact on the health status of older persons. Shanas (1978), for example, conducted a national probability survey on the health status and health care activities of the American older population in 1962 and again in 1975. The only change she found in this 13-year period was that the percentage of older persons who had not seen a doctor in over a year had dropped from 32 percent to 19 percent. But she did not find any change in the health status of older persons, whether aggregated for all persons 65 and older or disaggregated for different age groups within that population.

The contemporary challenges of providing adequate health care to the elderly are enormous. The probability of any person being institutionalized at some time after the 65th birthday is 25 percent or one in four (Kastenbaum and Candy, 1973). And we are much too familiar with the uneven, often scandalous nature of institutional care, as well as the feckless pattern through which our national and state governments deal with abuses in nursing homes and other long-term care institutions. We have seen often enough the cycle through which media exposure of nursing home conditions engenders a sense of public outrage. A commission is appointed to investigate conditions and to recommend legislation to deal with them, and reasonably strong regulatory standards are enacted. Nonetheless, the nursing home industry is able to remain remarkably immune to regulation by neutralizing or capturing the machinery of regulatory implementation (see Mendelsohn and Hapgood, 1975).

The highly touted alternatives to institutional care—home health care and homemaker services—are still touted, but not implemented on a substantial scale. One major reason they have not been fully developed is because neither Medicare nor Medicaid provides for most elements of home service that do not involve a skilled nursing component (U.S. Comptroller General, 1979). Consequently, a great many of the theoretically viable alternatives to institutional care remain financially impracticable.

Whether or not institutionalization is required, the social implications of ill health are significant and wide ranging. It is well established by now that an individual's health status affects his or her: self-esteem, social status, capacity for work, level of income, range of social contacts, and overall life style. We also know that the health status of an aging individual has a direct impact on the total family: on each member's own physical health; on the nature of family relationships; on the number of contacts within the family; on its living arrangements; on its economic status; and on its social and instrumental activities (Brody, 1980). This clearly emerging picture of the social implication of health is why we have come to speak of a "continuum of health and social services" or a "continuum of care" in which we recognize the need for support throughout the range of these overlapping areas of concern.

❖ Can we look to biomedical research to help reduce the challenges of providing supportive care? Not very likely. Biomedical research may make some progress in prolonging life by eliminating cancer, heart disease, and stroke; but if so, this would lead to more survivors at later ages, adding to the number of persons who might be expected to have disabling physical and mental health conditions (see Hayflick, 1976, and Pfeiffer, 1976). We can hope that research will lead to elimination of organic brain syndromes and other disabling conditions, but this seems even less likely at the moment than progress in eliminating the major fatal diseases. It is for this reason that many forums have begun to address issues concerning the quality of an extended life span.

The Politics of Aging

In briefly reviewing the results of federal programs for the aging, I have applied what some persons may regard as a severe or unrealistic standard of judgment—namely, whether those programs solve or substantially alleviate problems that our national government is officially committed to solving. But when we are allocating a quarter of our federal budget to combat those problems it may not seem an unrealistic criterion, and certainly should be an instructive one. By spending $132 billion on the elderly we are helping a great many people in a great many ways. Yet about nine million older persons, well over one-third of the elderly pouplation, are in severe financial distress. We have not improved the health status of the aged population since the introduction of Medicare and Medicaid. And a great many other problems of aging have only been met by token responses.

Many advocates for the severely disadvantaged aging, recognizing the limited effectiveness of our current policies, have comforted themselves with the notion that "senior power" will sharply increase federal expenditures and administrative efforts to improve the income security, health, and social problems of older persons. Looking to the ever-growing proportion of older voters in the population, they cling to images of the aging as a powerful or soon-to-be powerful voting bloc and organized interest.

Journalists and scholars of subjects other than politics have reinforced this image of a powerful, nationwide older persons' vote. Noting increased programs and expenditures for the aging, they portray politicians as being bullied by senior power. Inspired by demographic trends, the American Association for the Advancement of Science went so far as to sponsor a symposium in 1974 to address, seriously, the issue of whether the United States would become a gerontocracy in the 1990s or in the early 21st century.

Can we, in fact, expect that senior power will augment and/or redirect our expenditures of collective resources in a fashion that will redress the problems of the severely disadvantaged aged? If we heed the conventional wisdom the answer would seem to be yes. But if we carefully examine the political attitudes and behavior of individuals as they age, and the political behavior of aging-based organizations, we find that the popular images of senior power are inaccurate. The politics of aging is hardly likely to become focused on the problems of the severely disadvantaged.

Both those who cherish the image of senior power and those who fear it have been misled. Although older persons do cast 15 percent or more of the vote in national elections, they do not all vote the same. The population of older persons is politically heterogeneous, just as it is economically and socially heterogeneous (Hudson and Binstock, 1976).

Even if we accept the problematic assumption that voters are swayed by issues favoring their self-interest, most older voters do not primarily identify themselves, and hence their self-interest, in terms of aging. When a person reaches 65 or enters retirement status, he or she does not suddenly lose all prior self identities—sex, race, education, peer group and community ties—and the self interests that can be derived from them. Take the case of a 73-year-old Caucasian, Catholic widow in Chicago, living comfortably on income from capital gains and dividends, who is deeply involved in advocacy for children's programs. Given a candidate who takes positions on race relations, abortion, urban affairs, tax reform, day care for children, and on senior issues, which self-interests are decisive in influencing the vote of this senior citizen?

In short, the notion that the elderly are a homogeneous political constituency is an artificial and simplistic construct. Analyses of age as a variable in political attitudes and voting patterns have consistently shown that the differences within age groups are greater than the differences between age groups (Campbell, 1971). No sound evidence has been assembled showing an instance in which an "old-age interest" or an "old-age candidate" can be presumed to have shifted older persons' votes as a cohesive force.

Although the commonly purveyed images of the aging as a political force are inaccurate, the images, in themselves, provide resources·for some limited forms of power. The image of an aged voting bloc leads many politicians to support propositions that seem favorable to older persons, and to attend sizable meetings that involve older persons and their presumed interests. They do not wish to be listed among the missing, when the rolls of supporters of the aging are compiled. On the other hand, the image of the aging as a voting bloc is not sufficiently powerful to evoke than more than moderate, incremental, and symbolic support.

The relatively few politicians who make a heavy investment (even a symbolic one) in support for the aging, relative to their support for other constituencies, learn regretfully about the inaccurate image of the aging voting bloc. Most sophisticated politicians make sure that they are counted as sympathetic to the aging, but give relatively low priority to the elderly among the constituencies from which they seek votes.

❖ The Opportunities for Social Change

Because of the contrast between the images and facts concerning the aging as a political force, continuing attention to the notion of senior power may very well be a source of danger to disadvantaged older persons rather than a source of opportunities for change. In the years ahead the aging-based organizations will strive to maintain their resources and political legitimacy by claiming as large a constituency as they can. In doing so they will undoubtedly suggest that incredible number of citizens, tens of millions of older persons, can be mobilized by them as a cohesive voting bloc in response to old-age issues. The media will disseminate the suggestion because it will make good—that is, dramatic—copy. But, in fact there will be no such bloc.

It is not at all improbable that within the next decade or two older persons will come to be viewed as a controlling or decisive electoral force, despite their diverse voting behavior. And as slower rates of economic growth force us to reconsider explicitly many of the allocative decisions our nation has made, our frustrations will mount and could very well be displaced onto the mythical power of seniors. We have already seen a number of articles about the "social security ripoff" and other exercises in hyperbolic castigation of politicians for being "bullied" by the aging. One hopes that these are not portents of an era in which the aging will become a collective scapegoat for economic and political frustrations. But even if they are not, a serious danger lies ahead.

Simply put, the danger is that the people of our nation will find it convenient to assume that an imaginary political force of older persons has obtained all that is needed, perhaps more than a fair share, of public resources and assistance for the aging. As a consequence, those older persons who are in fact helplessly subject to severe deprivations will not be likely to receive significant attention from our government. Several journalists, for example, have discovered that 25 percent of the federal budget is currently spent on benefits for the aging. They have already begun to suggest that the country cannot afford to carry forward its social policy commitments to older persons; yet, they do not address, for example, the issue of how nearly 9 million poor among 24 million older Americans are to have minimally adequate incomes.

If the notion of senior power is more of a danger than a hope, where do the opportunities lie for redressing the economic, health, and social problems of the severely disadvantaged aging? A first step is the need to frame issues that will disaggregate the political, economic, and social images of aging, so as to focus on policies that can affect specific subgroups of older persons. To be sure, this will require a measure of political courage. We prefer to view the world in terms of the distortions purveyed by aggregate images because they are convenient and comforting. They help us to live with complex matters by making them seem simple. They allow us to evade issues of scarce resource allocation by redefining them as issues of economic growth. They enable us to measure health and income in terms of averages, and thereby to ignore the difficult cases.

❖   The most optimistic prospects would seem to lie in the crises that exist in the lives of individuals and that are felt profoundly in local communities. For these are crises that provide unmistakable incentives to those who can undertake to solve them, namely, the people who are affected by them. It was the randomization of disaster throughout almost all the strata of our society that provided a coalition for the political leverage leading to the Social Security Act and other ameliorative measures of the New Deal. And it was the extreme impact of sudden and large waves of immigration in the latter half of the 19th century had led to the development of genuinely effective public services—police services, fire protection services, and public health services—designed to solve extreme local crises. I believe that, similarly, it is through national political crises engendered by coalitions of the severely deprived that we will achieve adequate income transfers and adequate public regulation to meet the challenges of aging. And it is through local crises resulting from the absence of local service support systems, that we will achieve adequate services to meet the challenges of aging. Both prospects—national coalition and local service crises—are unlikely unless active efforts are undertaken to bring them about. But the active efforts required do not have to await the accidental emergence of a political leader or the impact of larger economic, social, and technological forces. The prospects lie among us and in our hands.

The forging of an effective coalition requires us to abandon the boundaries of artificial constituencies—such as "the aging," "the poor," "the handicapped," "the unemployed," "the minorities,"—which hide the heterogeneous conditions within all these categories, including many persons who are quite comfortable and many who are moderately comfortable. The very heterogeneity found within each of these categories precludes any one of them from serving as a foundation for the vigorous political organization and goal pursuit that is necessary to solve social problems. In their places we must build coalitions formed on common conditions of severe deprivation that transcend age, race, and other conventional categorizations. Effective advocacy through political organizations is built upon constituencies that are held together through a common set of incentives (see Wilson, 1973). The chronologically aged are not such a constituency. It is true that our focus to date on this large but artificial category has brought attention to aging as a social issue. But if we are to meet the priority needs generated by the trends of aging, it is time for us to shift gears and to focus attention on the commonalities of deprivation experienced by persons of all ages.

To the extent that such a coalition of the severely disadvantaged could be successful in engendering a political crisis at the national level, it might be effective in shaping federal income and regulatory policies that can solve priority problems. But given the fragmentation of power and authority in our political system, it is most unlikely that any comprehensive, coordinated health and social service delivery systems can be launched at the national level and effectively implemented at the local level (see Binstock and Levin, 1976). Any services that have developed effectively in our nation have begun in single communities as responses to local crises.

Again, I suggest that it is our own direct actions that can meet the challenge of developing effective service policies. If we wait for the crises of absent supportive services to emerge through natural evolution we will witness an enormity of human suffering. But we do not have to wait if we are willing to abandon our conventional approaches and undertake direct, militant action in our local communities. Our political history is replete with numerous models of effective political protest strategies that create a sense of crisis in local communities and elicit satisfactory responses from local governments. We can look to the tactics of Saul Alinsky (1971), the strategies of Martin Luther King, Jr. (1963), and to rent strikes and welfare sit-ins (Lipsky, 1968).

We hardly lack effective models for success in local political action. What we seem to lack is the motivation and commitment to undertake the onerous tasks required. Even as it is convenient for our public officials to hide behind aggregate indices and symbolic policies, it is convenient for us to simply blame them or to reassure ourselves that some form of technology, or coordination, or senior power will magically bring forth what is needed. In my view, the policies that are needed to cope with the trends of aging in America will not be forthcoming unless great numbers of us undertake direct political action to make them come forth.

References

Alinsky, S. D. *Rules for radicals: A pragmatic primer for realistic radicals.* New York: Random House, 1971.

Binstock, R. H. Interest-group liberalism and the politics of aging. *Gerontologist,* 1972, *12,* 265–280.

Binstock, R. H. Aging and the future of American politics. *The Annals of the American Academy of Political and Social Science*, 1974, *415*, 199–212.

Binstock, R. H., and Levin, M. A. The political dilemmas of intervention policies. In R. H. Binstock and E. Shanas (Eds.), *Handbook of aging and the social sciences*. New York: Van Nostrand Reinhold, 1976.

Brody, E. M. Women's changing roles, and care of the aging family. In *Aging: Agenda for the eighties*. Washington, D.C.: National Journal Issues Book, 1979.

Brody, E. M. Health and its social implications. In M. Marois (Ed.), *Aging: A challenge to science and social policy*. London: Oxford University Press, 1980.

Brotman, H. D. The aging of America: A demographic profile. *National Journal*, 1978, *10*, 1622–1627.

Califano, J. A., Jr. U.S. policy for the aging—a commitment to ourselves. *National Journal*, 1978, *10*, 1575–1581.

Campbell, A. Politics through the life cycle. *Gerontologist*, 1971, *11*, 112–117.

Hayflick, L. Human aging in 2025 A.D.: A prospective analysis. In *2025 A.D.: Aging in America's future*. Somerville, N.J.: Hoechst-Roussel Pharmaceuticals, Inc., 1976.

Hudson, R. B. The "graying" of the federal budget and its consequences for old-age policy. *Gerontologist*, 1978, *18*, 428–440.

Hudson, R. B., and Binstock, R. H. Political systems and aging. In R. H. Binstock and E. Shanas (Eds.), *Handbook of aging and the social sciences*. New York: Van Nostrand Reinhold, 1976.

Kastenbaum, R., and Candy, S. E. The 4% fallacy, a methodological and empirical critique of extended care facility population statistics. *International Journal of Aging and Human Development*, 1973, *4*, 15–21.

King, M. L., Jr. *Why we can't wait*. New York: Harper and Row, 1963.

Laslett, P. The comparative history of aging and the aged: With particular reference to the household position of aged persons. In M. Marois (Ed.), *Aging: A challenge to science and social policy*. London: Oxford University Press, 1980.

Lipsky, M. Protest as a political resource. *American Political Science Review*, 1968, *62*, 1144–1158.

Lowi, T. J. *The end of liberalism*. New York: W. W. Norton & Company, 1969.

Lowi, T. J. Interest groups and the consent to govern. *The Annals of the American Academy of Political and Social Science*, 1974, *413*, 86–100.

Mendelsohn, M. A., and Hapgood, D. The political economy of nursing homes. *The Annals of the American Academy of Political and Social Science*, 1974, *415*, 95–105.

Pfeiffer, E. Health care and well-being of older Americans in the year 2025. In *2025 A.D.: Aging in America's future*. Somerville, N.J.: Hoechst-Roussel Pharmaceuticals, Inc., 1976.

Pratt, H. *The gray lobby*. Chicago: University of Chicago Press, 1976.

Riemer, Y., and Binstock, R. H. Campaigning for "the senior vote": A case study of Carter's 1976 Campaign. *Gerontologist*, 1978, *18*, 517–524.

Shanas, E. *Final report: National survey of the aged*. Washington, D.C.: DHEW, OHD-90A-369, August, 1978.

Siegel, J. S. Demographic aspects of aging and the older population in the United States. *Current population reports* (special studies series p. 23, No. 29). Washington, D.C.: U.S. Department of Commerce, Bureau of the Census, 1976.

Truman, D. B. *The governmental process: Political interests and public opinion*. New York: Alfred A. Knopf, 1951.

U.S. Comptroller General. *Entering a nursing home—costly implications for Medicaid and the elderly*. (Pad-80-12.) Washington, D.C.: U.S. General Accounting Office, November 26, 1979.

U.S. House of Representatives Select Committee on Aging. *Federal responsibility to the elderly: Executive programs and legislative jurisdiction*. Washington, D.C.: U.S. Government Printing Office, 1976

U.S. House of Representatives Select Committee on Aging. *Poverty among America's aged*. Washington, D.C.: U.S. Government Printing Office, Comm. Pub. 95–154, 1978.

U.S. Senate Subcommittee on Aging of the Committee on Human Resources. *Older Americans Act of 1978*. Washington, D.C.: U.S. Government Printing Office, 1979.

Wilson, J. Q. *Political organizations*. New York: Basic Books, 1973.

v. Programs for Larger Social Change

This section is concerned with programs for larger social change as prevention. In many ways these articles illustrate the power of forces that resist changes in the larger society. If prevention efforts are to be successful then narrow religious views that defend a Divine Plan will often be melded with conservative views that oppose social change. Not all religious views are opposed to freer sexual expression. But efforts to liberalize sexual attitudes and behavior, as well as efforts to change the structure and content of our schools, reflect the existence of strong resistance to change. Attempts to improve neighborhoods and dark ghettos reflect a need for change the origins of which are in the social system. The articles in this section allow us a glimpse of the larger agenda for prevention.

The Role of Religion

James B. Nelson

Religion is a terribly ambiguous human enterprise, and it ought never to be confused with God. Religion is the patterning of human responses to what is *perceived* to be the divine, responses that take shape in doctrine, moral instruction, patterns of worship, styles of piety or spirituality, and religious institutional life. The power of religion for good is that the divine life does indeed break through these human forms in ways that fulfill persons, create life-giving human relationships, and transform social structures. But the power of religion for evil is just as great. The religious enterprise, that most dangerous of human enterprises, is always tempted to claim ultimate authority and sanction for its humanly constructed doctrines and precepts. Nowhere is all of this ambiguity more apparent than in sexual matters.

While I write here as a Christian, I believe that these observations will have considerable applicability to Judaism as well. Somewhere in the first few centuries of the Christian church, the patristic era, there arose two lists: the seven deadly sins and the seven virtues. As I attempted to formulate my observations about the religious dimensions of sexual health, two things occurred. First, I could not talk about the positive elements without talking about the ways in which Western religion has contributed mightily to sexual disease. Second, I discovered that my points fell, quite miraculously, into two groups of seven. Although these make no attempt to reflect the early Christian lists, I submit seven deadly sins which Western religion has contributed to sexual disease, countered by seven virtues (or positive resources) which the Judeo-Christian tradition offers to sexual health.

All of this is predicated upon certain assumptions about sexual health. The definition offered by the World Health Organization (WHO) (1975) is useful: "Sexual health is the integration of the somatic, emotional, intellectual, and social aspects of sexual being, in ways that are positively enriching and that enhance personality, communication and love" (p. 6). That is a remarkable definition, not only because it affirms the multi-

From James B. Nelson, "Religious Dimensions of Sexual Health," in George W. Albee, Sol Gordon, and Harold Leitenberg (eds.) *Promoting Sexual Responsibility and Preventing Sexual Problems.* Copyright © 1983 by the Vermont Conference on the Primary Prevention of Psychopathology. Reprinted by permission.

dimensional and relational aspects of sexual health, but also because it is (to the best of my knowledge) the first time any major health organization has used the concept of love in a health policy statement. Not incidentally, the WHO definition reflects the best in the Judeo-Christian tradition concerning sexuality and leaves out the worst! Now to the sins and virtues.

The first two deadly sins—spiritualistic dualism and sexist dualism—are the most basic, fundamental sins, and they are counterparts of each other (Ruether, 1975). Yet, for the moment they can be viewed separately. Any dualism is the radical breaking apart of two elements which belong together; it is seeing the two dimensions of life coexisting in uneasy truce or open conflict.

Spiritualistic dualism, the first deadly sin, was quite foreign to the Jewish Old Testament heritage. However, through the impact of the Greco-Roman culture and its Hellenist philosophy, it found its way into early Christian life and thought. The spirit was viewed as eternal and pure, while the physical body was seen as temporal, material, corruptible, and corrupting. Whatever salvation meant, it somehow involved escape from the distractions and temptations of bodily life into the realm of the spirit. Although, as we shall see in a moment, this spiritualistic dualism ran counter to the most basic insights of both Jewish and Christian traditions, it had an enormous impact, particularly upon Christian life, which is still with us.

Such dualism has multiple results. The body is viewed with suspicion, and its sexual feelings must be denied in favor of the higher life. A ladderlike image of true spirituality emerges, with celibacy reserved for the higher rungs. The alienated body produces a mind detached from the depth of feelings. Dichotomized thinking emerges from the mind-body dissociation; we become resistant to ambiguity, seeking simple and single reasons for understanding things. Both the body and its sexuality are depersonalized; the body is seen as a physical object to be possessed, controlled, and used by the self. Such are the wages of this deadly sin, spiritualistic dualism.

But what of the positive resources? Israel of the Old Testament knew nothing of this body-spirit split. It regarded the person as all of one piece. With a strong doctrine of the goodness of all of creation, Israel could not denigrate the body and its pleasures. They were gifts of God.

And what of Christianity? In spite of the fact that Hellenistic dualism made dramatic inroads, Christianity nevertheless remains a religion of incarnation. In its central affirmation, Christianity claims that the most decisive experience of God comes to us not principally in doctrine, not in philosophic abstraction, not in mystical otherworldly experiences, but *in flesh*. Even if ancient heresies (Gnostic and Docetic) still cast suspicion upon the goodness of material, bodily life and still question the full humanity of Jesus of Nazareth, the mainstream of Christianity has attempted to say that the most decisive, memorable, revelatory meeting place of God with humankind is in the meeting of flesh with flesh. And that has something to do with our sexuality.

So, the good news, the virtue (as opposed to this first sin) is this: the fully physical, sweating, lubricating, ejaculating, urinating, defecating bodies that we are are the vehicles of the divine experience. God continues to be most decisively experienced in the fleshly, embodied touching of human lives. The Word still becomes flesh and dwells among us, full of grace and truth.

Word becoming flesh: this is the mystery of communication and communion. The secret of our sexuality is our need to reach out to embrace others physically, emotionally, spiritually. The good news of a Jewish creation-affirming faith and a Christian incarnationalist faith is that our body-selves with all of their rich sexuality are God's way of inviting us into authentic humanness, through our need to reach out and embrace. Our sexuality is the divine plot to tease us into becoming "body-words of love." Our sexuality is both the physiological and the psychological grounding of our capacity to love. It is that basic. We who take these core religious affirmations seriously are bidden to celebrate the body as a means of grace. That is good news from religion for sexual health.

The second deadly sin is sexist or patriarchal dualism. It is the twin of spiritualistic dualism in some basic ways. For centuries men have assigned to themselves the primary characteristics of spirit and mind, and have labeled women as body and emotion, hence inferior and needing to be subdued by the higher powers.

If spiritualistic dualism was foreign to the Hebraic Old Testament culture, sexist or patriarchal dualism was not. Women were second-class citizens in the community of faith and much of the time looked upon as male property. The patriarchal culture continued its influence into the Christian era and is still pervasive. The essence of sexist dualism is the systematic and systemic subordination of women by men in institutional life and in interpersonal relations.

That this is a deadly sin in regard to the health of women hardly needs elaboration. That it is a deadly sin for males, also, is true. Unquestionably, women have borne the brunt of the manifold forms of injustice. For both women and men, the sexist estrangement takes its toll in patterns of dominance and submission. Women compete with women for male acceptance, which they have been taught is essential for their self-worth. Men find emotional intimacy and tenderness with other men to be threatening to the masculine, heterosexual image. Spouses find it difficult to speak honestly with each other about their sexual needs and anxieties, and performance fears invade their sexual love making.

What is the good news, the virtue that Western religion might contribute here? The Apostle Paul expresses it: "There is neither Jew nor Greek, there is neither slave nor free, there is neither male nor female, for you are all one" (Galatians 3:28).

The internalization of this reality makes possible the growth of our androgyny. (I realize that "androgyny" is an ambiguous term, inasmuch as it trades upon the very sexual stereotypes which it attempts to overcome. Nevertheless, it is a useful interim word, reminding us that societal sterotypes do not define our authentic being.) None of us is intended to be either rational or emotional, either assertive or receptive, either cognitive or intuitive, either strong or vulnerable, either initiating or responding, but all of these. A core religious affirmation is the *oneness* of human being and human becoming. Actually, we do not have to become androgynous, for each of us essentially is. We only need to be allowed to be actually what we are essentially, and the religious affirmation is important here (Singer, 1976, p. 333).

Moreover, the Judeo-Christian understandings of God are crucial to our own self-understandings. Stereotypically, masculine language and images have shaped that perception: God is "He" and "Him." Masculine titles have predominated: God is King, Lord, Master, Father. But, one of the best kept secrets in the Bible (particularly the Old Testament) is the abundance of feminine images for God. God is there likened to a woman in childbirth, bringing forth new creation; God is there as a nursing mother drawing humanity to her full breasts; God is there as a seamstress clothing her children with garments in the wilderness (Russell, 1973, pp. 97ff).

If this kind of religious imagery is internalized and experienced, it can lead to a more androgynous experience of the self. It might lead, also, to a more androgynous spirituality. A masculinized imagery and spirituality has emphasized God as structure, judgment, law, order, intellect, and logic. A feminist imagery would lead to the experience of God as nature more than society, as mystical oneness more than cognitive analysis, as flow and change more than structure, as immanence more than transcendence. Both dimensions are needed for sexual health, for each of us is created with androgynous capacities destined to be realized in unique ways.

The third sin is homophobia. The word was coined a few years ago to denote an irrational fear of homosexuality (Weinburg, 1973, Chap. 1). It has been, tragically enough, part of the Judeo-Christian legacy. Nevertheless, the antihomosexual bias simply cannot be justified by careful biblical interpretation (Boswell, 1980, Chap. 4; Nelson, 1978, Chap. 8). The Bible does not actually deal with homosexuality as such. This understanding of a psychosexual orientation toward those of one's own sex is distinctly modern. Furthermore, when the Bible deals with homosexual acts (as distinguished from orientation), it deals with them in the context of lust, idolatry, rape, and with the notion of leaving, giving up, or turning away from one's natural orientation. Thus, heterosexual orientation is presupposed. There is no biblical guidance on the matter of same-sex expression for those so oriented, within a context of mutual respect and love.

If the biblical legacy does not explain our persistent homophobia, misogyny (male distrust, fear—even hatred—of women) does. Patriarchal control idealizes a disembodied, detached rationality and enforces compulsory heterosexuality for both men and women. The only respectable alternative to heterosexuality is either celibacy or asexuality. Harrison (1981) writes:

More than anything else we now need a clearer historical appreciation for the ways in which this long-standing and deeply rooted antipathy toward women in the Western Christian tradition interfaced and interacted with anti-body and anti-sensual attitudes. The fact is that the stigma of homosexuality in this society incorporates and encompasses all of the power dynamics of misogyny. Until we recognize this fact, we will not even begin to grasp why homophobia is such an intense and 'nutty' madness among us. (p. 8)

The antihomosexual attitudes of the dominantly Christian West thus cannot be explained simply by historical influences. As Boswell's (1980) careful study has pointed out, misogyny is a more consistent trend in Christian history than is homophobia. The connection, however, is quite clear. In male homosexual activity there is the stigma that some men must be passive, act like females, that is, like "failed males."

If both Jewish and Christian cultures have been dominantly homophobic, there are, nevertheless, positive resources for sexual health within these traditions. First, there is biblical affirmation of same-sex loving relationships. This material is usually overlooked by the antihomosexual proof texters, but it is there. For example, the close emotional bonding of David and Jonathan, of Ruth and Naomi, of Jesus and the beloved disciple are celebrated by the biblical writers. These are not, I assume, accounts of genital expression, but that is not the point. The point is that careful biblical scholarship simply cannot sustain the sweeping condemnation of all deep same-sex feeling which often has been asserted in the name of the Bible.

Another religious resource follows upon the recognition that the Bible does not deal with the issue of same-sex genital expression in the context of mutual respect and love. That resource is the affirmation that the morality of homosexual genital acts must be judged by the same fundamental criterion as the morality of heterosexual genital acts. To this theme I will return later.

In terms of the psychodynamics of homophobia, there is a more basic religious resource still. It is the message of God's radical affirmation of each and every person. In both Old and New Testaments this is called grace. It is the spontaneous, unmerited acceptance of the self by God. Here is the foundation for a sense of personal security in the self.

One of the strong dynamics of homophobia seems to be insecurity about one's own sexual identity and, hence, the tendency to condemn in another what is feared in the self. For the one, however, who has discovered a basic sense of inner worth through the divine acceptance, there is less need for fear. As a male I need not fear "the woman" within. As one predominantly heterosexual, I need not fear the homosexual feelings within. Nor need I be envious of the apparently greater sexuality of gays and lesbians (for our stereotypes constantly draw our attention to what they do in bed).

A common dynamic of what the religious tradition calls "sin" is thus false security. It is a false security rooted in an inner insecurity which then attempts to punish those who seem to threaten the self. That the security-creating divine acceptance, grace, can undercut this destructive dynamic is good news, indeed.

The fourth deadly sin which contributes to sexual disease is guilt over self-love. Christian theology has not had a good record in dealing positively with self-love. The dominant interpretation has seen self-love equivalent to self-centeredness, hence incompatible with the religious life. Self-love has been interpreted as acquisitive, individualistic, concerned with the self's private satisfactions, and prone to use others as tools for one's own desires. Thus, a sharp disjunction has been drawn between *agape* (selfless, self-giving love perceived in God and held normative for the faithful) and *eros* (human desire for fulfillment). Although, to be sure, a more positive appreciation of self-love has been present in certain elements of the tradition, the negative evaluation has been dominant.

When a suspicion about self-love combines with a suspicion of the body and of sexual feelings, there is a sure formula for sexual disease. The self-hate which emerges is usually of an indirect sort, but it *is* a rejection of one's actual self. Alongside this is often an idealized image of the self, but, since this is unattainable, hurt pride and self-hate emerge together.

In sexual expression, such self-rejection (or rejection of self-love) finds guilt in spontaneous sexual pleasure. Masturbation is an obvious arena of guilt, simply because giving oneself sexual pleasure is understood as sheer self-centeredness. But there is also a "works-righteousness" syndrome which becomes performance anxiety in sexual relations with the partner. In performing I always split myself into two people—one doing the performing, the other watching both the performance and the audience response. Such self-conscious splitting, watching, and judging further nurture my anxiety and undermine my capacity to commune with the other.

If guilt over self-love is a deadly sin, the good news from the religious heritage is that love is indivisible and nonquantifiable. Jesus said, "Love your neighbor *as* yourself," not "instead of yourself." It is not true that the more love we save for ourselves the less we have for others. Authentic self-love is not narcissism nor is it a grasping selfishness. Rather, it is that self-acceptance which comes through the affirmation of one's own graciously given worth and (in spite of all our distortions and flaws) our creaturely fineness.

Self-love is not only basic to personal fulfillment, but also to the capacity for authentic sexual intimacy with the partner. If I cannot say yes to myself, I cannot offer myself fully to another. I can surrender to the other, but I will have lost the gift I was asked to bring. True sexual intimacy depends upon a solid sense of identity in each of the partners. The entanglements in which identity is confused and diminished become symbiotic relationships in which one person becomes an extension of the other.

Sexual intimacy is love's communion, not unification. Sexual intimacy, then, rests in some large measure upon each partner's sense of personal worth. Without this we easily elevate the other into the center of our lives, hoping that the other's affirmation of us will assure us of our own reality. But this is too large a burden for the partner, for then the beloved has become idolatrized and confused with the divine.

Genuine self-love, furthermore, personalizes the body. When we can love ourselves as body-selves, we are aware of bodily tensions and their causes. There is more spontaneity of the body-self, for when we find the security not to demean ourselves we need not deaden any aspects of ourselves or dissipate our energies in useless rituals. Self-acceptance brings with it the profound sense that I am the body which I live, the sense that I have a real self with which to relate to others. I do not desire to absorb or be absorbed by another. I am a unique self interested in communication and communion, not in conquest and dependency. And that points to sexual health.

The fifth deadly sin is a legalistic sexual ethics. Legalism is the attempt to apply precise rules or laws to actions regardless of the unique features of the context. Legalism is the assumption that an objective standard can be applied in the same way to whole classes of actions without regard to the meanings those actions have to persons.

Many adherents of both Jewish and Christian faiths in our society have fallen into more legalism about sexual morality than virtually any other arena of human behavior. If one looks at such issues as masturbation, homosexual expression, and, in fact, virtually any form of genital expression outside heterosexual marriage, it is easy to find the legalistic posture in Orthodox and Conservative Judaism, in the official natural law stance of Roman Catholicism, and in a variety of conservative Protestant groups.

Adding to the confusion of this ethical scene is that some of the stringent sex rules of traditional orthodox religion have been based, at least in some significant measure, upon erroneous biological assumptions. Jews and early Christians alike made the biologically inaccurate and patriarchal assumption that the male semen was the carrier of life, the woman furnishing only the ground into which the seed was planted. Furthermore, it was frequently assumed that in any one male the total amount of semen was limited. Add to these assumptions the quite understandable concern of these early religious peoples for reproduction and the survival of the tribe in a threatening environment, and it is not difficult to understand why any deliberately nonprocreative male sex act was anathema.

The virtue which speaks to this deadly sin of legalism is love. Our sexuality is intended to be a language of love. Our sexuality is God's way of calling us into communion with others through our need to reach out, to touch, and to embrace—emotionally, intellectually, physically. It is God's beckoning us into the communion of love.

Since we have been created with the will to communion, the positive moral claim upon us is to become what we essentially are: lovers—in the richest, most inclusive sense of that word. The negative side of this, sin, is not basically a matter of breaking moral codes or disobeying laws (though it may involve that). More fundamentally, it is the failure to become what we are. It is the alienation which inhibits fulfillment and communion. It is the failure of love.

The values which emerge from love are several, and they become those criteria by which specific sexual acts might be measured in a nonlegalistic manner (Kosnick, Carroll, Cunningham, Modras, and Schulte, 1977, pp. 92-95). These values apply equally, I believe, to both heterosexual and homosexual expression. First, love is self-liberating. In a sexual act it expresses one's own authentic selfhood and yearns for further growth. Moreover, such love is other enriching; it has a genuine concern for the well-being and growth of the partner. Also, sexual love is honest; it expresses as candidly and truthfully as possible the meaning of the relationship which actually exists between the partners. Further, it is faithful; love expresses the uniqueness of the relationship, yet without crippling possessiveness. In addition, sexual love is socially responsible, aware of, and concerned for the larger community to which the lovers belong. It is life serving; the power of renewed life is shared by the partners. Finally, true sexual love is joyous, exuberant in its appreciation of love's mystery and life's gift.

An ethics centered in this kind of love will not guarantee freedom from mistakes in the sexual life, but it will serve the sexual health of persons crippled by legalism. It will serve their human becoming and their maturation as lovers after the image of the Cosmic Lover by whom they were created.

The sixth deadly sin of which our religious traditions are often guilty is a sexless image of spirituality. This has been more a bane of Christianity than of Judaism, for the church far more than the synagogue has been influenced by the Hellenistic, Neoplatonic split between spirit and body. Consequently, in the early Christian era a ladder image of spirituality emerged. True virtue was associated with movement upward, away from the earth.

Bodily mortification and celibacy were elevated as particularly honorable. Even among married Christians, those who abstained completely from sex were deemed more virtuous than those who had intercourse with the intent to procreate. And those who made love in order to express affection and because they enjoyed it were least meritorious of all.

The good news, however, is that a sensuous, body-embracing, sexual spirituality is more authentic to both Jewish and Christian heritages. A clue is found in an Old Testament book, the Song of Songs. Here is a biblical love poem celebrating the joys of erotic love between a woman and a man. Although much of Christian interpretation over the centuries allegorized this poem into a symbol of "the purely spiritual" relation of the soul and God, devoid of any carnal reality, it is, in fact, a sexual story. The setting is an erotic garden. The lovers delight not only in each other's embodiedness, but also in the sensuous delights surrounding them: flowers, fruits, trees, fountains. Here there is no body-spirit split. Here there is no sexist dualism, no hint of patriarchy, no dominance or submission. The woman is fully the equal of the man. She works, takes initiatives in their meetings, and has an identity of her own apart from her lover (Nelson, 1981, pp. 90-91).

It is true, there is another garden story in our religious heritages, the Garden of Eden. Here the sexual dualisms have become apparent. There is shame in nakedness. Childbirth and daily work alike are cursed by pain, and the woman is derivative from the man. While the erotic garden of the Song of Songs represents a creation-centered spirituality, the Garden of Eden in Genesis represents a sin-and-redemption-centered spirituality. While the latter type has clearly dominated the notions of Western Christian spirituality, it is not the only (or perhaps even the most authentic) type.

We are beginning to realize that repressed sexuality "keeps the gods at bay" and that repressed human development does not bode well for the human-divine relationship. We are beginning to see that the bodily dimensions of feeling and emotion, longing and desire, are not foreign to but rather essential to a healthy spirituality. Such a spirituality will help men and women "discover that their flesh and its desires are not inherently evil, but are sharings in the passionate longings of God...to relate to creation, sharings in God's own lust for life. Spirituality must show forth that God who is shamelessly, even scandalously, in love with earth" (Deschene, 1981, p. 33).

The seventh deadly sin of our religious traditions has been the privatization of sexuality. Here, my pun is intended. Sexuality has been located essentially in "the privates," and hence our understandings of its dynamics have been restricted to the domain of private, interpersonal morality. But such a genitalization of sexuality in itself is a mark of sexual sin and alienation. For our sexuality is far more than genitals; it is our way of being in the world as female or male persons, our capacity for sensuousness, our self-understanding as body-selves, that deep inner drive toward communication and communion with the earthiness of earth and earth's Creator-Spirit. As such, our sexuality pervades the whole of life, including all of our social and institutional relationships.

To the extent that we can transcend a narrowed privatization in our understanding of sexuality, we can also comprehend the fact that an enormous range of social justice issues are at stake. Some are more obvious than others: justice for women, gays, and lesbians; commercialized sex; sexual abuse of women and minors; abortion; population control; the sexual rights of the aged, the handicapped, and the institutionalized. Moreover, a wholistic view of sexuality can help us all see more clearly and respond more effectively to those sexual dimensions present in social issues which appear to have little to do with our subject.

White racism in American society is one such issue. Historically, the schizophrenic attitudes of white males toward women ("there are two kinds—the good ones and the bad ones") were organized along racial lines. The white woman was elevated as the symbol of purity, and the black woman ("the other kind") was used for economic and sexual purposes. Then white male guilt was projected onto black males, who were fantasized as dark sexual beasts never to be trusted around white women. Further, the insecurity of many white people with their own flesh (for the respectable notion of religious virtue does not seem to accommodate many body feelings) frequently led to a "dirty body" image of those whose skin is so obviously different. These sexual dynamics, unfortunately, are still virulently alive in white racism.

Social violence is another issue with important sexual dimensions. The fact that violent crime in this society is overwhelmingly a male phenomenon is no accident. Nor is it an accident that men are directors of an insane global arms race ("my rocket is bigger than your rocket"). The machismo cult of competitiveness, toughness, superiority, potency, and homophobia is terrifyingly present. We are also beginning to learn about the interconnection between the deprivation of body pleasure and tendencies toward physical violence.

The list could be extended. The links between a Western white culture's inability to live in ecological harmony with the earth and our proneness toward self-body dissociation may be significant. The connections between a pervasive consumer mentality and our sexual alienation might also need more understanding.

Religion, then, is an ambiguous human enterprise. There are at least seven deadly sins, and perhaps even more, which certain elements in the Judeo-Christian heritage have contributed to our sexual disease. But speaking from faith's perspective, I am even more convinced of the positive resources of this religious tradition for sexual health. For, God the Cosmic Lover has a passionate love for this earthy creation and has made our sexuality a fundamental dimension of our own passion for wholeness, health, and love. This God somehow keeps breaking into our ambiguous religious ways with fresh resources for our healing.

References

Boswell, J. *Christianity, social tolerance, and homosexuality.* Chicago: University of Chicago Press, 1980.

Deschene, J. M. Sexuality: Festival of the spirit. *Studies in Formative Spirituality,* 1981, *2* , 25-38.

Harrison, B. W. Misogyny and homophobia: The unexplored connections. *Integrity Forum,* 1981, 7, 7-13.

Kosnick, A., Carroll, W., Cunningham, A., Modras, R., and Schulte, J. *Human sexuality: New directions in American Catholic thought.* New York: Paulist Press, 1977.

Nelson, J. B. *Embodiment: An approach to sexuality and Christian theology.* Minneapolis: Augsburg, 1978.

Nelson, J. B. Between two gardens: Reflections on spirituality and sexuality. *Studies in Formative Spirituality,* 1981, 2, 87-97.

Ruether, R. R. *New woman, new earth.* New York: Seabury Press, 1975.

Russell, L. *Human liberation in a feminist perspective.* Philadelphia: Westminster Press, 1973.

Singer, J. *Androgyny: Toward a new theory of sexuality.* Garden City, N.Y.: Anchor Books, Doubleday, 1976.

Weinberg, G. *Society and the healthy homosexual.* Garden City, N.Y.: Anchor Books, Doubleday, 1973.

World Health Organization. *Education and treatment in human sexuality: The training of health professionals.* Geneva: World Health Organization, 1975.

A Behavioral Settings Approach

Phil Schoggen

❖   In the study of behavior settings, the focus is upon particular situations or concrete contexts of molar behavior. The ecological psychologist studies consistencies in behavior which are associated with specific place-thing-time constellations regardless of which persons are involved. Just as the student of personality seeks to identify regularities or consistencies in behavior of single individuals over time related to such personal characteristics as genes, prenatal conditions, early experience, and child-training practices, the student of behavior settings seeks to identify regularities or consistencies in behavior across individuals over time related to the particular concrete situations in which the behavior occurs. The concepts, theories, and research methods of personality psychology may be required to understand why a particular 13-year-old boy is fascinated with fire and loves to light matches, but they are neither needed nor appropriate to understand why lighting matches and making fires among 13-year-old boys in general occur more often on Boy Scout cook-outs than in Sunday School classes: the cook-out setting requires match-lighting and fire-making but the Sunday School class setting resists them, requiring instead such behavior from 13-year-old boys as Bible reading, discussions between teacher and class members, and praying, regardless of the identities or individual personality characteristics of the people involved. The pressures and constraints of settings are so clear and strong that occupants of the settings must conform or face vigorous sanctions, as a boy who lights matches in Sunday School or reads the Bible on cook-outs will certainly find out. The behavior setting survey is essentially a method for studying, systematically and quantitatively, the environments that place situational coercions on people's molar behavior. The study of settings is the study of the concrete environmental situations with respect to which people direct their molar behavior—having lunch in the Pearl Cafe, buying groceries at Reid's Grocery Store, worshiping at the Methodist Church Worship Service, working on academic activities in the fifth grade, rooting for the home team at the high school basketball game. The behavior patterns in these examples represent the behavior of people in general in the settings. Having lunch, buying groceries, worshiping, and so on are stable, extraindividual patterns which regularly and consistently occur in the settings specified and are independent of the behavior of any particular person.

The behavior setting method, therefore, is a peculiar approach to psychology, an approach that focuses not on individual behavior or even on social interaction, but rather on the behavior of persons en masse associated with particular environmental settings. Deliberate exclusion of the individual personality is the basis for the not completely tongue-in-cheek reference to the method as "the psychology of the absent organism."

The concept of the behavior setting has been carefuly defined and precise operations for behavior setting identification and description have been published (Barker, 1968; Barker and Schoggen, 1973). For the present purpose, it will suffice to define a behavior setting as a cluster of *standing patterns of behavior* of people en masse occurring within a *particular part of the milieu* (a specific place-thing-time constellation)—where there is a *synomorphic relation* between the behavior patterns and the milieu. That is, the behavior and the milieu part fit together; there is a similarity of shape between the behavior and the environment.

❖ These and similar data obtained in several of the ecological studies over the years (Barker and Wright, 1955; Barker, 1960; Barker and Barker, 1961; Barker and Gump, 1964; Barker and Schoggen, 1973) led Barker to develop behavior setting theory with special reference to the consequences of undermanning on inhabitants' behavior. The main point of the theory, presented in detail elsewhere (Barker, 1968), is that undermanned settings—settings with unfilled habitat-claims—exert more pressure on potential participants to enter and take part in the operation and maintenance of the setting than adequately manned or overmanned settings. If the junior class play has parts for 12 actors and there are only 15 members of the class, no member is likely to be exempt from pressure to take a part, or at least to help backstage; but if there are 50 juniors, only the more talented or highly motivated are likely to become involved. Concretely, the theory predicts that Midwest's habitat, with its relatively undermanned settings will generate the following differences in the behavior output of Midwesterners as compared with Dalesmen: Midwesterners, on the average, will (a) spend more time per person in the public settings of the town; (b) more frequently assume positions of responsibility in operating the town's behavior settings; and (c) carry out many more actions of highest leadership responsibility.

The findings of the study (Barker and Schoggen, 1973, chapter 8) strongly support all three of these predictions: (a) the average Midwesterner spent 125 percent as many hours per year in the public behavior settings of the town (Midwest, 1,356 person-hours per year per person, Yoredale, 1,089); (b) the average Midwesterner occupied positions of responsibility 250 percent as frequently as Dalesmen (Midwest, 8.0 positions per year per person, Yoredale 3.2); (c) the average Midwesterner carried out 257 percent as many actions of highest leadership responsibility (Midwest, 1.8 leader acts per year per person, Yoredale 0.7).

The theory of undermanning has also been tested in studies of high schools differing in size (Barker and Gump, 1964). One of these studies (Gump and Friesen, 1964) compared a large high school (2,287 students) with four small ones (83–151 students) in Eastern Kansas in terms of student participation in voluntary nonclass behavior settings. They found that, as expected, the settings of the small schools were in fact undermanned by comparison with those of the large school (mean number of persons per behavior setting: 12 in small schools, 36 in the large school).

The results showed that students in the small schools participated in just as many extracurricular settings as large school students despite the fact that the large school had more such settings available. Also consistent with theoretical expectations was the finding that on the average small school juniors occupied positions of responsibility in twice as many behavior settings as did large school juniors (small school, 8.6; large school, 3.5 positions per student):

	Large	*Small**
Total Number of Juniors	794	23
Total Number of Settings	189	48
Mean Positions per Junior	3.5	8.6

*Average data from four small schools.

Thus, while the large school provided a richer habitat in terms of total number of settings available, the small schools much more often co-opted students into positions of responsibility in operating their settings.

In a follow-up study, Willems (1964) attempted to assess the psychological effect on the students of the differences in behavioral participation. Juniors were interviewed, using both open-ended and card-sorting techniques for identifying psychologically experienced forces toward participation in the nonschool settings. The data are reported in terms of own forces (attractions) and induced or external forces (pressures) reported by the students as reasons for participating in the voluntary activities. Results are given for both *regular* (ordinary, average) students and for students designated *marginal* (at high risk for dropping out because of low academic aptitude and other background factors).

Both the card-sort and the open-ended data showed that small school regular students reported significantly more forces, both own and foreign, toward participation in settings than did large school students. Regular students and marginal students in the small schools did not differ appreciably in either the number of pressures or the number of attractions reported. In the large school, on the other hand, marginal students reported both fewer attractions and fewer pressures, though only the latter difference was statistically significant. Willems comments on these findings as follows:

> The data on forces and responsibilities are relevant to the question of the comparative efficacy of personal variables and ecological variables in influencing behavior. The absence of differences between regular and marginal students in the small schools and the presence of such differences in the large school indicates that school size, as well as the kind of person, is a

determinant of forces toward participation. The fact that marginal students of the small schools reported more forces than did the regular students of the large school is relevant too. In the large school, the academically marginal student appeared to be truly an outsider, while in the small schools being marginal made no apparent difference on the experience of pressures, attractions, and responsibilities. (Willems, 1964)

In an altogether independent investigation, Baird (1969) subjected the central hypothesis of the *Big School, Small School* report to critical examination and obtained relevant new data from a very large national sample of 21,371 students drawn randomly from the 712,000 who took the ACT (American College Test) and Student Profile for college admission. High school size was studied in relation to number of high school achievements and activities. Baird reports that, consistent with behavior setting theory, students in small schools participated to a greater extent in a variety of areas than did students in large schools.

Wicker and his students have addressed the theory of undermanned behavior settings in a series of studies of churches varying in size (Wicker, 1969; Wicker and Mehler, 1971) and report findings that are generally consistent with the theory.

Beyond the derivations from behavior setting theory reported and documented above, a number of probable psychological consequences of undermanned behavior settings have been suggested (Barker, 1968; Barker and Gump, 1964; Barker and Schoggen, 1973). While not derived from the theory of undermanning in any strict sense, these are psychological consequences on inhabitants of undermanned ecological environments which it seems reasonable to expect on the basis of common observation and some empirical evidence.

(a) Persons in undermanned habitats have *less sensitivity to and are less evaluative of individual differences*; they are more tolerant of their associates. When the supply is short and the demand is high, those who are available to do the job must be accepted even if their skills and experience are limited. In Midwest, with its severe manpower shortage relative to Yoredale, less experienced and less able persons (children, adolescents, and old people) are accepted into settings and given leadership responsibilities more commonly than their English counterparts. Discrimination on the basis of appearances and superficial traits is less likely in undermanned settings. When there is a manpower surplus, on the other hand, competition among many possible contenders for the limited number of available opportunities to participate sometimes becomes so keen that many persons with appropriate experience and excellent functional skills are excluded, sometimes on the basis of superficial personality traits or other largely irrelevant considerations.

(b) Persons in undermanned habitats *see themselves as having greater functional importance*. The relative scarcity of setting inhabitants makes them more important people and they experience this directly without needing to be told. It is obvious to all that a setting, to operate, must have a minimum number of participants, and each person's contribution therefore is seen as more valuable. In a small church choir with only two tenors, both feel a strong obligation to attend rehearsals and performances because they understand the serious consequences for the tenor section and the threat to the choir as a whole of their absence. Small school students expressed similar feelings about being needed to help make the setting go.

(c) Persons in undermanned habitats have *more responsiblity*. Responsibility is experienced by a person when a behavior setting and the gain it provides to others depend upon his actions. A setting that is optimally populated does not burden itself with indispensable personnel; the people are too unreliable, so substitutes, vice presidents, a second team are regular features of optimally manned or overmanned settings.

(d) Persons in undermanned habitats have *greater functional identity*: they are seen in terms of what they can do in the setting. A person with an essential function is seen as more than a person—as a person-in-context. The concern is with getting the job done, not what kind of person he is.

(e) Persons in undermanned habitats *experience greater insecurity*. Faced with the need to perform more difficult and more varied actions often without proper training or appropriate experience, a person in an underpopulated setting is in greater jeopardy of failing to carry through his tasks. The problem is exacerbated by the lack of reserves to turn to for help. This amounts to increased dependence upon every other person to carry through on their responsiblities. But the risk of failure also implies the opportunity for success, and this gives meaning and personal significance to the activity.

The implications of the theory of undermanning for the primary prevention of psychopathology should now be apparent. The evidence sketched above from studies of small towns and institutions suggests that ecological environments with surplus manpower exert stultifying and debilitating pressures on their human inhabitants, while undermanned ecologies tend to enhance growth and development by providing opportunities and challenges for meaningful participation in important activities. High schools, churches, towns, and other ecological environments with manpower surpluses appear to be ruthless in excluding, or limiting primarily to spectator positions, all but the most able of the available inhabitants. But undermanned settings reach out to almost any potential participant with encouragement to enter and take an active part in operating the setting, even though his skills may be limited.

In more general terms, it would appear that the analysis of ecological environments in terms of behavior settings is a promising method of increasing our understanding of how environmental factors relate to psychological processes. Only through such improved understanding will it ever be possible to design, construct, and maintain environments that minimize psychopathology through providing environmental properties that are conducive to optimal mental health.

REFERENCES

Altman, Irwin. *The environment and social behavior.* Monterey: Brooks/Cole, 1975.

Baird, L. L. Big school, small school: A critical examination of the hypothesis. *Journal of Educational Psychology,* 1969, *60,* 253–260.

Barker, R. G. Ecology and motivation. In M. R. Jones (Ed.,), *Nebraska Symposium on Motivation.* Lincoln: University of Nebraska Press, 1960.

Barker, R. G. On the nature of the environment. *Journal of Social Issues,* 1963, *19,* 17–38. (a)

Barker, R. G. *The stream of behavior.* New York: Appleton-Century-Crofts, 1963. (b)

Barker, R. G. *Ecological psychology: Concepts and methods for studying the environment of human behavior.* Stanford: Stanford University Press, 1968.

Barker, R. G., and Barker, L. S. Behavior units for the comparative study of cultures. In B. Kaplan (Ed.), *Studying personality cross culturally*. New York: Harper and Row, 1961.

Barker, R. G., and Gump, P. V. *Big school, small school*. Stanford: Stanford University Press, 1964.

Barker, R. G., and Schoggen, P. *Qualities of community life: Methods of measuring environment and behavior applied to an American and an English town*. San Francisco: Jossey-Bass, Inc., 1973.

Barker, R. G. and Wright, H. F. *One boy's day*. New York: Harper, 1951.

Barker, R. G., and Wright, H. F. *Midwest and its children*. New York: Harper and Row, 1955. Reprinted by Archon Books, Hamden, Connecticut, 1971.

Gump, P. V., and Friesen, W. Participation in nonclass settings. In R. G. Barker and P. V. Gump (Eds.), *Big school, small school*. Stanford: Stanford University Press, 1964.

Newton, M. R. A study in psychological ecology: The behavior settings in an institution for handicapped children. Masters Thesis, University of Kansas, 1953.

Schoggen, M. Characteristics of the environment of three classrooms: An exploratory study. Peabody College, J. F. Kennedy Center, Nashville, Tennessee, 1973 (mimeographed).

Schoggen, M., and Schoggen, P. Environmental forces in the home lives of three-year-old children in three population subgroups. *Catalog of Selected Documents in Psychology*, Journal Supplement Abstract Service, 1972, *6:* 8.

Schoggen, P. Environmental forces in the everyday lives of children. In R. G. Barker (Ed.), *The stream of behavior*. New York: Appleton-Century-Crofts, 1963.

Schoggen, P. An ecological study of children with physical disabilities in school and at home. In R. Weinberg and F. Wood (Eds.), *Observation of pupils and teachers in mainstream and special education settings: Alternative strategies*. Leadership Training Institute in Special Education, University of Minnesota, Minneapolis, 1975.

Wicker, A. W. Size of church membership and members' support of church behavior settings. *Journal of Personality and Social Psychology*, 1969, *13*, 278-288.

Wicker, A. W., and Mehler, A. Assimilation of new members in a large and a small church. *Journal of Applied Psychology*, 1971, *55*, 151-156.

Willems, E. P. Forces toward participation in behavior settings. In R. G. Barker and P. V. Gump (Eds.), *Big school, small school*. Stanford: Stanford University Press, 1964.

Changing the Schools

Henry M. Levin

Next to our jails and the military, the workplace is the least democratic institution in America. Few constitutional protections apply to a worker as any ardent practitioner of free speech would quickly find out if he or she were to use the workplace to test the First Amendment. No Bill of Rights prevails in the workplace, for within a wide latitude the owners of capital and their managers make the basic decisions that affect not only our employment status, remuneration, and possibility of promotions, but the fine detail of our working lives is determined largely by the organization of production and the nature of the work environment. Although all of these matters have a crucial impact on the quality of our daily experiences and our well-being (see House, 1974; Kasl, 1974; and Margolis and Kroes, 1974), they are not based upon a democratic process in which we participate. Rather, they are predicated on the dictates and needs of those who own and manage the workplace (see Tawney, 1931, for a discussion of the prerogatives of private property).

But, if citizens have a right to a participatory role in the political affairs of their societies, why are they refused such a role in the workplace? Most of us have never asked this question, for as the fish is the last to discover the water, so are we the last to question the basic facts of life that have dominated our experiences and formed our consciousness. The major premise underlying this presentation is that the tyranny of the workplace is not legitimate and that every employee ought to have a right as a "citizen" of a workplace to participate in those affairs that impact on his or her life. Economic democracy then, refers to the democratic participation of workers in the decisions that affect their working lives. For illustrations and further discussion see Jenkins (1974), Zwerdling (1978), and *The Annals* (1979). How social change might make this possible is the focus of this paper.

I wish to thank Sharon Carter for her help in preparing the manuscript.

From Henry M. Levin, "Economic Democracy, Education, and Social Change," in Justin M. Joffe and George W. Albee (eds.) *Prevention Through Political Action and Social Change*. Copyright © 1981 by the Vermont Conference on the Primary Prevention of Psychopathology. Reprinted by permission.

441

In the following pages, I will attempt to demonstrate the existence of a dialectical relation (see Ollman, 1971, chap. 5) between the educational system and the workplace that both reinforces and—at the same time—undermines the structural relations between employers and employees. Most major social institutions have the properties of both reinforcing the existing social order and at the same time creating the conditions for changing it. Probably in few cases is this as clear as in the historical relation between education and work. The next section provides a picture of the nature of work and of schooling and their connections. Following this presentation I will describe and analyze some of the responses to the present "difficulties" of the workplace that have been raised by young and overeducated workers. Finally, I will address the prospects for economic democracy and their educational implications. The purpose of this paper is to describe a rather unconventional view of social change with respect to a concrete issue, the quest for democracy in the workplace.

A Brief Synopsis of the Relation between Work and Education

For our purposes perhaps the most important single fact about work is that the vast majority (over 90 percent) of the labor force work for corporations, government agencies, and other organizations in exchange for wages and salaries rather than working as their own bosses. That is, most persons are dependent for income primarily on their own labor, which is purchased by those who own the facilities and tools that are needed for production. At the time of the founding of the nation, some four-fifths of the nonslave population worked as self-employed farmers, artisans, or merchants while owning the land, property, or tools needed for their calling. By 1880 this proportion had been reversed with some 80 percent of the population working for firms that owned the means of production and that "hired" their labor.

A second and related aspect of work is the size and centralized nature of the workplace. Rather than the small workshops, farms, and commercial establishments that characterized the late 18th and early 19th centuries, most employment became concentrated in large, bureaucratic firms by the late 19th century (see Nelson, 1975, for details). These entities have come to dominate the markets for their products as well as the demand for labor in the areas where they operate. Thus, most individuals in the labor market do not face a large number of employment opportunities among large numbers of employers, but rather there are relatively limited employment prospects concentrated among relatively few potential employers. Further, the size of these economic entities prevents new competitors from arising, since the former dominate their markets and can practice various types of anticompetitive practices. Moreover, their cozy relationships with both the government regulatory agencies as well as such large government entities as the Pentagon enable them to utilize the power of government for ensuring their profitability (see Baran and Sweezy, 1966).

A third aspect of work is its organization. A historical picture of changes in work organization is provided by Edwards (1978), Braverman (1974), and Marglin (1974). Typically the workplace is organized in a hierarchical fashion with a large number of relatively low-paid workers at the bottom, a smaller number of more highly skilled and supervisory level workers in the middle, and even fewer persons representing the various levels of management at the top. This pyramidal form of organization is based upon an extremely fragmented division of labor, where work tasks have been divided into minute and routinized functions that permit the use of relatively unskilled workers at the bottom where most of the employees are situated. Even at higher levels, there is often such a fragmentation of the productive process, that only at the very top of the organization are a few managers or executives able to relate to the entire production operation. That is, most workers, whether blue collar or white collar, are required to perform repetitive and routinized activities. They are ignorant of the larger production process, and they do not experience the satisfaction of producing a whole product. Further, their activities are highly restricted and regularized by the nature of the job, and there is little opportunity to learn new skills or to make independent judgments. Thus, most workers have very little control over the process of their work activity and have little or no opportunity to express their own ideas, insights, and individuality. While workers at higher levels and managers have increasingly more independence as one moves up the organizational hierarchy, restriction of activity is characteristic even at these levels.

A fourth important aspect of work related to the preceding ones is that given the lack of intrinsic satisfactions, most workers toil for the external rewards. Especially important in this respect is the income that is received and that can be used for consumption of goods. Thus, most workers are forced to relinquish control over the nature of their work activities as part of the wage labor contract, and the wages and salaries become the focus of their work effort. Further, because most employees do not see any possibility of receiving satisfaction from their work activity, they place their hopes in rising levels of consumption of goods and services. Thus, work is looked at as necessary drudgery that must be carried out in order to obtain a meaningful life in the sphere of buying and consumption. In short, it is the prospect of high levels of consumption that provides the major motivation for work rather than factors internal to the work process.

It is little wonder that biographies of workers (see Terkel, 1974; U.S.

Department of Health, Education, and Welfare, 1973, for example) suggest that work is stultifying to personal growth, injurious to the health, and for most persons a very disappointing experience. Most work lacks any intrinsic meaning that makes it worth doing for its own sake. While persons born into such a world must necessarily take this for granted as a requisite for a modern society that is based upon the technology that yields our high "standard of living," a number of sources of evidence argue increasingly in terms of a different interpretation. These studies argue that technology and organizational practices grew to reflect the need for domination of the workplace by its capitalist owners and for extracting profits from the workforce (see Marglin, 1974; Gintis, 1976; and Edwards, 1978). A highly centralized and bureaucratic workplace in which jobs are fragmented into repetitive and routinized tasks simplifies the extraction of labor from workers. Each employee need only follow a specific set of functions at a prescribed speed, which will depend upon the overall rate of production set by the organization and its machinery. Supervision is simplified, since productivity can be readily observed. And the simple nature of the tasks means that workers can be easily replaced if they do not do what is expected. This "efficiency" in production is often associated with the organizational dictates of Weber (1946) and the "scientific management" of F. Taylor, whose approach is analyzed by Haber (1964) and Edwards (1978).

Thus, the internal discipline and control of the workplace by the few at the top of the organization is cemented by both the hierarchy and by the extreme division of labor. Further, the worker is set apart not only from those above and below him or her, but also from fellow workers at the same level. Under conditions of high unemployment, each worker sees himself or herself as fortunate to have a job or to have steady work. Further, the possibility of promotion up the pyramid depends on few rising, so workers are placed in a competitive and antagonistic position to each other. Not only has this mode of organization undermined the establishment of trade unions (where each worker sees his own individual possibilities of employment or promotion depending upon not getting involved in this type of activity), but it has also set groups of workers against each other. Thus, skilled workers are very jealous about maintaining their wage and other advantages over unskilled ones, and other antagonisms according to race and sex are also exploited and exacerbated as individual workers and groups are forced to compete with each other for jobs and benefits.

What is perhaps even more interesting are the recent studies that show that productivity would be higher (although not control of the work force and the extraction of profits through its labor) according to other modes of work organization. The recent study of *Work in America* carried out by a Task Force of the Secretary of Health, Education, and Welfare identified a large number of work experiments and practices that modified traditional work relations and increased productivity (U.S. Department of Health, Education & Welfare, 1973). Studies of industrial worker cooperatives have shown similar results (Carnoy and Levin, 1976a; Johnson and Whyte, 1977). That is, the owners of capital have been able to organize production to meet their needs to control the workplace in behalf of maximizing the rate at which profits could be extracted. While capital accumulation on behalf of the owners of productive property has expanded at a rapid historical rate from this process, the vast majority of workers have been subject to conditions of work that do not permit a healthy personal or social development or productive work experiences.

FUNCTIONS OF SCHOOLS

One can best understand many of the functions of the schools by viewing their roles in terms of preparing workers for the social and skill requirements of the workplace. As the workplace became increasingly centralized and work became fragmented under the practice of scientific management, so did the schools move from a highly decentralized form of lay control to a bureaucratic and centralized institution dominated by professionals (Tyack, 1974; Katz, 1971; Bowles and Gintis, 1976). As work became increasingly subdivided into minute tasks to be allocated to workers according to their capabilities, schools adopted practices for curriculum tracking and for testing students to assign them to tracks. The schools became highly standardized with a system of age-grading and a common set of instructional materials for each grade and curriculum. And many of the "modern" factory practices became embodied in the operations of schools.

Further, schooling became organized into an institution in which rules and regulations dominated educational life. Students learned to work for extrinsic rewards such as grades and promotions and the avoidance of demotions or failures rather than for the intrinsic value of the educational process. And teachers, like the bosses in the workplace, determined which students were following the rules and carrying out their activities in the manner prescribed by the curriculum and the need for maintaining order. Thus, the schools developed in a manner parallel to the workplace with similar modes of organization and values.

The process by which the socialization of the labor force by the educational system tended to follow the transformation of work under monopoly capitalist control is very complex. It has been documented—in part—by a number of researchers (see Bowles and Gintis, 1976; Levin,

1976), and it has been termed the correspondence principle. This principle can be viewed as the tendency for the educational system to follow the organization and content of the workplace as its principle agenda. It can be shown that the inequalities of the workplace are also reproduced by the schools and that the social relationships of capitalist work in its evolving forms were soon emulated by the educational systems. Indeed, the present schools cannot be fully understood without an understanding of the nature of work roles for which the young are being prepared. Alternatively, educational reforms such as those of the War on Poverty that attempted to change these functions have not been successful because of their lack of correspondence with the larger society generally and the workplace specifically. Details of this argument are provided by Carnoy and Levin (1976b) and Levin (1978).

Historically, the relationship of the schools can best be understood by looking at the functions of schools and those of the workplace. The alienating qualities of the work process have been strongly evident in the educational one as well. Students have little control over the process and product of their educational activities, and they are placed in antagonistic relations to one another in the grading and educational selection process. Since those who will do best in school will also do best in the workplace, students see themselves in competition with their fellow students in much the same way that they will experience this relation during their working lives. The concept of correspondence is a very powerful way for integrating an understanding of dominant school practices with those of the workplace.

Threats to the Educational and Work Processes

Although correspondence between educational and work processes is very helpful in understanding the stability of each, the principle is not useful for understanding change. At the present time both the workplace and the school are threatened with disruptions to the existing modes of activity. In this section we will develop briefly some of the dynamics of change that will tend to alter both the workplace and the educational system.

Although the logic of correspondence between education and work and the forces that sustain it are powerful, the reproduction of any social institution that is in contradiction to itself is not smooth. Both the educational system and the system of production and work are characterized by internal contradictions or structural antagonisms such that they operate in ways in which forces that will oppose their smooth operation will arise (see Carter, 1976; Levin, 1978). In the system of work that we described, the owners of the firms and the workers who are hired by the firms have opposing interests. The owners wish to maximize their profits and capital accumulation, while the worker wishes to obtain as large a wage as possible while minimizing his contribution to a labor process that is alien to his personal needs. But maximum profits depend upon the extraction of surplus from the employee, maximizing the amount of labor obtained from him or her while paying the worker only the minimum necessary to reproduce his or her labor power.

As we noted, through the hierarchal division of labor and the development of the educational system to produce socialized workers for the capitalist mode of production, it was possible to mediate these contradictions between the opposing interests of workers and capitalists. Moreover, such conditions as high unemployment further mediate the labor-capital contradiction, for the worker realizes that he or she can be easily replaced by a presently unemployed person if he or she does not do what the capitalist owners and managers require. This is particularly true when there are no alternatives to work for survival.

But over time the success of these mediating forces has tended to decline so that the contradictions have become manifest. In part this is due to the independent dynamics resulting from the internal contradictions in the mediating institutions themselves. For example, the educational system has traditionally provided diplomas and other certificates to reward those who complete particular levels. These certificates could be used, in turn, to obtain jobs at appropriate levels in the economic system. But as students learn to work for rewards external to themselves, such as certificates, rather than for the intrinsic satisfaction of learning and inquiry, the certificates become an end in themselves, and the student will tend to minimize the effort to obtain the reward. Thus, students look for easy teachers, try to guess what the teacher will ask for on exams to minimize studying, and cram for examinations to perform well in the short run while discarding the knowledge after the exam. Obviously, such students have learned behaviors that enable them to minimize work effort in the labor process and that might even provide insights into disrupting that process.

Historically, the correspondence of the schools with the workplace has tended to overshadow the underlying dynamics of the educational system. One of the most important of these is the present tendency of the educational system to provide more educated persons than the economic system can absorb. An important incentive for families and individuals to emphasize more schooling for themselves and their offspring has been the expectation that with additional schooling comes greater life success. The more education that a person attains, the higher the occupational status and earnings that could be obtained. Economists even viewed this process as tantamount to an investment in human capital, where the investment return generally exceeded that for investment in physical capital (Becker, 1964).

As long as the economic system expanded in the aggregate and moved from agriculture to production to the services, there was an expansion of the occupational structure at the levels that could absorb a more and more educated labor force. At each level of education it was possible for workers to view a set of occupational prospects and earnings that was better than the prospects for less-educated persons. And, in general, those with college educations were able to achieve technical, managerial, and professional positions, while those with less education had to settle for lower earnings and less prestigious careers. Thus, the training and socialization provided by the schools at each level also seemed to dovetail relatively well with the eventual demands of the workplace at the appropriate occupational level.

In recent years, though, the rate of economic growth has diminished at a time when there is an unusually large number of persons of college age and when a very high proportion of those entering the labor force have obtained at least some college-level training. The reduction in the rate of economic expansion and the maturation of the structure of the economy have resulted in an inability of the economy to absorb the increase in the number of persons with college training; this is the focus of the work of Freeman (1976) and Rumberger (1978). A more extensive analysis is found in Levin (1978) and Carnoy and Levin (in press). Instead of the economy providing greater opportunities for those with college education, it appears that young persons with college training will increasingly have to accept those jobs that were traditionally filled by persons with much lower educational attainments.

What is evident is that the same incentives that stimulated the expansion of enrollments in the schools for socializing a growing labor force for capitalist and government production will continue to operate even when the opportunities to employ more educated persons do not expand at a commensurate rate. The so-called private returns on educational investment depend not only on the earnings for the additional education, but also on the earnings that would be received without further education. Even if the earnings for college graduates grow slowly over time or decline when adjusted for rises in the price level, a college education may still represent a very good investment if the opportunities for high school graduates decline at an even greater rate. Evidence of this phenomenon is found in Grasso (1977) and Rumberger (1980).

Further, education represents one of the few hopes for most families and individuals for social mobility from generation to generation, so as the ideology of educational attainment continues to persist, the quest for more education as an instrument of status attainment will also persist. The existence of an ideology of education as a path of social mobility—as well as the fact that as opportunities for college graduates decline, there is an even greater deterioration for high school graduates—leads to the following conclusion: The educational system will continue to turn out more and more educated persons regardless of the inability of the economy to absorb them.

On the economic side, there is little on the horizon to suggest that the long-run prospects for economic growth will improve much. First, problems of high energy costs and rising costs of other natural resources run counter to technologies that have been predicated on cheap and unlimited energy and other natural resources. Second, to a large degree the government cannot use either fiscal or monetary policy to increase the economic growth rate without triggering various shortages, bottlenecks in production, and price increases in markets that are dominated by the monopolistic elements characterizing the economic system. Third, the costs of labor and the stability of production in many of the Third World countries promise much greater profits than further investment in the United States. Many countries in Latin America and Asia are characterized by dictatorships that promise enormous profits to foreign investors by preventing their workers from organizing and by refusing to provide child labor laws or meaningful, minimum wage protection for the labor force. While local elites receive substantial rewards from these practices, the majority of the workers are subjected to arduous work at subsistence wages with far greater profits for investors than would be derived in the United States. Accordingly, future economic growth rates in the United States are not likely to approach those of the post–World War II period.

To further aggravate the situation, many existing jobs are being transformed by technology and capital investment into ones that are becoming more and more routinized and devoid of the need for human judgments and talents. Studies of automation have suggested that the critical skills and judgments that are associated with particular jobs are eliminated by greater use of technology and capital (Braverman, 1974; Bright, 1966). Even many traditional professions have become increasingly proletarianized in this way as the expansion of professional opportunities has shifted from self-employment to corporate and government employment. Under the latter forms of organization, the professional is given a much more specialized and routine function, rather than choosing for himself or herself the types of clients, practices, hours, and work methods to be employed.

Thus, not only do the alternatives for the educated person seem to be deteriorating in both quality and quantity, but an analysis for the longer run suggests that the forces that are creating this deterioration will continue to prevail. Thus, young and educated persons are likely to find themselves in situations where their expectation and skills exceed those associated with available jobs. Since most jobs will not have the intrinsic characteristics that would keep such persons engaged, the inadequate nature of the extrinsic rewards will operate to make it more and more difficult to integrate such persons into the labor force. That is, the lack of opportunities for promotion and the limited wage gains in conjunction with the relatively routinized nature of most jobs will tend to create a relatively unstable work force. It is also important to note that the availability of public assistance in the form of food stamps, medical care, and other services, as well as unemployment insurance, tends to cushion the impact of losing employment, so the negative impact of losing or quitting one's job is no longer as powerful a sanction for job conformance.

As the *Work in America* report noted, these phenomena may have rather severe repercussions for labor productivity (U.S. Department of Health, Education, & Welfare, 1973). The dissatisfactions that result from frustrated expectations with respect to the quality of work and its extrinsic rewards can create threats to productivity in a variety of ways. Most notable among these are rising absenteeism, worker turnover, wildcat strikes, alcoholism and drug usage, and deterioration of product quality. Even rising incidences of sabotage are possible responses by young workers who feel that they are overeducated for the opportunities that have been made available to them and who do not see the possibilities of major improvements in their situations.

But the overproduction of educated persons relative to available opportunities is not only creating disruptive potential for the workplace, it is also suggesting difficulties for the educational system. As the exchange values of a college degree and high school diploma have fallen, there are a number of indications of a relaxation of educational standards. For example, there is considerable evidence that average grades have risen at the same time that standardized test scores in basic skill areas have fallen (Wirtz, 1977).

While there are many possible causes for these phenomena, one of the most intriguing is that these are natural responses to the falling commodity value of education. Thus, the educational system seems to be providing higher grades for relatively poorer quality work, and students no longer seem willing to put in the effort to acquire the various cognitive skills. This explanation fits our overall framework in that, to a large degree, existing educational activities will be undertaken for their extrinsic values rather than for their intrinsic worth. As the extrinsic value of education falls in the marketplace, the grades given for any level of effort must rise to ensure a given performance. Moreover, the effort that a student will put in to acquiring an education will also decline as the financial and prestige rewards decline.

A further example of this type of disruptive potential of the schools is reflected in the increasing problem of discipline. To a great extent, the discipline of workers is maintained through the promise of good pay, steady work, and possible promotion for those who conform. Since the work is intrinsically without value to the worker, it is these incentives that must be used to ensure appropriate working behavior. A similar situation has existed in the school, where the fear of failure and of low grades and the attractions of promotion and high grades has helped to maintain discipline among students. These systems of extrinsic rewards have served to ensure that students see it in their best interests to "follow the rules." But, as the job situation and possibilities of social success from education have deteriorated, even the grading system is no longer adequate to hold students in check. In fact, recent Gallup Polls of problems in the schools are consistent in implicating discipline as the most important difficulty (Gallup, 1977).

In summary, there exists a constellation of relations between the schools and the workplace that can provide either reinforcement or disruptive potential. While historically the operations of schools cannot be understood without an examination of their correspondence with the requirements of the capitalist workplace, the independent dynamic of schools and their internal contradictions also represent forces for challenging the institutions of the workplace. The result of these forces is that it is becoming more and more difficult to integrate students into either school life or working life than it has in the past. And the disruptive aspects of this situation are stimulating various responses in both the educational and work setting.

Workplace and Educational Responses

No social institution can continue to function and reproduce itself when the result of its functioning is the creation of obstacles to its further reproduction. This is the present quandary faced by both the workplace and the schools, and substantial efforts are being made in both sectors to create reforms which will avoid the current problems. While I will mention some of the efforts that are being made in the educational sector, I will place most of my emphasis on the changes in the workplace. The reason for this is that our historical analysis suggests that while the educational system can trigger change in the workplace through the workings of its independent dynamics, the changes in the education-work relation will first occur in the workplace. Subsequently, they will be transmitted to the schools in a new pattern of correspondence. That is, the workplace lies at the center of gravity in this interdependent system as reflected in the historical development of the schools.

This means that by looking at present educational reforms we may be observing only a reaction to present educational disruptions rather than a longer-range solution. In contrast, by looking at workplace reforms of a long run and stable nature, we may be seeing the basis for structural changes in the schools that will support the new working relationships. In order to apply this interpretation, it is only necessary to review the three most prominent educational reforms for attempting to improve the articulation of schools and workplaces: career education, life-long learning or recurrent education, and "back to basics." Each of these can only be understood in light of the increasing difficulties in integrating young and relatively educated persons into the workplace.

CAREER EDUCATION

Career education represents a rather diverse set of approaches that seems to focus on integrating more closely the worlds of education and work (Hoyt et al., 1972). Particular strategies include attempts to increase career guidance on the nature of and attributes of existing job positions, to improve the career content of curricula, to intersperse periods of work and schooling as part of the regular educational cycle, and to provide a more "realistic" understanding of the nature of work and available job opportunities. Obviously, an important aspect of this approach is to reduce the "unrealistically high" expectations for high-level careers and to guide students into preparing for more attainable ones. But there is virtually no evidence that such an approach will make students more "realistic" and offset the historic quest for social mobility through the educational system. Without supportive changes in the workplace, it is unlikely that this traditional function of the educational system can be altered by the introduction of career education.

LIFE LONG LEARNING AND RECURRENT EDUCATION

Concurrent with the press for career education has been the movement towards altering traditional educational patterns through life-long or recurrent education (Mushkin, 1974; Peterson et al., 1979). This effort is aimed at reducing the present high social demand for formal education—particularly at the college level—by breaking the traditional educational cycle in favor of one in which students can take instruction at times in their lives when they perceive the need. It is presumed that the young will obtain jobs at existing employment levels, and they will undertake additional instruction only when there is a need to upgrade their skills or when they wish to satisfy some nonvocational curiosity or interest.

The problem with this approach is that there is a dearth of employment positions even at lower levels of educational attainment, including high school graduates. This relative lack of productive work for young persons who leave the educational system will tend to work against their taking the recurrent educational approach seriously. Further, those jobs that are available without college training will rarely permit upward mobility into new careers that will benefit from recurrent education. More specifically, most careers require a minimum educational level for entry to higher positions (see Thurow, 1975; Edwards, Reich, and Gordon, 1975). College-educated executive trainees, engineers, lawyers, and other managerial and professional employees have very high probabilities of maintaining these positions and at least some probability of rising to higher levels. But high-school-educated stock clerks and similar workers have almost no chance of rising to managerial or professional levels through recurrent education. Whatever else their merits, recurrent and lifelong education are not likely to alleviate the problem of overeducated persons in the job market. Again, there is the shortcoming of using an educational strategy to address what is essentially a noneducational problem.

BACK TO BASICS

The back-to-basics movement refers to the attempt by parents, taxpayers, and educators to focus educational institutions on the teaching of basic cognitive skills within a highly structured curriculum. In part, this trend is work oriented in that its advocates assert that the young are unable to do well in the job market because of a failure to learn basic skills and self-discipline. The evidence of declining test scores and rising discipline problems is thought to give testimony to this claim. Even if the dearth of challenging jobs or employment is recognized, it is assumed that a young person with good basic skills and discipline will have an edge over persons without these attributes.

But, again, there is a problem in altering cognitive achievement and discipline through the back-to-basics movement if these problems derive from the falling value of education in job markets themselves. That is, to the degree that students and educators might be more lax with respect to both basic skills and discipline as a result of their declining importance in terms of life opportunities, forces more basic than school curriculum and organization are responsible for the quandary. Thus, it is predicted that career education, recurrent education, and back to basics will not resolve the dilemmas of disruption and breakdown in the traditional functioning of both school and workplace. Unless there are basic alterations in labor markets and the workplace that support changes in the educational setting, the latter are not likely to make much of a difference.

WORK REFORMS AND ECONOMIC DEMOCRACY

Both historical evidence and its extension through our overall approach suggest that the disruptive influences of overeducation in job markets is more likely to be resolved through alterations in the workplace. In particular, the fact that the extrinsic aspects of work can no longer be made attractive enough to fulfill the higher expectations of the more educated job holder means that an emphasis must be placed upon improving the intrinsic qualities of work. The most important class of reforms for enhancing the intrinsic attractiveness of the workplace are those which increase the participation of workers in decisions affecting the work process, that is, attempts to democratize the workplace. Broadly speaking, we refer to these as the implementation of economic democracy, a notion that is discussed by Bernstein (1976), Blumberg (1968), Greenberg (1975), and Jenkins (1974).

The democratizing of the workplace, then, represents an attempt to increase the involvement and commitment of the worker to his or her employer through increasing his or her participation in decision making. It is expected that by increasing involvement and commitment, the traditional rewards of wages, possibilities of promotion, and steady employment will become less important for motivating workers. To a certain degree employees will be willing to trade off these benefits in place of an increased level of satisfaction and participation in the workplace. There are many ways that approaches to economic democracy can be implemented.

Some of the most successful efforts have relied upon the use of work teams or autonomous work groups (Susman, 1976). Instead of dividing the work into fragmented and repetitive tasks that are assigned to individuals, an entire work process or sub-assembly is assigned to a team of workers. Such a process could be the accounting function of a small firm, or the responsibility for a sub-assembly of a large piece of machinery. The work team is given responsibility for most of the work process. That is, the group must schedule the activity, assign particular team members, organize and execute the work activity, and inspect the results for quality control. Thus the team would be responsible, collectively, for its own activities, and these would be determined in a participative fashion.

These approaches have been tried in such diverse enterprises as automobile assembly (Volvo) and the manufacture of pet foods (Gyllenhammar, 1977; Walton, 1975). In almost all cases, the productivity of labor increases as worker turnover and absenteeism decline and product quality rises. In essense, workers relate to a community of colleagues, and they share decision making jointly. To a large degree, the work becomes intrinsically more interesting and meaningful as the worker experiences more of an influence over his or her working life and a greater camaraderie with his or her fellow workers.

While the use of work teams or autonomous work groups represents one form of industrial democracy, there are many other forms. For example, the use of a policy of codetermination in which governing boards of firms are composed of representatives of both capital and labor is prevalent in West Germany and is being considered as part of company policy for the United Kingdom and for the Common Market countries (Jenkins, 1974, Chap. 8). There is some question whether this particular policy will increase participation on the shop floor. A more decentralized approach is the use of worker councils of elected workers who advise management on workers' interests. These functions can also be established through trade unions as in Sweden, where the workers have been given the rights in recent years to share decision making with respect to hiring, firing, distribution of work, and work safety (Schiller, 1977). That is, Swedish managers cannot make these decisions without approval by the workers, and workers are legally entitled to leave their jobs if safety hazards exist.

A more extensive version of industrial democracy is that of worker self-management itself. This mode of control can take many forms, but the Yugoslavian experience is most instructive because of its relatively long establishment in that country (Vanek, 1971). The Yugoslavian model is based upon workers' councils that make the major policy decisions for the firms. In small enterprises (less than 30 employees), all of the workers are members of such councils and in larger enterprises, the councils are elected by the workforce. The council holds all formal power, and it makes decisions regarding hiring and firing, salaries, investment, and other operations of the firm. Under this arrangement, the management is accountable to the workers. Such managers are appointed by the elected representatives of the central board of management. The personal income of the workers is dependent both upon the overall success of the enterprise as well as the contribution of the individual toward that success, although a minimum income is guaranteed to all workers.

While the Yugoslavian approach has particularly broad implications for the democratization of work in public enterprises, its counterpart in the private sector is the producer cooperative. Producer cooperatives are both owned and operated democratically by their members. In these cases, the worker-members exercise control of both the internal organization of work and the levels of remuneration, product planning and development, marketing, pricing, and other functions. Any surplus that is generated is allocated to investment or distributed among the members, so the workers benefit not only from a more democratic form of working life, but also from the financial success of the cooperative. In some cases, firms that might have otherwise closed their doors have been successfully transformed into producer cooperatives by their workforce (Bernstein, 1976; Carnoy and Levin, 1976a).

These examples of increased worker participation and democratization of work or industrial democracy all have one factor in common. By increasing the participation of workers and their intrinsic attachment to the job, it is expected that workers will become better integrated into the workplace. This integration should result in improved productivity through lower worker turnover and absenteeism and higher quality workmanship. A fairly large number of actual cases and experiments have tended to confirm the expectation of higher productivity in the more participative setting (Blumberg, 1968; U.S. Department of Health, Education, and Welfare, 1973).

EDUCATIONAL IMPLICATIONS OF ECONOMIC DEMOCRACY

If these forms of economic democracy will increasingly become evident in the workplace as a means of integrating the "new" worker, surely they will have repercussions for education. Such organizational modes set out rather different educational needs, and if the pattern of correspondence between the school and workplace is to be reestablished there must be changes in the schools. What are some of the new worker requirements that the schools will need to attend to?

Based upon previous analyses (Carnoy and Levin, in press; Levin, 1978), it appears that there are at least five dimensions of economic democracy that would require changes in the educational system. These include: (1) the ability to participate in group decisions; (2) capacity for increased individual decision-making; (3) minimal competencies in basic skills; (4) capacity to receive and give training to colleagues; and (5) cooperative skills.

The ability to participate in group decisions is an obvious prerequisite for the democratized workplace. Educational reforms that might be consonant with this requirement include greater democracy in school organization; more emphasis on group projects and teamwork; greater integration of schools and classrooms by race, ability, and social class; heavier reliance on team teaching; and a focus on group dynamics for improving interactions among student colleagues in problem-solving.

Individual decision making is important in the economic democracy mode because of the increase in decisions that the individual must make in the workplace in comparison with the present situation. That is, a democratized workplace tends to require a greater amount of individual judgment as well as collective decision making. An educational approach that might respond to this need is the construction of a curriculum with greater emphasis on problem solving than that which is found at present.

Minimal competencies for all students become important as workers are presumed to have the aptitudes to rotate jobs and share in decision making. Under existing systems of work, it is expected that workers will have widely different competencies, so that some workers will need very nominal skills and others will need very complex ones. A flattening of job hierarchies, especially through the use of teams and autonomous work groups, would necessitate much greater equality in worker skills and competencies. This requirement suggests that mastery learning types of approaches and criteria-based testing would become more important (see Bloom, 1976).

The emphasis on collegial training, where workers train their fellow workers as members of work teams or groups, would require the ability of most workers to assist others in learning job skills. The fact that workers would need to both train others and receive training themselves suggests that new forms of instruction for the schools might emphasize to a greater extent the use of peer-teaching approaches. We might expect, then, a much greater use of students for assisting other students in learning particular skills.

Finally, most forms of industrial democracy require greater cooperative skills. The movement from a highly competitive form of work organization to a cooperative one will necessitate greater attention to cooperative forms of learning in the schools. Possible educational responses include a greater emphasis on group assignments and problem-solving (Slavin, 1978).

Summary

This paper started with the view that just as democratic participation is a desirable property for our political life, it is also an important goal for other areas of our social and economic existence. Indeed, as Carole Pateman (1970) has suggested, political democracy might not be fully attainable without economic democracy in work organizations. To the degree that considerable pathology in our society is created by the stressful conditions of existing work, a movement toward economic democracy can reduce the incidence of psychopathology.

But one must obviously be wary about predictions of such profound change as the democratization of the workplace. "If wishes were horses, then beggars would ride," is an old saw. Most beggars lack transportation, and in a similar way we find that many of our dreams are delusions at best. Accordingly, one must leap beyond wishes and posit a view of social change that would seem to be useful for predicting the nature of future alterations of those institutions under scrutiny.

In this paper, I proposed a dialectical understanding of the change process in which the structural contradictions of capitalism initiate changes in both the workplace and the educational sector. The dynamics of this dialectic were presented, and specific forms of economic democracy and educational reform that would mediate the contradictions were posited.

The overall conclusion of the paper is the assertion that economic democracy is a very likely prospect for the future, and that it may have the effect of democratizing to a greater extent such other institutions as the school and family. For those of us who abhor the present tyranny of the workplace, our hopes are heightened by this reading of the future. However, we should acknowledge that the forces of domination have been with us for a considerable part of our history as evidenced by the following quote from a secret diary of Marcus Aurelius (c.100 B.C.), which was said to have guided him in his daily dealings with his fellow man:

TESTES SOURS VIRILITER APPREHENDE, DEINDE COR ET MENS SEQUENTER

Translated liberally, this means "Once you've got them by the testicles, their hearts and minds are sure to follow." This has certainly been an important assumption of the development of capitalist work organizations and state bureaucracies alike. Whether these forms of control are in their twilight years is still to be contested, but the preceding analysis gives substantial cause for optimism.

References

The Annals, Special Issue on "Industrial democracy in International Perspective." Vol. 431, May, 1977.

Baran, P., and Sweezy, P. *Monopoly capital*. New York: Monthly Review Press, 1966.

Becker, G. S. *Human capital*. New York: Columbia University Press, 1964.

Bernstein, P. *Workplace democratization: Its internal dynamics*. Kent, Ohio: Kent State University Press, 1976.

Bloom, B. S. *Human characteristics and school learning*. New York: McGraw-Hill, 1976.

Blumberg, P. *Industrial democracy: The sociology of participation*. New York: Schocken, 1968.

Bowles, S., and Gintis, H. *Schooling in capitalist America.* New York: Basic Books, 1976.

Braverman, H. *Labor and monopoly capital.* New York: Monthly Review Press, 1974.

Bright, J. The relationship of increasing automation and skill requirements. In *The employment impact of technological change,* Report of the National Commission on Technology, Automation, and Economic Progress, Appendix Volume 2. Washington, D.C.: U.S. Government Printing Office, February 1966, pp. 207–221.

Carnoy, M., and Levin, H. 'Workers' triumph: The Meriden experiment. *Working Papers,* 1976, winter, 47–56. (a)

Carnoy, M., and Levin, H. *The limits of educational reform.* New York: David McKay, 1976. (b)

Carter, M. Contradiction and correspondence: Analysis of the relation of schooling to work. In M. Carnoy and H. Levin (Eds.), *The limits of educational reform.* New York: David McKay, 1976.

Edwards, R. C. *Contested terrain: The transformation of the workplace in the 20th century.* New York: Basic Books, 1978.

Edwards, R., Reich, M., and Gordon, D. M. *Labor market segmentation.* Lexington, Mass.: D. C. Heath, 1975.

Freeman, R. B. *The overeducated American.* New York: Academic Press, 1976.

Gallup, G. H. Ninth annual Gallup Poll of the public's attitudes toward the public schools. *Phi Delta Kappan,* 1977, September, 33–48.

Gintis, H. The nature of labor exchange and the theory of capitalist production. *Review of Radical Political Economics,* 1976, *8,* 36–54.

Grasso, J. *On the declining labor market value of schooling.* Paper prepared for the Annual Meeting of the American Educational Research Association, New York City, April, 1977.

Greenberg, E. S. The consequences of worker participation: A clarification of the theoretical literature. *Social Science Quarterly,* 1975, September, 191–209.

Grubb, W. N., and Lazerson, M. Rally 'round the workplace: Continuities and fallacies in career education. *Harvard Educational Review,* 1975, *45,* 451–474.

Gyllenhammar, P. G. *People at work.* Boston: Addison-Wesley, 1977.

Haber, S. *Efficiency and uplift: Scientific management in the progressive era, 1890–1920.* Chicago: University of Chicago Press, 1964.

House, J. S. The effects of occupational stress on physical health. In J. O'Toole (Ed.), *Work and the quality of life.* Cambridge, Mass.: MIT Press, 1974, pp. 145–170.

Hoyt, K., Evans, R. N., Mackin, E. F., and Mangum, G. L. *Career education: What it is and how to do it.* Salt Lake City: Olympus, 1972.

Jenkins, D. *Job power.* Baltimore: Penguin Books, 1974.

Johnson, A., and Whyte, W. F. The Mondragon System of worker production cooperatives. *Industrial and Labor Relations Review,* 1977, *31,* 18–30.

Kasl, S. V. Work and mental health. In J. O'Toole (Ed.), *Work and the quality of life.* Cambridge, Mass.: MIT Press, 1974.

Katz, M. B. *Class, bureaucracy and schools: The illusion of educational change in America.* New York: Praeger, 1971.

Levin, H. M. A decade of policy developments in improving education and training of low income populations. In R. Haveman (Ed.), *A decade of federal antipoverty programs: Achievements, failures, and lessons.* New York: Academic Press, 1977.

Levin, H. M., and Carnoy, M. *The dialectic of education and work*. Stanford, Calif.: Stanford University Press, in press.

Levin, H. M. Educational reform: Its meaning? In M. Carnoy and H. Levin (Eds.), *The limits of educational reform*. New York: David McKay, 1976.

Levin, H. M. *Workplace democracy and educational planning*. Paris: International Institute of Educational Planning (UNESCO), 1978, in press.

Marglin, S. A. What do bosses do? *The Review of Radical Political Economics*, 1974, *6*, 60–112.

Margolis, B., and Kroes, W. Work and the health of man. In J. O'Toole (Ed.), *Work and the quality of life*. Cambridge, Mass.: MIT Press, 1974.

Mushkin, S. (Ed.). *Recurrent education*. Washington, D.C.: U.S. Government Printing Office, 1974.

Nelson, D. *Managers and workers: Origins of the new factory system in the United States, 1880–1920*. Madison, Wis.: University of Wisconsin Press, 1975.

Ollman, B. *Alienation: Marx's conception of man in capitalist society*. New York: Cambridge University Press, 1971.

Pateman, C. *Participation and democratic theory*. New York: Cambridge University Press, 1970.

Peterson, R. E., Cross, K. P., Valley, J. R., Powell, S. A., Hartle, T. W., Kutner, M. A., and Hirabyashi, J. B. *Lifelong learning in America*. San Francisco, Jossey-Bass, 1979.

Rumberger, R. W. The economic decline of college graduates: Fact or fallacy? *The Journal of Human Resources*, 1980, in press.

Rumberger, R. W. *Overeducation in the U.S. labor market*. Unpublished doctoral dissertation, School of Education, Stanford University, July 1978.

Schiller, B. Industrial democracy in Scandinavia. *The Annals*, 1977, *431*, 63–73.

Slavin, R. E. *Cooperative learning*. Report No. 267, Center for Social Organization of Schools. Baltimore: Johns Hopkins University, 1978.

Susman, G. I. *Autonomy at work: A sociotechnical analysis of participative management*. New York: Praeger, 1976.

Terkel, S. *Working*. New York: Pantheon Books, 1974.

Tawney, R. H. *Inequality*. London: Allen and Unwin, 1931.

Thurow, L. *Generating inequality*. New York: Basic Books, 1975.

Tyack, D. B. *The one best system*. Cambridge, Mass.: Harvard University Press, 1974.

U.S. Department of Health, Education, and Welfare. *Work in America*. Cambridge, Mass.: MIT Press, 1973.

Vanek, J. *The participatory economy*. Ithaca, N.Y.: Cornell University Press, 1971.

Walton, R. E. Criteria for quality of working life. In L. Davis and A. Cherns (Eds.), *The quality of working life*, (Vol. 1). New York: The Free Press, 1975.

Weber, M. Bureaucracy. In H. H. Gerth and C. W. Mills (Eds.), *From Max Weber: Essays in Sociology*. New York: Oxford University Press, 1946.

Wilcox, K. *Schooling and socialization: A structural inquiry into cultural transmission in an urban American community*. Unpublished doctoral dissertation, Department of Anthropology, Harvard University, 1977.

Wirtz, W., et al. *On further examination: Report of the advisory panel on the Scholastic Aptitude Test score decline*. New York: College Entrance Examination Board, 1977.

Zwerdling, D. *Democracy at work*. Washington, D.C.: Association for Self-Management, 1978.

A Community Action Program

Kenneth B. Clark

This paper is an attempt to look back on some of my involvements and experiences in the area of minority status, social power, and problems of social therapy or social change. The paper, therefore, is divided into three sections: (1) general rationale, or my conceptual frame of reference; (2) a diagnosis of the social problems and pathology of a particular community in which I have spent a great deal of time living and studying; and (3) a suggested remedy in the form of a proposal for community action that became the prototype for the Johnson administration's War on Poverty. I shall conclude this presentation with a sort of summary epilogue.

Traditionally, mental health has been perceived and approached in terms of individuals. The discipline of psychiatry emerged from the practice of medicine, and this fact probably accounts for the tradition of dealing with personality disturbances in terms of the one-to-one physician/patient relationships that characterize the diagnosis and treatment of physical diseases. Furthermore, mental diseases, or mental problems, like physical disease, inflict pain and discomfort on individuals. It is understandable, therefore, that attempts to deal with emotional, personal, or social instability, which are not essentially medical problems, would imitate the medical model. Up to the present, the psychodynamic theories that have significantly influenced practice in the field of psychiatry and psychotherapy have been concerned primarily with the motivation, the conflicts, and the aberrations of individuals. At times it seems to those of us in the field of social psychology as if this preoccupation with individuals tends to obscure the profound truth that the individual personality is a product of and functions only within a social milieu. So often has this rather simple fact been ignored, that the theory and practice of psychiatry seemed to be predicated upon the assumption that all problems of individual adjustment could be adequately understood by studying and treating the individual. The belief that neurotic conflict was self-

From Kenneth B. Clark, "Community Action Programs—an Appraisal," in Justin M. Joffe and George W. Albee (eds.) *Prevention Through Political Action and Social Change*. Copyright © 1981 by the Vermont Conference on the Primary Prevention of Psychopathology. Reprinted by permission.

generating, and either had its origin within the individual or reflected some peculiar, unique constellation of development forces, or sometimes forces within the family structure, was the prevailing dogma in the therapeutic field. This was probably reinforced by direct observation of the symptoms of psychoses. Psychosis is manifested by individual aberrations, sometimes dramatic behavioral deviance and stark or sudden breaks with reality. The obvious need to diagnose, treat, hospitalize, and protect the psychotic patient certainly contributed to the postponement of the development of a social psychological approach to the understanding and treatment of non-psychotic individuals. The belief that the distinction between neurotic maladjustment and psychotic deviance was merely one of degree led to treatment of both types of problems by the same general methods and interpretations by the same basic theories.

This parallel between the approach to problems in mental health and problems of physical health extends to the recent emphasis on control and prevention of diseases through public health medicine. I believe this is a very positive development. As I understand public health medicine, it is not primarily concerned with the diagnosis and treatment of individuals but is concerned with the general problem of environmental control and public hygiene. The rationale is that this method, if successful, would reduce the incidence of infectious disease, epidemics, and other afflictions of individuals.

I use public health medicine as a model for all attempts to protect individuals by creating a healthier social environment. Understandably, this approach had to take root in the sphere of physical medicine before its rationale and effectiveness could be tested in the area of mental health. I believe that it is now long past time for us to start thinking about mental and emotional problems in terms of a preventive, sociological approach. The basic rationale of the Harlem Youth Opportunities Unlimited (HARYOU) study, which I founded and directed in 1963, was to examine the general problems of minority status and psychopathology as a basis for understanding and controlling juvenile delinquency in the Harlem community at that time. I hoped to test my belief that a high proportion of non-psychotic aberrations of the human personality can be understood and treated in terms of the social power complex and social pathology that affect individual human beings. Most of what is presented in this paper comes from my HARYOU research and some general observations during the past 25 years or more working with my wife, Mamie P. Clark, and as research director at Northside Center for Child Development, which is located in Harlem. The observations and ideas dealing with the relationship among community pathology, personal pathology, and social power come primarily from the study of the Harlem community and the problems of its youth both from the HARYOU study and my research director role at Northside Center.

The final HARYOU report was presented to the President's Committee on Juvenile delinquency in 1964 under the title, *Youth in the Ghetto: A Study of the Consequences of Powerlessness.* The HARYOU document became the prototype for the Johnson Administration's Community Action–War on Poverty program.

Let me tell you a little about the background of the HARYOU study, what was in our minds, and what we tried to accomplish. And I will conclude by telling you of our failures. In its planning stage, HARYOU conducted research on the nature and the dynamics of the community. Before attempting to design a realistic program for Harlem's youths, we simulated and observed the process of community participation and confrontation. The HARYOU staff was directly involved in many of the problems of the community that it was trying to understand. Senior staff members were required to become involved observers. Essentially, HARYOU was an experiment in community psychiatry. It operated on the assumption that the emotional problems of the bulk of the youth in Harlem must be understood in terms of the pervasive pathology that characterizes our society and that makes the ghetto possible.

If individuals were to be helped we would have to remedy the problems of the community in which they lived—and they would have to be involved in seeking the realistic remedies. The unresolved problems of the ghetto spawn human casualties in such great numbers and in such varying forms that one could not hope to increase the effectiveness of the vast number of individuals who need help by any therapeutic procedure that depended upon a one-to-one relationship.

When I looked at the waiting list at the Northside Center and thought of the hundreds and thousands of youngsters who were not even referred to the waiting list, I felt terribly frustrated. One had to work with blinders, to pretend that what was being done within the walls of that and similar clinics was very effective in itself and should not be judged against the tremendous unfulfilled needs outside. It would be impossible within the foreseeable future to train sufficient numbers of clinicians to salvage the number of human beings who are being wasted daily in the Harlems of this nation. The enormity of this problem is staggering for those who refuse to accept the cyclic relationship between social injustices and human degradation as God-given and irremediable.

The fundamental challenge that must be faced and resolved successfully is one of determining the most effective means of bringing about desirable social change. How does one bring about community mental health? How does one persuade a society to develop and maintain social environments that are conducive to health rather than to dehumanization?

Let me make a brief theoretical digression. The problem as I saw it, at that time, was a problem of power. One cannot understand the pathology, the dehumanization, the continued destructiveness of human beings without first understanding something about how those with power use their power to affect the destiny of those who are seen as powerless. Certain aspects of social power are relevant to the problem of providing psychotherapy for oppressed people and depressed humans. As I thought about this, it became more and more clear to me that the problem of power is really not alien to the field of psychology. The psychodynamic theory of Alfred Adler was an early attempt to explain human motivation and problems of social interaction in terms of striving for power. According to Adler, the desire for power comes out of basic feelings of inferiority, which, says he, are inevitable concomitants of childhood impotence and dependence upon adults. Indeed Adler points to interpersonal levels of power when he insists on the universality of various forms of compensation that dominate the ongoing struggle for a sense of personal worth and dignity. The implications of Adlerian theory for the problems of personality development in infancy, childhood, and adolescence, I thought, could or might provide a bridge for understanding and testing the relationship between interpersonal and intrafamilial struggles on the one hand, and social intergroup power conflicts and accommodations on the other.

I am aware of the fact that there is a real risk of overpsychologizing and oversimplifying complex social and political problems. It is all too easy to assume that complex problems of social power, as these are reflected in the perpetuation of social injustices and inequities, can be understood simply by understanding a child's struggle for a positive sense of his or her own worth and his or her conflicts with punitive or overindulgent parents. I therefore had Adler in the back of my mind but tried desperately not to explain what I was observing in Harlem too easily in terms of existing psychological or psychodynamic theory. I went and tried to deal with the problem, by gathering evidence, not ignoring theory totally, but recognizing that theory could only be a starting point or a frame of reference that would enable me to interpret the empirical evidence.

What follows now are the symptoms of social pathology in the form of the data gathered in that study. I present them to you, not as in any way unique, but as indicators of the persistent injustices and inequities tolerated, accepted, justified, perpetuated by people like ourselves in this society.

What are some of the realities of the American racial ghettos? The basic reality in these ghettos is that they are the institutionalization of American racism, racial discrimination, involuntary subjugation, and restriction of freedom of movement; the ghettos reflect and maintain the powerlessness of their victims. Ghettos exist because those with power use their power to perpetuate, not to remedy them. The powerlessness of the victims of the ghettos is reinforced by deteriorated housing, overcrowding, inferior economic status, a high incidence of disease and infant mortality, pervasive physical drabness and ugliness. The HARYOU study revealed the extent to which the physical neglect and mental degradation of the ghetto dehumanizes its victims. A comparative analysis of the indices of social pathology and disorganization in the ghetto revealed that central Harlem ranked high on six of seven indices of social pathology. Its rate of juvenile delinquency was consistently twice, and in recent years, two to three or more times as high as the rate for New York City as a whole. For the past seven, ten, fifteen years the proportion of habitual narcotic users has been from three to eight times that of the city as a whole. Even these figures do not reveal the full extent of the wastage of human potential through narcotics since the accuracy of the statistics seems to be influenced by class and status factors. What is known, however, is that in the Harlem ghetto at the time of the HARYOU studies drug addiction was widespread, and there is no evidence that the situation has improved in the intervening years. The sale of drugs is comparatively blatant; police are obviously accepting this. There seems to be a conspiracy to permit this in Harlem and, I suspect, to make the Harlems a source of whatever economic benefits there are for those who traffic in drugs.

Infant mortality is twice as high in Harlem as in the rest of the city. Proportionately three times as many youths under the age of 18 in Harlem are supported wholly or in part by Aid to Dependent Children Funds as compared with the rest of the city.

The homicide rate of the community is more than six times as high as that of the rest of the city. Only with respect to suicide is the rate in Harlem no higher than the rate for the rest of the city. But contrary to the general belief that suicide rates are lower among low socioeconomic groups, the suicide rate for Harlem is approximately the same as the suicide rate for the city as a whole. And what is even more surprising is the fact that three health areas in the central Harlem community have recorded suicide rates twice as high as the rate for the City as a whole, and these three areas are bounded by Columbia University. I often wonder whether there is a morbid psychological spillover from Columbia University to these parts of Harlem.

In spite of the attempt of Americans, middle class, white and black Americans, to deal with this fundamental problem of morality and conscience by denying it, the social pathology of the American ghetto is real, and it is stark. The new technique for avoiding this reality is containment: nobody can go into Harlem, nobody should go into ghettos because unfortunately these are horrible places. So we wall them off. We try to pretend they do not exist. Yet we cannot wish away the ghettos or the destructive cycle they perpetuate. The powerless victims of American ghettos seem unable to mobilize and sustain their efforts to change the conditions of their lives.

The criminally inferior education provided by the ghetto schools continues to produce hundreds of thousands of functional illiterates each year and makes it impossible for these young people to compete for the types of jobs that would raise their economic status. And do not be misled by pilot programs or special enrollment. These programs are at best palliatives. They address themselves to a comparatively small percentage of the casualties. The majority of the children in ghetto public schools are still victims of educational neglect and in such large numbers that it amounts to educational genocide. Not only must they cope with underemployment and unemployment, but some of the most sensitive of them are doomed to self-destructiveness.

One of these days I would like to write something about suicide in the ghettos; suicide, not in the sense of an absolute, abrupt act of self-destruction, but rather the slow process of prolonged suicide. Self-destruction over a period of time—prolonged symbolic suicide. Like most middle class observers I have often been perplexed by what might seem to be mindless acts of hostility and aggression on the part of some young people in our ghettos. My intuition is that the acts that seem mindless to the middle class are in fact acts of suicidal depression and self-destruction. The individual seeks to destroy himself by destroying others and incurring the wrath of a society which will then retaliate and then become honest enough to destroy him for his aggressiveness.

So much for diagnosis. What did we seek to do about it? It is interesting that after the study and diagnosis, some very realistic individuals suggested that this condition could be a terminal illness and that it was just an act of wishful thinking to think in terms of social therapy. Some "objective" social scientists did not and do not now share our diagnosis. Some observers of American racial problems continue to believe and assert that the pathologies of American ghettos reveal the inherent inferiority of the victims. Others contend that the cycle of cultural deprivation and personal deterioration is difficult if not impossible to remedy. My HARYOU associates and I rejected these perspectives and insisted that our diagnosis was not only self-validating but also remediable. We did have a difficult diagnostic problem in trying to understand the nature of the disease that we were confronted with in the larger community; what was there about the larger community that made it possible for social pathology and cruelty to exist and persist in this society? We tried to understand the insidious, latent, pervasive, epidemic of immorality in the larger society. But our primary task was to try to come up with a program, something that we thought might help some of the children and young people in Harlem.

We did not have time to engage in a definitive diagnosis of the disease of the larger society that was so flagrantly dehumanizing in those youngsters of privileged people who could not accept others who differed from them, and therefore became accessories in their destruction. While we were concerned about the moral schizophrenia, the ethical ineffectiveness and instability of the privileged and the protected, we did not have time to seek the answers to these questions. We were obsessed by the pervasive plague, the chronic epidemic that we were studying in Harlem. Given this fact, it may be that one of the reasons for the failure of this prototype community action program was that it was designed and presented as if it were possible to tackle Harlem's pathology in isolation from the privileged pathology of the larger society. In this regard, I would like to share a comment made by one of the young people with whom we worked during the HARYOU Study. Near the end of the study we discussed some of the findings and the program recommendations with the professional staff and with some members of the community and the HARYOU Associates, the teenagers from whom we learned a great deal, and who joined us in trying to understand the realities of Harlem. During one of the last discussions before we submitted the report to the federal government, this young man who was a high school dropout looked at me and my associates and said: "Dr. Clark, how can you seriously expect to impose this program for our benefit, this design for social change, when the sources of your support are governmental agencies which do not give a damn about us." And he continued with deep feelings: "You know, if they were going to do anything that this program suggests we probably wouldn't have needed the program in the first place." He said: "These people don't want to help us." Unfortunately, his comment was prophetic. By the way, I should tell you one other thing that this young man said. As he finished prophesying that the HARYOU community action program was not going to be given the opportunity to work, he said: "I hate my parents. I hate my parents for bringing me in a world that treats me like dirt." He cried.

Every clinician in the room said: "Look—you have to fight." The HARYOU-type community action programs, are based upon the premise that concerned citizens have to fight and struggle to change the power relationships between those who inflict injustices and inequalities upon human beings and those who are the victims. We thought that we would increase the chances of effective social change if we involved the individuals who are the victims of the pathology and saw that they learned to develop and use rational techniques for change.

In the federal government community action/antipoverty program, that rationale for HARYOU became known as MAXFEAS—maximum feasible participation of the poor. We thought that this was necessary because it would change the self-image of these individuals. To the extent that these passive, dependent, powerless young people could be involved, they could act. They could help to establish objectives and goals and methods and could fight intelligently for their objectives. The tantalyzing question remains unanswered: Is it possible to cure the ills of the ghetto without curing the pervasive moral pathology of the larger society? The dehumanization inherent in the ghetto is merely a symptom of the presently undiagnosed systemic sickness of the whole society.

Let me conclude with an account of what happened. First, the HARYOU experiment failed. The indices of pathology, which were enumerated at the beginning of this presentation, reveal that the sickness of the ghetto is self-perpetuating. The antipoverty programs have not succeeded in alleviating the predicament of the poor and the powerless. If it had not been for wishful thinking, we would have seen the clues to this failure in the early days of HARYOU. In the early days of HARYOU there was successful political domination of the program. It was not possible to keep these programs out of the clutches of local, state, and federal political officials. The main reason that it was not possible was because the government was a source of funding, and it is an inviolable law that the political official who controls the purse strings will not give up control of the programs that he finances. A political official like Adam Powell, who was the first honest and direct political opponent of an independent community action program in his district, rightly understood that if a community action program were permitted to develop and become strong without his control from the beginning or at sometime during the critical process, it could be a political liability. As Roy Wilkins told me at the time, I was most naive to believe that even the best community action program could be brought into a district where there is an effective congressman, if that program were not controlled directly or indirectly by that congressman from the very beginning. The people in the Harlem community were in no position to counter this basic fact of life.

Second, the failure of community action programs reflected the naiveté of those who planned them. By naiveté I mean our belief that if we just explained to the victims the nature and determinants of their victimization, then by coming together, by organizing, by discussing, by mobilizing their alleged power, they would be able to confront and deal with the realities of their victimization. This did not happen. We did not take into account the fact that these individuals lacked the skills to plan and negotiate for their rights. They were themselves so much the victims, they were easily coopted by more sophisticated political officials and professionals. They imitated the worst characteristics of those who were initially in control. They were manipulated; and they sometimes used the community action apparatus as a vehicle for legitimizing hustles and seeking to justify nonrational actions.

The most disturbing thing I observed was that too often when the indigenous members of the community were placed in decision-making positions, they were no more sensitive than the more privileged to the basic human needs of their brothers and sisters. The human memory is a fragile thing—particularly when human beings are seeking to escape from the traps of degradation.

The failure of community action programs tended to give additional support to the contention that the victims of this society's injustices are themselves responsible for their own predicament.

I conclude by saying to you that if we—and some of us are incorrigible optimists—are going to have effective community action programs in the future, the following conditions will have to be met:

1) Genuine commitment to social, racial, and economic change on the part of the decision makers of our society. There is very little evidence of genuine rather than just verbal commitment to these goals.

2) Social and economic priorities must reflect this commitment. At the moment, defense and balanced budgets determine how this society spends its money.

3) We must train low-status, low-income people in the skills and techniques that will enable them to participate in the process of social change. We must do so while they are actually becoming involved in social-change activities, confrontations and conflicts.

4) We must train a group of professionals in our colleges and universities, in our social work schools, in our urban study programs, in our social science departments, in our public policy and our clinical psychology programs who are able to work with and for those who our society has neglected and rejected and dehumanized. We must train young people to have the empathy and the respect for potential and the humanity of these victims of social inequities. Work with rejected human beings must have the clear objective of providing them with the skills and personal security and psychological strength that are essential for

them to continue the struggle on their own toward the goals of democracy and justice.

These things must be done if we are serious about primary prevention of psychopathology—the theme of this conference. I do not know whether we are able or will do these things that must be done to remedy the problems of our ghettos. But the alternative to effective community action programs is self-perpetuating dehumanization and intensified moral insensitivity. Or, what may be even worse, passive acceptance of and accommodation to injustice, cruelty, and inhumanity as the norms of our "democratic society." This would be a terminal form of moral schizophrenia.

References

Clark, K. B. HARYOU: An experiment. In J. H. Clarke (Ed.), *Harlem: A community in transition.* New York: Citadel Press, 1965.

Clark, K. B. *Dark ghetto: Dilemmas of social power.* New York: Harper and Row, 1965. (Reprinted and distributed in paperback ed. by *Christianity and Crisis,* 1965; Harper and Row Torchbook, 1967.)

Clark, K. B. "No gimmicks, please, Whitey." *Training in Business and Industry,* 1968, 5, 27–30.

Harlem Youth Opportunities Unlimited, Inc. *Youth in the ghetto: A study of the consequences of powerlessness and a blueprint for change.* New York: HARYOU, 1964.

Neighborhood Change

Sharland Trotter

Old neighborhoods are newly fashionable among the young middle-class professionals who grew up in the suburbs. We can debate whether the cause of this trend is economics, changing tastes, or a quest for roots. It is happening—sometimes at the expense of poorer communities which, having withstood waves of urban renewal and highway construction, now find themselves being pushed out—or priced out—by changing fashion.

Old neighborhoods are also newly fashionable among social scientists and policy makers. After more than a decade of ambiguous and often misguided "community" programs mandated by the federal government, there is a new and welcomed focus on self-defined neighborhoods, on voluntarism, and on self-help. Thus, in mental health policy discussions, we hear a lot these days about community support systems and natural helping networks—that is, friends, relatives, spouses, co-workers, and neighbors—and the importance of people's attachments to local, small-scale associations based on mutual aid.

Recommendations abound—from the President's Commission on Mental Health, among others, about how to link professional service providers and programs with these so-called "natural" helpers—by, for example, giving natural helpers more information about formal services, bolstering their helping skills by providing consultation and training, and by capitalizing on the inherent strengths of existing social networks (Warren, 1976).

Without in any way denigrating the importance of these insights or the goodness of these intentions, much of what is being called for by mental health advocates has a disquietingly abstract ring to it. Neighborhoods are clearly in vogue, but there is a latent danger that professionals will be tempted to jump on the neighborhood bandwagon, just as they jumped on the community mental health bandwagon more than a decade ago, romanticizing and idealizing neighborhoods without paying sufficient attention to their social and political dynamics.

From Sharland Trotter, "Neighborhoods, Politics, and Mental Health," in Justin M. Joffe and George W. Albee (eds.) *Prevention Through Political Action and Social Change.* Copyright © 1981 by the Vermont Conference on the Primary Prevention of Psychopathology. Reprinted by permission.

In terms of primary prevention, what a good neighborhood provides is a supportive contextual backdrop—not a deliberate or self-conscious helping system. It is important to remember that neighbors are not primarily or necessarily friends, confidants, or surrogate therapists; in fact, they are frequently valued precisely because they mind their own business. Suzanne Keller (1968), who has examined the art of neighboring as thoroughly as anyone, observes that:

> The neighbor is one to whom a person turns because of proximity, not because of intimacy, and because he or she provides resources for dealing with "real trouble." Small-scale, transitive, and emergency problems, perhaps—but not therapeutic encounters.

> Essentially, the neighbor is the helper in times of need who is expected to step in when other resources fail. These needs range from minor routine problems to major crises, and the help requested may be material or spiritual. Moreover, the help asked for and given is not unlimited. It is called forth in situations that spell danger to a group or community as in times of natural disasters or unforseen calamities, or that routinely afflict any and everyone so that the help you give today you may ask for tomorrow. (p. 58)

There is mounting evidence that those who have adequate social supports tend to be better protected, especially in times of crisis, from a wide variety of pathological states, both mental and physical, than those who lack such supports (Kaplan, Cassell, and Gore, 1977). Gerald Caplan has observed, for example, that often, even the superficial links with neighbors add up to a significant support system which directly affects treatment outcomes for people in crisis (Caplan, 1974).

A vital city neighborhood manages to achieve a remarkable balance between public and private realms, respecting people's demands for privacy while providing endless opportunities for human contact. It is a balance made up of hundreds of "small, sensitively managed details, practiced and accepted so casually that they are normally taken for granted" (Jacobs, 1961, p. 59).

How is such a mixture created? In part, it has to do with the richness and diversity of street life in a city neighborhood, and the gradual accretion of a sense of public respect and trust. On the surface, the public contacts provided in a healthy neighborhood are casual, unplanned, often associated with errands, and usually trivial: people stopping for a moment to chat; admiring or admonishing one another's children or dogs; getting advice from the butcher; giving advice to the druggist on where to get a home improvement loan; trading jokes with the owner of the local dry cleaning establishment. The details are inconsequential, but they add up to an atmosphere of trust that is significant. The absence of public trust is devastating to any neighborhood, and its markers are easy to identify: crime, blight, fear, anonymity, and apathy. Its presence helps fasten people to a social mainstream without implying personal commitments. Read this description by Jane Jacobs (1961), one of our most prophetic urban critics:

> . . . Consider the line drawn by Mr. Jaffee at the candy store around the corner— a line so well understood by his customers and by other storekeepers too that they can spend their whole lives in its presence and never think about it consciously. One ordinary morning last winter, Mr. Jaffee, whose formal business name is Bernie, and his wife, whose formal business name is Ann, supervised the small children crossing at the corner on the way to P.S. 41, as Bernie always does because he sees the need; lent an umbrella to one customer and a dollar to another; took custody of two keys; took in some packages for people in the next building who were away; lectured two youngsters who asked for cigarettes; gave street directions; took custody of a watch to give the repair man across the street when he opened later; gave out information on the range of rents in the neighborhood to an apartment seeker; listened to a tale of domestic difficulty and offered reassurance; told some rowdies they could not come in unless they behaved and then defined (and got) good behavior; provided an incidental forum for half a dozen conversations among customers who dropped in for oddments; set aside certain newly arrived papers and magazines for regular customers who would depend on getting them; advised a mother who came for a birthday present not to get the ship-model kit because another child going to the same birthday party was giving that; and got a back copy (this was for me) of the previous day's newspaper out of the deliverer's surplus returns when he came by. (pp. 60–61)

To identify Bernie as an "informal caregiver" or a "natural helper" and attempt to make his role more explicitly therapeutic, to talk about him as some sort of "gatekeeper" to the mental health or social service system is to miss the point utterly. Indeed, Bernie would no doubt be dismayed at such a suggestion—precisely because he understands so well the importance of maintaining that invisible line between public and private lives. A good neighborhood, in other words, encourages casual offers of help without the threat of unwelcome entanglements, and provides a supportive context that can be taken for granted.

The development of a supportive social context depends on a perceived sense of permanence, which in turn requires a core of long-term residents with a shared affection for the place, who have forged neighborhood networks that operate through churches, PTAs, ethnic clubs, civic associations, and the like. A number of recent surveys have demonstrated that the most important factor in an individual's attachment to a neighborhood is length of residence—the capacity to stay put (Kasarda and Janowitz, 1974). To be sure, a good urban neighborhood can tolerate a certain amount of transcience, and can absorb newcomers into its midst with relative ease. But the increments have to be gradual or "community," in the sense of the social, human capital of a neighborhood, is irretrievably lost.

Historically, public policy, in its obsession with buildings and roads, has destroyed countless thousands of once-solid neighborhoods. By now the gross physical assaults are legendary; an $80 billion interstate highway system, acres of expensive and ill-planned subsidized housing, grandiose "urban renewal" schemes that have left havoc, instability, and helplessness in their wake. Harrison Salisbury, in a series of articles for the *New York Times* a few years ago, said it very well.

Even a ghetto [he quoted a pastor as saying] after it has remained a ghetto for a period of time builds up its social structures and this makes for more stability, more leadership, more agencies for helping in the solution of public problems.

But when slum clearance enters an area, it does not merely rip out slatternly houses, it uproots the people. It tears out the churches. It destroys the local businessman. It sends the neighborhood lawyer to new offices downtown and it mangles the tight skein of community friendships and group relationships beyond repair. (p. 137)

In addition to the gross physical assaults, there have been subtler assaults on neighborhoods, including private sector disinvestment, housing policies that have favored single-family suburbs, redlining by banks, credit allocation policies, and, more insidiously, federal tax policies. As our society has become more mobile and fluid, the preconditions for small-scale community life have been increasingly undermined.

Clearly, the price of modernization and mobility has been alienation, a dominant theme in literature and a major concern of social scientists for most of this century. There is disagreement in the scholarly literature about just how seriously neighborhoods as primary communities have been weakened, but the gross indicators suggest that the weakening has been substantial. The classic study of the upwardly mobile organization man of the postwar years, who uprooted family and home to climb the corporate ladder, concluded: "If by roots we mean the complex of geographical and family ties that knitted Americans to local society, these young transients are almost entirely rootless" (Whyte, 1955).

For the sons and daughters of the immigrant generations who made it into the middle class, exchanging the confining if supportive ties of the old neighborhoods for the more anonymous amenities of suburban life may have been a reasonable trade. But with the slowing of the American economy and the apparent hardening of class lines, the new urban immigrants—blacks and Hispanics, primarily—as well as the old white working class, may well face the worst of both worlds: a society more fluid and anonymous but less mobile. They have neither the traditional supports nor the compensating opportunities.

One striking finding of recent research is that poor and working class people tend to be more dependent on informal support systems such as family networks, at the local level than are the more affluent. For example, a Harvard–MIT study found that 15 percent of upper and 19 percent of middle class respondents to a survey indicated that they had relatives in their immediate neighborhood. But 43 percent of the white working class and 61 percent of the white "lower class" lived within easy reach of relatives. For blacks of all classes the figure was 44 percent. For Hispanics it was 59 percent (Coleman, 1978).

A wealthy suburb or an in-town high-rise may score high on all the indicators of alienation: people not knowing their neighbors; few relatives in the area; atomized transportation through the automobile; regional shopping centers rather than neighborhood stores; little if any street life; double-locked doors. But members of the middle class suffer less because they can, after all, afford to purchase some semblance of community.

A car (or two) can overcome the physical isolation. Long distance telephone calls can contact relatives. Housekeepers can be hired to provide child care. Holidays and cultural excursions are taken for granted. The family can join a country club to provide a social life. A buzzer system and security guards can reduce crime and the fear of crime. And if all else fails, a private psychotherapist can be consulted.

But the poor cannot purchase these facsimilies of community. If the neighborhood networks they depend on break down or are destroyed, they simply do without.

Research also indicates that social support networks are somewhat more intact in white working class neighborhoods than in poor black ones. There are many reasons that this might be so. For one thing, the dislocating consequences of urban renewal have been felt almost entirely by poorer neighborhoods. And the housing projects that have taken over streets that once throbbed with casual public life are every bit as alienating as luxury high-rise apartment buildings, and probably more so. When there is little opportunity for natural, public contact, people tend to isolate themselves from one another to a remarkable degree. And when there are the additional burdens of poverty and discrimination, when you cannot be as choosy about who your neighbors are as the upper middle class can be, then suspicion and fear of trouble are likely to far outweigh the need for neighborly advice and help. The irony, of course, is that the people most in need of effective social supports (because they are the most susceptible to the stresses of poverty and racism) often have the least effective supports to fall back on.

But income alone by no means tells the whole story. In a study of the "human ecology" of child abuse and neglect, James Garbarino and Deborah Sherman (1979) did an in-depth analysis of two neighborhoods that were matched on socioeconomic characteristics but which presented dramatically different social environments for child rearing.

Parents in the low-risk area, which was perceived as a stable neighborhood where people had put down roots and where houses were well maintained, were much more inclined to use the neighborhood as a resource for their children. There was more exchanging of child supervision and more parentally sanctioned play among children in the neighborhood. Notably, the parents in this neighborhood, and particularly the mothers themselves, also assumed more exclusive and direct responsibility for child care than did parents in the high-risk area, which had a high percentage of "latchkey" children.

It was found, in other words, that families in the low-risk area were basically able to take care of themselves. It was only in the context of relative self-sufficiency that they could call upon others and make use of informal support networks. That is, they could afford to become involved in neighborly exchanges without fear of exploitation.

In contrast, the picture that emerges from the high-risk area is one of a neighborhood facing disruptive change and deterioration, threatened, among other things, by the imminent construction of an interstate highway through its center. In this neighborhood, the researchers found, there was more transience, less self-sufficiency, less reciprocal exchange, and generally less adequate provision of child care. Instead, very needy families· were clustered together in a setting they considered hostile, where they were forced to compete for scarce social resources.

In such a stressful environment, people are inclined to take advantage of one another whenever possible by "getting all they can from others while giving as little as they can get away with." In short, there is a widespread conviction that the neighborhood exerts a negative influence on families and that a family's own problems are compounded rather than ameliorated by the neighborhood. It would thus seem that socially impoverished families may be particularly vulnerable to socially impoverished environments.

It is terribly important to begin to study families, as these researchers have done, *in context*; that is, to examine the social surroundings that help to shape family life, making the difficult business of child rearing easier or that much more difficult.

Families, of course, are also being rediscovered as a topic of popular debate, scholarly research, and public policy discussion. Long and lively arguments go on in the pages of academic journals and popular magazines, as well as in living rooms and across kitchen tables about whether the family is falling apart or continuing to thrive.

Some have voiced a fear that the present concern with families mirrors a current mood of privatism, a retreat from collective responses to social problems, and an inclination to look for personal, psychological solutions to problems that are at bottom public and political (Featherstone, 1979). Maybe so. But while they are perhaps less in vogue among intellectuals, neighborhoods represent a growing political force that evokes precisely the opposite mood—one of collective strengths and social connectedness.

In cities all over the country, the anti-neighborhood policies and trends noted above have begun to generate their own antibodies, in the form of community advocacy organizations, anti-highway coalitions and the like. Even in some of the hardest hit communities, with the most depressing economic and demographic statistics, there is resurgent energy, creativity, and ingenuity.

The city of St. Louis offers a striking example. It stands number one under distressed city criteria (Urban and Regional Policy Group [URPG]—Carter Urban Policy Document, 1978); number one in per capita vacant land and building abandonment; number one in absolute population loss; number one in infant mortality and lead poisoning rates; and number one in commercial/industrial tax abatement. Pursuing a strategy of downtown development at untold costs to its neighborhoods and their residents, St. Louis is best defined as a downtown commercial district, surrounded by what Martin Mayer (1978) has described as "a zone of devastation that must be experienced to be believed" (p. 151).

In the middle of this "zone of devastation," in an all-black neighborhood that many had considered beyond restoration,* emerged the Jeff-Vander-Lou Community Development Corporation. Its immediate impetus was a city urban renewal plan that would have dislocated many residents for the second or third time in their lives. With strong local leadership, a fiercely determined community self-help group, and seed money from neighborhood churches and a few local businessmen, Jeff-Vander-Lou not only stopped the city from intervening, but has rehabilitated several hundred housing units, operates an extensive array of human services, including day care, and has attracted a new Brown Shoe Company factory into the area, providing more than 400 new jobs.

The St. Louis (or, more properly, the Jeff-Vander-Lou) experience is a

---

*In fact, a consulting firm retained by the city of St. Louis actually recommended a plan of radical triage to withdraw services from what were euphemistically termed "depletion areas." When a public outcry forced city officials to scrap the plan, the experts were bewildered and offended (National Commission on Neighborhoods, unpublished paper).

potent reminder of the skills and resources that ordinary people possess and how much can be accomplished through collective action at the neighborhood level.

Local voluntary self-help networks—what people can do for themselves—are of course nothing new. The United States has always been renowned for its multitudes of small, local institutions; indeed, American democracy was founded on the principle of self-determination. There has been an abundance of research and observation, dating from de Tocqueville, that attests to the historical importance of voluntary neighborhood organizations and institutions in the lives of individuals.

For example, an extensive behavioral study of civic participation in five countries showed that in comparison with Britons, Germans, Mexicans, and Italians, Americans were the most likely to belong to local voluntary associations; most likely to rely on those associations to represent their interests in local disputes; and most likely to believe that such associations were important (Almond and Verba, 1965).

The authors of this study concluded that "voluntary associations are the prime means by which the function of mediating between the individual and the state is performed. Through them, the individual is able to relate himself effectively and meaningfully to the political system. . . .

"If the citizen is a member of some voluntary organization, he is involved in the broader social world but less dependent upon and less controlled by his political system" (p. 245).

More recently, local, small-scale organizations have been invoked as a significant means of empowering communities against large, centralizing institutions and insensitive bureaucracies. The major function of such groups is to empower poor people to do the things the more affluent can already do, to spread the power around a bit more, and to do so where it matters—in people's control over their own lives (Berger and Neuhaus, 1976).

In this era of giantism—and privatism—the fact that significant numbers of people are banding together to shape the destinies of their own communities is very hopeful indeed. The community that gave rise to Jeff-Vander-Lou is not so exceptional as it might appear to be. The decade of the seventies has seen the proliferation of a host of local activist groups, whose roots are to be found in the social movements of the 1960s, in the early Alinsky organizations of the 1950s, and in the union struggles of the 1930s and '40s.

Although for the most part they avoid the revolutionary rhetoric of the 1960s, these groups have arisen largely because of the obvious failures of both representative democracy and governmentally mandated citizen participation to meet the needs of the non-rich. Their strategies reflect an increasingly sophisticated blend of confrontation and cooperation woven around such issues as health, housing, schools, public safety, utility rates, and property taxes. If they are initially successful, and as they mature, such groups often evolve from single-issue to multi-issue organizations and move from "protest to program" (Perlman, 1976). For example, Baltimore's Southeast Community Organization (SECO) began as a single-issue (anti-highway) group, gradually became a multi-issue advocacy organization, and has recently branched out into economic and housing development.

Within a neighborhood, each new victory, no matter how small, can feed a sense of possibility that is more important than any specific project, and can be an important force for liberating local energy, pride, and confidence. We need small victories.

In many ways, that is precisely what the new emphasis on neighborhoods is all about—small-scale solutions to problems that are locally defined and collectively implemented.

Let me give a few examples.

Neighborhood Housing Services is a program that identifies a small neighborhood with run-down housing and a lack of confidence in its future, and aims to upgrade every house in the neighborhood, not for middle-class newcomers but for the present residents. While the federal government pays the salaries of a small staff and helps to capitalize a high-risk loan fund, the program is controlled locally, and local residents develop strategies appropriate to their perceived needs. The hallmark of NHS is that in every city where it operates (and there are now about 80), community residents, local bankers, and city officials work together to restore a neighborhood on the edge of decline and to do so before gross deterioration sets in. Besides physically fixing up houses, this approach builds important political alliances and rebuilds neighborhood confidence and pride.

❖ A community group in Southeast Baltimore (SECO) received NIMH funds to analyze their community's needs and resources and to plan appropriate mental health strategies. People in the neighborhood canvassed other residents, community leaders, doctors, pharmacists, school and human service personnel. When they discovered that families were breaking up, that people were moving out of what had once been a stable neighborhood, and that ethnic pride was often an obstacle to help-seeking, they began to turn obstacles into strengths by developing neighborhood resource directories, family communications workshops, advocacy hotlines, and so forth. The programs themselves are not particularly novel, but the way they were developed is.

The common thread among these programs is that their focus is on every-day, immediate, and immediately recognizable problems *as those problems are defined by the people involved.* Defining the problem means owning it, and that is the first step in taking collective responsibility for dealing with it. Pre-packaged remedies are not dictated by distant bureaucrats; clients are not "serviced" by experts and professionals. Instead, in the process of working through the problem, experts come to be seen not as threatening, disruptive, insensitive meddlers, but as additional valuable community resources, and technical advice is sought when and as it is needed. (This has the added side-effect of improving the self-image of the experts as well.)

More important, the problem-solving process, with its emphasis on local ownership, creates important spillover benefits that are probably more significant than the solution of the ostensible problem. As people learn new skills they acquire competence, confidence, and a sense of mastery. Increasingly, ordinary people in ordinary neighborhoods are coming to grips with the issues and problems that affect them and their families, beginning to see how power and politics operate, and are gaining a new sense of self-esteem.

Because this kind of problem-solving demands communication among neighbors, the fabric of the community is strengthened. Through collective action, alliances are forged, leaders are created, and passivity is sharply challenged. This is prevention in the best sense. The resources and networks that are developed to tackle one problem will be there to tackle the next one.

This approach to social policy suggests a powerful analogy to individual therapy. Clinicians have long known—and their patients have long been impatient with the fact—that psychotherapy requires the patient to do most of the work. Hearing the doctor diagnose the problem does not help. Passively following the doctor's orders does not help. And while drugs are sometimes part of the process, there is no magic pill. The patient must work through the problem in his or her own way, and gain a sense of ownership, both of the problem and its resolution. All successful therapy builds on existing strengths.

So it is with neighborhoods. There are very few communities that do not have some latent strengths on which to build, yet policy makers have largely ignored what good mental health professionals know so well. Instead, they have defined neighborhoods in terms of their defects and weaknesses (a habit that is as destructive to neighborhoods as it is to people). The prevailing model is still one of providing categorical services through massive national programs, and this is frequently both demeaning and futile, because it denies the recipients the experience of working out their own solutions.

This is not to suggest that government should bear all the blame for all of our problems, or that government is totally incompetent to share in the solutions. Each of the small local programs described above was bolstered with federal dollars. But the dollars came with very few strings attached, so that local people were in command from the beginning. And that has much to do with their success.

Moreover, the strings that *were* attached tended to knit various sorts of people together rather than to unravel tenuous relationships as government programs so often do by inspiring political bickering and competition. In a time when public policy seems to reflect a fundamental loss of faith in social sympathies, these programs have deliberatley brokered social empathy and political collaboration by insisting on strategies that require people to work together.

This is a rather remarkable exception to the general rule of federal assistance, to be sure, but it does suggest that aid be sensitively delivered and that government can be effective in helping to provide contexts in which people can help one another.

A successful neighborhood can be defined as one that keeps sufficiently abreast of its problems so that it is not destroyed by them. An unsuccessful neighborhood is one that is overwhelmed by its problems and defects and is progressively more helpless before them.

Once a neighborhood has reached the point of being overwhelmed, once it is beset with a multitude of problems that are beyond the capacity of its residents to deal with, it is clear that preventive action will not make much difference. But if public policy can learn to anticipate trends that are emerging but not yet at the crisis point, carefully targeted government aid can be a powerful inducement to collective action, and that is probably the best preventive medicine there is.

References

Almond, G., and Verba, S. *The civic culture.* Boston: Little, Brown, 1965.

Berger, P. L., and Neuhaus, R. J. *To empower people.* Washington, D.C.: American Enterprise Institute for Public Policy Research, 1977.

Caplan, G. *Support systems and community mental health: Lectures on concept development.* New York: Behavioral Publications, 1974.

"Cities and People in Distress" (Carter Urban Policy Document), Washington, D.C., 1978.

Coleman, R. P. *Attitudes toward neighborhoods: How Americans choose to live.* Working Paper #49. Cambridge, Mass.: Joint Center for Urban Studies of MIT and Harvard University, 1978, 20–21.

Featherstone, J. Family matters. *Harvard Educational Review,* 1979, 49, 20–52.

Garbarino, J., and Sherman, D. *High-risk neighborhoods and high-risk families: The human ecology of child maltreatment.* Unpublished manuscript, Boys Town Center for the Study of Youth Development, Boys Town, Nebraska, 1979.

Jacobs, J. *The death and life of great American cities.* New York: Random House, 1961.

Kaplan, B. H., Cassell, J. C., and Gore, S. Social support and health. *Medical Care*, 1977, *15*(s) Supplement, 47–58.

Kasarda, J. D., and Janowitz, M. Community attachment in mass society. *American Sociological Review*, 1974, *39*, 328–340.

Keller, S. *The urban neighborhood: A sociological perspective.* New York: Random House, 1968.

Mayer, N. *The builders.* New York: Norton, 1978.

Perlman, J. E. Grassrooting the system. *Social Policy*, 1976, 7, 4–20.

Salisbury, H. Quoted in J. Jacobs, *The death and life of great American cities.* New York: Random House, 1968.

Warren, D. I. Public policy and the balance between formal and informal problem coping systems in urban communities (USPHS grant 3ROI-MH-24982). Rockville, Md.: Center for the Study of Metropolitan Problems. National Institute of Mental Health, 1976.

Whyte, W. *The organization man.* New York: Doubleday, 1955.

VI. Sources of Resistance and Opposition to Prevention

History teaches us not only that power corrupts, but that power is sweet, as sweet to the powerfully corrupt as it is bitter to the powerless. Power, we are told, is never relinquished voluntarily. Predictably, proposals for social change that would result in the redistribution of power will be opposed by those who hold it with all the force necessary to discredit or eliminate the threat.

Sometimes the arguments in opposition to social change are subtle, and often opponents play tunes that are familiar, tunes that we all like to sing. Goldenberg reminds us that the War on Poverty took as its principal theme the task of individual remediation, of changing people rather than changing society. Many mental health professionals, and others interested in doing something helpful about the oppressed, found individual remediation (which was supported by massive federal funding of intervention programs) to be in keeping with their biases. The professions have long valued individual treatment over primary prevention efforts, and the promise of major funding for individual treatment programs had wide appeal. It blinded the middle-class professional to the truth that the system is the oppressor and that the victims are not to blame for their powerlessness. Trying to empower victims without changing the systems that oppress them was doomed to failure.

Another subtle way of avoiding action to eliminate oppression as a way of reducing psychopathology is to take the Olympian libertarian position espoused by Szasz. By arguing that mental illness does not exist, he concludes that programs to prevent mental illness are not needed. In many ways Szasz attempts to develop his thesis that everyone is responsible for his or her own life circumstance, that people are free to choose their behavior, or at least should be treated as if they are free to choose. While his arguments have had a positive effect in correcting many of the irrationalities of psychiatric imperialism, he has neglected to concern himself with the reality of oppression, the fact that people can be seriously, and even irreparably, damaged by exploitation and resulting feelings of powerlessness. Nowhere does he deal with the damaging effects of pathological child rearing, sexual exploitation of children, or institutional racism. His arguments and our responses are included to try to clarify this issue.

Also included in this section is a debate between one of us (Albee) and a psychiatrist (Lamb) on questions involving the appropriateness of prevention efforts as these relate to explanatory models for psychopathology. Because many of the issues that are raised by conservatives in opposing prevention efforts are stated quite clearly by Lamb and Zusman, the debate is included to alert readers to standard arguments against prevention—forewarned is forearmed.

The Politics of Timidity

I. Ira Goldenberg

Popular myth has it that time and distance make for increased clarity. Objectivity, so the guiding fiction goes, is a function of our ability to remove ourselves from events initially perceived as either too ambiguous or complex for balanced analysis. When this distancing is accomplished through conscious effort it is seen as evidence of heroic self-discipline or, at the very least, effective professional training. When it is simply the result of the passage of time, it is perceived as both inevitable and uncontrollable.

❖ Is it possible then, within this altered context, to understand the past without succumbing to the lures of nostalgia or self-righteousness? Probably not. Our penchant for alternately romanticizing or denigrating the past is matched only by our ability to rationalize either course of action. We have become masters of the art of writing our own epitaphs.

Nevertheless, we must try, if for no other reason than to provide our heirs with a perspective within which the struggle for liberation retains its meaning in the face of those whose unremitting hostility or insatiable idealism toward all such struggles leads only to resistance, apathy, or cynicism. Let us at least be one with Yevtushenko (1963) when he wrote:

> I hate the cynics with their lordly view of history, their scorn for the heroic labors of my countrymen, whom they try to represent as a lost flock of sheep, their skills for lumping the good with the bad and spitting on the whole thing, and their utter inability to offer any constructive alternative. (p. 40)

And if objectivity is beyond our ken, let us surely leave to the next generation a clearer understanding of the contradictions that both limit and define attempts at social intervention in a postindustrialized society bereft of a true revolutionary history. The purpose of this paper is to contribute to that understanding by focusing attention on an issue that has consistently interfered with or undermined our efforts to create a society more worthy of those whose labors built it: It is the issue of our own timidity in the face of contradictions—and the manner in which that timidity has influenced both the ways in which we have conceptualized problems and the actions we have undertaken to deal with them.

On Timidity

According to the venerable Mr. Webster, to be timid is to be lacking in courage, boldness, and determination. But it is much more than that. It is a revulsion over the prospects of dealing directly with the vicissitudes of personal action in an unpredictable and often irrational world. To be timid is to look at the world and purport to see rationality "just around the corner" or a light "at the end of the tunnel." The timid are eternally optimistic about the progress and potential of humankind, and so long as that progress and potential demand taking no personal risks, the timid will be in the forefront of every battle for human dignity and freedom. To be timid is to cultivate a lifestyle in which struggles are forever occurring "out there" in a depersonalized world that could easily be transformed if only the forces of oppression could be tempted, educated, or impressed (often by research results whose findings are either redundant or could have been predicted long before the studies were undertaken) to listen to the muted cries of the disenfranchised and disaffiliated. But the timid will not put themselves "out there," for they have seen what often awaits those who have accepted the responsibility of first being what they want others to become (need we mention again the fate of the Kennedys, Martin Luther King, and Malcolm X?). And so, the timid always seek to fulfill their visions and needs by continually creating two separate worlds for themselves. The first is a world of ongoing concern for a generalized and often abstract humankind, a concern bordering on genuine passion for both the oppressed and their oppressors. The second, however, is a world so constructed as to prevent themselves from ever having to change or give anything up, a world in which the timid do not risk exposing themselves or their own interests to the very same society from which they demand a commitment to self-reflection and renewal.

More than anything else, however, being timid is being unable to free oneself from one's own conditioning; it is being unwilling, even in the face of the most obvious of contradictions, to scale the walls of our own personal and professional prisons; it is being incapable of forging an identity between our own sense of incompleteness and the social, economic, and institutional imperfections that currently define the conditions under which most of our brothers and sisters struggle to survive.

Any serious attempt at a retrospective analysis of the events of the past 15 years must begin with an appreciation of the consequences of our collective timidity. Perhaps a few examples will suffice.

The War on Poverty

For all its accomplishments (some of them unintended), the War on Poverty remains the single best example of the sacrifice of impact on the altar of consensus. In retrospect we can see that the late-lamented War on Poverty was never intended to be a war at all. At its very best it was a painfully timid and overly self-conscious assault on the consequences, rather than the causes, of human misery. It was the kind of program whose philanthropic appeal was from the very beginning basically devoid of the threat that would have accompanied it had its creators touted it as a crusade against the social, economic, and institutional foundations of our society. Consequently, the initial consensus that surrounded the War on Poverty was one of the unthreatened and the unembittered. They saw their lives, not as indictments of the "American dream," but rather as testaments to its validity. Unlike the "target populations" for whom it was intended, the War on Poverty was created by people whose faith in America and its institutions was as unshaken as their belief that poverty could be eliminated through the development of a massive program of individual remediation.

And that is the key: "individual remediation." The War on Poverty was both an expression of and, more important, a vehicle for the perpetuation of the view that poverty was basically traceable to individual shortcomings on the part of poor people themselves. Thus, whatever limited resources the War on Poverty had at its disposal were almost entirely devoted to "fixing up" individuals. Poverty was to be eradicated through more personalized forms of counseling, training, and education, through programs specifically aimed at "Pygmalionizing the poor," however varied and lofty the accompanying rhetoric. What was not stated was the obvious: that people were poor because they had no money, goods, or power in a society that judged human worth specifically in those terms. What was not acted upon was equally obvious: that the barriers to possessing either goods or power were not created by the victimized, but by the institutional sources of their victimization. And so the War on Poverty, whatever its accomplishments, actually served to extend and reinforce the doctrine of personal culpability. As Cloward (1965) put it in his testimony before the Senate Select Subcommittee on Poverty:

The chief target of the federal anti-poverty program is the victim of poverty, not the sources of victimization.

If fundamental institutional change is not the primary object of the anti-poverty program, massive individual remediation is, and this is the sense in which the program does not constitute a plan to attack longstanding social and economic inequalities in our society.

Nothing being said should be taken to mean that casualty programs are not needed. No humane society can abandon those who have already experienced the ravages of prolonged deprivation. The point is, however, that low-income people as a class cannot expect to benefit from the anti-poverty program as it is currently conceived. But if we fail to make a broad spectrum of institutional changes, new casualties will steadily fill the vacuum left by individuals who are helped by the anti-poverty program, for the causes of economic deprivation will continue to be at work.

The broad consensus favoring the current anti-poverty program is hardly proof of a national determination to wipe out economic deprivation. The very breadth of this consensus, however, merely lays bare the fact that no vital institutional interests are threatened by the program. (p. 231)

Were we timid in settling for a not-so-massive program of individual remediation? Of course. Was it politic, good sense, and expedient to settle for so much less than was needed? Probably. Were we ignorant or naive about the consequences of accepting programs whose ultimate intent was to perpetuate a blaming the victim mentality? Absolutely not. We chose, for whatever reason, to disregard or, by our very muteness, to weaken Cloward's argument and position.

The Social Technicians

Timidity takes many forms. In the case of the War on Poverty it manifested itself as a willingness to accept and work within a conceptual and programmatic framework of unquestioned mischief-making potential. At other times it has surfaced in the form of tolerating reactionary practices within the helping profession itself, practices parading under the umbrella of "social change agentry," but clearly oriented toward systems maintenance.

During the past 15 years (as has probably been the case throughout recorded history), we have seen similar symbols and rhetoric employed by people with apparently opposing social intentions. Both Richard Nixon and Huey Newton spoke of "power to the people," but they surely meant different kinds of power for different groups of people. Even today, living as we are in a period of obvious retrenchment, it is stylish for almost anyone, independent of how directly or indirectly he or she may be involved in the basic issues of change, to refer to him or herself as "social change agents." Thus, we now find change agents tilling the soil on organic farming communes in Vermont, "Rolfing" each other at the Esalen Institute in California, or just plain trying to "make it through the night." They all proclaim that "my life is a political statement" and profess a deep and unabating kinship with various movements for human liberation. So be it. But at some point we must begin to call into question those individuals and practices whose rhetoric, however appealing, serve to mask a set of patently reactionary motives.

We have not done so in the past, more than likely because of a misguided and conditioned reluctance to expose our own profession (and colleagues) to the judgment of social history. Nowhere has this been clearer than in our unwillingness to publicly disavow ourselves from the "social technicians" masquerading as change agents, who have enriched themselves at the expense of the people.

Unlike social interventionists, social technicians function as guardians of the system. The results of their work generally show up as systems' maintenance rather than systems' change, regardless of the rhetoric that usually accompanies their styles or techniques. Social technicians appear in many forms, maintain that their orientation and skills are "value-free," and often claim to be solely interested in increasing the sense of well-being and overall competence of those who inhabit the setting to which they are ministering. In fact, the results of their efforts are to mute discontent, "cool out" the situation, or otherwise inhibit the transfer of power and resources from those who control them to those who are controlled by them. The social technician identifies strongly with the employing institution's values, sees little need for any basic change, and encourages the adaptation of low-status/low-income members to the system's needs through the application of a variety of techniques derived from research in the social and behavioral sciences.

A few instances. Following the ghetto riots of the late 1960s, many mental health professionals undertook (with NIMH and HEW support monies) the training of so-called nonprofessionals in the application of individual and group techniques for use in instances of "community crisis intervention." Upon closer examination, especially by local community groups, such projects often were revealed to be rather elaborate attempts to employ inner-city people as defusers of community discontent in their own neighborhoods (CRRC, 1971). In the field of organizational behavior, much of Argyris's (1967) work, particularly with the State Department during the American military buildup in Vietnam, could be viewed as consistent with a social technician's orientation. Finally, in the fields of education and criminal correction, one cannot help but be frighteningly impressed with the upsurge in the use of mental health professionals to either isolate and remove troublesome students/inmates or to run longterm training programs designed to better equip school/prison line personnel and administrators to deal more efficiently with problems of discipline. These activities are geared to focus attention away from the broader and more basic ideological and political issues which are at the root of much of the current unrest in our public educational and correctional institutions (Goldenberg, 1973; McArthur, 1974). Have we really arrived at a point where we seriously equate the implementation of token economies and behavior modification programs with the requirements for social justice?

Let us finally be clear about the fact that the social technician, whatever his or her status and presumed membership in the helping professions, is no ally in the struggle for a more equitable society. The social technician is generally called into a situation when there is a problem as defined by those who control the setting. Such problems usually involve decreasing profits and efficiency, client or consumer unrest, or an increased questioning of the setting's values by those, usually the majority, who are most directly and adversely affected by the setting's policies. The social technician's job is to check the problem as quickly as possible. Like his or her employers who control the setting, the social technician is fundamentally afraid of basic change, perhaps for two reasons: first, because his or her own social and economic interests would be endangered; and second, because at some deep level he or she views the masses as inherently violent and destructive in nature, as in need of being controlled by a class more benignly virtuous and stable by disposition, and as being incapable of handling the responsibility for determining the direction of their own lives. With the social technicians as our comrades, we need never want for enemies.

"Separate-But-Equal" Formulations of Oppression

Any retrospective analysis of the past, especially one that finally enables us to uncover and expose the reactionary influences that reside within our own profession, should not delude us into thinking that we have been less timid in confronting the contradictions that exist among those with whom social interventionists have historically identified themselves.

We have recently been witness to revelations and have felt revulsion for a crypto-fascist clique in the White House that attempted to further subvert the quality of our national life. In its aftermath, beyond the time covered by the predictable euphoria that accompanies any exorcism, we have seen passivity, resignation, and even a newfound fearfulness take hold of the American people. But even more than this, we seem to be caught at a particular moment when poor people, minorities, and women—the groups historically most systematically excluded from the body politic—are more separated from each other and more fragmented than ever before. At a time when our country might once again be moved, however grudgingly and hesitantly, toward a reexamination of its collective consciousness, those whose unity is so crucial in that struggle appear newly estranged from each other's pain. To accept this situation without attempting to change it would be nothing less than a reaffirmation of our timidity, this time with respect to those with whom our own dreams and destinies have always been bound.

The problem is clear, and it is important that we recognize it for what it is: There is no semblance of a "united front" to pool the efforts and resources of those whose only real leverage lies in the weight of their numbers. The reason for this state of affairs is equally clear: Oppressed peoples hold mutually exclusive and antagonistic views on the nature and origin of their oppression. There are different realities, and the failure to acknowledge these distinctive realities is to succumb to fantasy. But even more so, the inability or unwillingness to transcend these realities is an exercise in stupidity, however conflict-ridden the process of transcendence might be.

Take the present author as an example. My own approach to the problems of oppression and social intervention is essentially a class-based approach. What that means, of course, is that the concept of economic class is the fundamental dimension around which I seek to understand both the original nature as well as the subsequent historical development of the exploitative process. But what that also means is that, since class is conceived as the unifying superordinate theme, questions of race and sex (not to mention age and sexual preference) are necessarily relegated to a subordinate position within the analytical framework. In short, issues of racism and sexism are both contained and subsumed below the imperatives of a class perspective. But that is my reality, and no matter how much I am committed to its essential validity, it is currently not the functional reality of other minorities and of women. For black people there is an incontestable experiential legitimacy that makes for a racial view of the world, a perspective within which questions of class and sex become subordinated to issues of race. For feminists, on the other hand, the essence of the oppressive experience is sexual in nature, with class and race assuming a secondary analytical role. While poor people, Third World peoples, and women are all oppressed, each group can separately and with compelling justification define the genesis of the oppressive experience in such a manner as to transform members of the other two oppressed groups into residents of the enemy camp.

Even among members of the "same" group there is tension and conflict that can only be understood as the result of multiple group identity. Describing the plight of politically active black females, Beal (1970) wrote:

Since the advent of Black Power, the black male has exerted a more prominent leadership role in our struggle for justice in this country. He sees the System for what it really is, for the most part, but where he rejects its values and mores on many issues, when it comes to women, he seems to take his guidelines from the pages of the *Ladies Home Journal*. (pp. 342–343)

The movement for women's liberation is a struggle whose most recent phase was largely initiated by middle and upper-class white women, but it seeks the active involvement of poor white and Third World women. It also functionally excludes (perhaps even views or speaks of as part of the "enemy camp") poor males, both black and white. Thus, of course, it presents low-income women, both Third World and white, with the problem of choosing between their economic class and their social caste, a choice as divisive and uninspiring as it is unfortunate. And the situation is not discernibly different with respect to struggles involving the self-determination of Third World peoples (both rich and poor) and poor people (both black and white). In each instance, because of the nature of the superordinate imperative around which the social order is analyzed, class versus race versus sex, members of one or another oppressed group will find themselves at best, left out or, at worst, identified as part of the oppressive process.

If we have learned nothing else from the history of liberation movements, we should at least appreciate the degree to which existing social orders have benefited from a disorganized and divided citizenry. When that disorganization is imposed from without it can be dealt with comparatively easily as an expected manipulation emanating from those whose vested interests are being threatened. When, on the other hand, the disunity has its origins among the oppressed themselves, the situation fast approaches the level of a catastrophe. We are currently at that point, and the "separate-but-equal" formulations of oppression should no longer be tolerated because of some misguided sense of symbolic loyalty to a nonexistent alliance.

The Consequences of Our Own Socialization in a Goods and Power Oriented Society

Thus far we have focused attention on the consequences of knowingly accepting limited definitions of the nature of longstanding social and economic inequities, of the need to finally purge our profession of systems-perpetuating practices, and the necessity of openly challenging our brothers and sisters in struggle to forge a new unity of purpose founded upon a collective analysis that transcends self-defeating parochialism. Having reviewed these issues, it is time that we point to a final variable in the change process, a variable that has too long gone unexamined: ourselves.

Let us begin by recognizing that we live (and have been socialized) in a society dominated by an ethos revolving around the acquisition and retention of Goods and Power. Let us also understand that the American ethos is predicated on the existence of three critical assumptions about Goods and Power. Simply put, these assumptions are that:

(1) Goods and power are not, either by definition or by their nature, limitless; (2) whatever goods and power exist at a particular point will, under no conditions, be shared equally among the people; and (3) it is the individual who is the major referent for any and all analyses concerning the manner in which goods and power are both acquired or not acquired and used or misused.

In a very real sense the assumptions given above, especially when taken together, provide the intellectual and perhaps the spiritual basis for the development of a socioeconomic system which, of necessity, must be exploitative in nature and competitive in design. It is a system in which one person's advantage ultimately depends on another's disadvantage, in which one person's success must be predicated on another's failure, and in which one person's rise must occur at the expense of another's decline. Add to this scenario the perpetuation of inequity across generations, and one can begin to appreciate the power of a system to both create the past and negate the future.

Given the above, it is much easier to become philosophically and even politically opposed to the assumptions underlying the social order than it is to be free of the effects of having been processed by that order. The years of socialization, of learning and internalizing the myths and cultural imperatives that come to govern one's life, are not easily overcome; they leave in their wake a powerful legacy of experiential and behavioral predispositions. These predispositions may well be at variance with the goals of social intervention. At their very best they can impede the process of social change; at their very worst they can disable it permanently.

For the social interventionist, the problem of transcending one's own socialization involves a great deal of unlearning, particularly in those areas having to do with status, security, and control needs. It can only be accomplished to the degree that one's capacity to be self-critical about one's own needs (and the social genesis of those needs) match one's commitment to the legitimate aspirations of those with whom one is working. However distasteful one may find the historical consequences of a system predicated on an exploitative individualism, one must acknowledge its subtle impact on one's life, particularly as that impact manifests itself in the manner in which one relates to the struggles of others.

Are we prepared to acknowledge the impact of having grown up, of even having "made it," in a social order we now need to change? I think we are, for we have seen and lived too long with the contradictions of not doing so. It is, I suspect, much less frightening to demystify our own existence than to continue to bear witness to the consequences of our own timidity.

Summary and Conclusions

The human drama continually unfolds, almost as if guided by the momentum of its own incompleteness. Its possibilities assume their meaning through struggle. Both the noblest and meanest moments of our collective history as a species have emerged through the struggles to alter the conditions of bondage. Indeed, the whole of humankind is the unfinished story of oppression and the attempts to undo its obscenities to the human spirit (Goldenberg, 1978).

The need for a radical reconstruction of American society is no longer a matter worthy of serious or extended debate. It will not be accomplished through a reenactment of predictably timid and overly self-conscious thrusts at the consequences, rather than the causes, of suffering. And it will certainly not be satisfied by equating social change with the momentary relief that may accompany the exorcism of Richard Nixon from the body politic.

What is required, at least as a beginning, is a thoroughgoing analysis of the contradictions and possibilities of a superindustrialized technocracy whose very power and existence depend on the perpetuation of the powerlessness and expendability of those whose labors built it. The historically oppressive character of the "American experience" is its own demon. It is not just our leaders who require the exorcist's touch, but also our institutions and ourselves. It is this that Otto Rene Castillo was telling us in his poem "Apolitical Intellectuals."

> One day
>   the apolitical
>   intellectuals
>   of my country
>   will be interrogated
>   by the simplest
>   of our people.
>
> They will be asked
>   what they did
>   when their nation died out
>   slowly,
>   like a sweet fire,

small and alone.

No one will ask them
    about their dress
    their long siestas
    after lunch,
    No one will want to know
    about their sterile combats
    with "the idea
    of the nothing."

No one will care about
    their higher financial learning.
They won't be questioned
    on Greek mythology,
    or regarding their self-disgust
    when someone within them
    begins to die
    the coward's death.

They'll be asked nothing
    about their absurd justification,
    born in the shadow
    of the total lie.

On that day,
    the simple men will come.

Those who had no place
    in the books and poems
    of the apolitical intellectuals,
    but daily delivered
    their bread and milk,
    their tortillas and eggs,
    those who mended their clothes,
    those who drove their cars,
    who cared for their dogs and gardens
    and worked for them, and they'll ask:
"What did you do when the poor
    suffered, when tenderness
    and life
    burned out in them?"

Apolitical intellectuals
    of my sweet country
    you will not be able to answer.

> A vulture of silence
>   will eat your gut.
>
> Your own misery
>   will pick at your soul.
>
> And you will be mute in your shame.

If there has been an overall theme to this paper, it has certainly been a simple one: that the reconstruction of our society (or any society) carries with it a very fundamental belief, not only that the dehumanizing aspects of a social order can indeed be changed, but also that the very process of changing the social order can be as ennobling of the human spirit as it is cleansing of the human condition. It is this belief—call it a guiding fiction if you will—that enables us, even in the face of our sometimes meager accomplishments, to recommit ourselves to the struggles that lie before us, to the "unfinished business" entrusted to us by our predecessors. It also enables us to reach out for the fabric that joins people together, to pursue the human chorus whose song will never be captured or contained.

As finite beings caught somewhere in the midpassage of civilization, we are a part of an evolutionary process whose beginning and end will never be a part of our direct experience. We were neither present at our inception as a species, nor will we hopefully be in attendance at our collective demise. It is through struggle that we come into contact with the meaning of our existential passage.

By their very nature, the problems of oppression and social intervention cut across the usual and often comfortable distinctions we seek to make between our public–professional roles and our private–personal missions. We cannot claim immunity from ourselves. This, I should like to believe, is what Alinsky (1971) meant when he wrote: "A major revolution to be won in the immediate future is the dissipation of our illusion that our own welfare can be separate from the welfare of all others" (p. 23).

References

Alinsky, S. D. *Rules for radicals*. New York: Vintage Books, 1971.

Argyris, C. How effective is the State Department? *Yale Alumni Magazine*, May 1967, 38–41.

Beal, R. M. Double jeopardy: To be black and female. In R. Morgan (Ed.), *Sisterhood is powerful*. New York: Vintage Books, 1970.

Castillo, O. R. Apolitical intellectuals. From *Let's go*. Translated and with an introduction by M. Randall ©. London: Cape, Golliard Press in association with Grossman Inc., New York, 1971.

Cloward, R. A. Poverty, power and the involvement of the poor. *Testimony before the U.S. Senate Select Subcommittee on Poverty.* Washington, D.C., June 29, 1965.

Community Research Review Committee of the Black United Front. *Review of the Laue Project entitled Community Crisis Intervention.* Boston: May, 1971.

Goldenberg, I. I. The problem of safety in our inner-city school: A view from the bottom. *Testimony before the U.S. House of Representatives General Subcommittee on Education.* Washington, D.C., February 26, 1973.

Goldenberg, I. I. *Oppression and social intervention: Essays on the human condition and the problems of change.* Chicago: Nelson-Hall, 1978.

McArthur, A. V. *Coming out cold.* Lexington, Mass.: D.C. Heath & Co., 1974.

Yevtushenko, Y. *A precious autobiography.* New York: E. P. Dutton, 1963.

"Prevention":
A Libertarian Analysis

Thomas Szasz

Before turning to a consideration of the subject of "preventing psycho-pathology," I should like to offer some remarks about two basic issues with which I have tried to wrestle for a good many years. One is the nature of so-called mental illness—lunacy, madness, psychosis, psycho-pathology, call it what you like. The other issue, which now seems quite separate from psychopathology, but which was very much a part of it in the early nineteenth century, is the nature of liberty—freedom, auton-omy, choice, responsibility, call it, again, what you will. In the course of the last century or so, these two concepts and the social problems to which they point have become separated. My contention is that unless we reunite them, we can make no sense out of the riddle "mental ill-ness"—and are likely to injure the cause of liberty.

For a quarter of a century, I have maintained that there is no such thing as mental illness (see Szasz, 1961). To many people this has seemed—and still seems—a very exciting and daring thing to do. Why? Actually, my assertion is no more daring than declaring (to a secular audience) that there is no God. Today, a lot of people no longer believe in God—at least not in the Hebrew, Christian, or Islamic version of a God that made the world in six days and gave mankind rules about what to eat and drink, how to have sex, and so forth.

This sort of disbelief in revealed religion does not mean that one must go out into the streets and tear down synagogues, churches, or mosques, kill the priests, burn the Bible or the Koran. It means only that we recog-nized these religions as culturally evolved conventions; and that we real-ize that moral codes—ethical systems—may exist and operate without a

This paper was adapted from a lecture delivered at the University of Vermont, Burlington, January 25, 1979.

belief in God or revealed religion. In fact, the Constitution of the United States guarantees our right to believe or not believe in religion.

Not so with mental illness. Mental illness, authorities now assert, is a fact, just like physical illness is. Saying that there is no mental illness thus sounds like saying that there is no cancer of the colon—which would indeed be a stupid thing to say. The point (which I have made in several of my early books) is that bodily illnesses are literal diseases, whereas mental illnesses are metaphorical diseases. This follows from the fact that we are human beings who *have* bodies and *display* behavior. Bodily abnormalities are physical, or literal, diseases. Behavioral "abnormalities" are mental, or metaphorical, diseases. For thousands of years, such "abnormalities" were viewed as religious problems. Then they were viewed as moral and philosophical problems. Only in the last two hundred years or so have some of these phenomena been viewed as "mental diseases." The fashionable contemporary contention that "mental diseases" are, or are due to, as yet undetected lesions in the brain need not detain us here. Perhaps some are; those that are, are real, bodily diseases (similar to neurosyphilis or brain tumor). The fact remains that the term "mental illness" is used to identify undesirable behaviors, an identification whose primary significance is perforce moral and political.

If a behavioral act is deemed undesirable, two questions about it arise immediately: 1) Who is the actor, and who judges his behavior? 2) Undesirable or not, should the behavior be allowed or should it be prohibited? Suicide is a good example. A person—say Ernest Hemingway—wants to kill himself. Psychiatrists say that that proves he is mentally ill, restrain him as insane, and "treat" him with electric shock against his will. The underlying question—which the psychiatric imagery and strategy helps to avoid and evade—is whether a person has a right to kill himself. That, briefly, is how the concept of mental illness connects with the concept of liberty.

It is generally believed that liberty—individual self-determination—is a much-treasured value in our society. That is both true and not true. Let us remember that most societies throughout history were based on the assumption that individuals have no rights. Ancient societies were tribal societies. The individual existed only as a member of a group. I cannot here trace the development of the idea of individual freedom. Suffice it to say that the idea is relatively recent, and, with a few exceptions, has not taken real root outside of English-speaking countries. The belief that individuals possess "inalienable rights" that the state has no "right" to take away from them is, of course, quintessentially American.

What, you might ask, has all this to do with the prevention of psychopathology? Just this: The enterprise we now call psychiatry rests on two major pillars—mental illness and coercion. "Mental illness," as I indicated, supplies the rhetoric for the so-called "medical model"; that is, it supplies the mechanism for medicalizing everyday human problems— problems of growing up, sexual and marital relations, bringing up children, adjusting to illness and old age, and so forth. Coercion, masquerading under the euphemism of "mental hospitalization" (which is classically involuntary), is the political intervention by means of which deviance is implicitly authenticated as disease. Coercion is essential to psychiatry. This is why there is an inexorable conflict between psychiatry and liberty. If psychiatric diagnoses could be attached only to individuals who ask for and consent to them; if, in other words, psychiatric interventions were restricted to consenting adults—the scope of psychopathology would shrink to near-nothingness, and psychiatry, as we know it, would disappear.

How, then, can we talk about the "primary prevention of psychopathology" if I am right that there is no such thing as psychopathology? If psychopathology is simply a misleading term—psychopathologizing, as it were, moral, legal, political, social problems? What now follows is my effort to address this problem—without getting entangled in the implications entailed by the vocabulary of psychopathology.

You know the proverbial wisdom that one man's meat is another man's poison. It seems to me obvious that, similarly, one man's psychopathology is another man's psychological normality—or, indeed, psychotherapy. The importance of this simple fact can hardly be exaggerated. It explains why all efforts to prevent psychopathology have been such utter failures—in free societies. It also explains why such efforts have been (or at least have officially been declared to be) such glorious successes—in totalitarian societies.

Free societies are characterized by their toleration of contradictory moral and political philosophies and hence by the existence, within their borders, of individuals and groups holding widely differing values. These differences affect attitudes toward both physical and (so-called) mental illness. For example, there are people in America who believe it is better to die of a hemorrhage than to receive a blood transfusion. Others believe that it is better to give birth to unwanted children than to practice contraception or resort to abortion.

When we turn to "mental illness" and look at it as a euphemism for personal conduct of which the psychodiagnostician disapproves, then it becomes immediately obvious that this is a matter to which the maxim about one man's meat being another man's poison applies quite literally. Did not Freud insist that religion was a mass psychosis? This was a crucial modification of Marx's condemnation of religion as the "opiate of the people," since Marx's phrase, unlike Freud's, was couched in terms that did not (yet) impart to the opinion the status of a scientific fact. Freud's imagery and terminology implied nothing less than that—which is why I think he was not just a genius but an evil genius. (I have touched on this subject in several of my recent books; see Szasz, 1976, 1978.) Suffice it to say now that the idea that Freud's great achievement was, so to speak, religious, and that, depending on our values, he was a genius for good or evil, has occurred to a number of persons long before I espoused this idea. For example, Arnold Zweig, who was in sympathy with Freud's moral and political aspirations, put it this way (in a letter to Freud):

> To me it seems that you have achieved everything that Nietzsche intuitively felt to be his task, without his really being able to achieve it. . . . He longed for a world beyond Good and Evil; by means of analysis you have discovered a world to which this phrase actually applies. Analysis has reversed all values, it has conquered Christianity, disclosed the true Antichrist, and liberated the spirit of resurgent life from the ascetic ideal. (December 2, 1930; in E. L. Freud, 1970, p. 23)

But the "true Antichrist" cannot be "disclosed." "He" can only be attributed. Such reflections bring us right back to my earlier remark about the prevention of mental illness. Although it is possible to believe that psychopathology is something objective, like a falling stone obeying the laws of gravity, or that psychiatric diagnoses of depression can be correct or incorrect like medical diagnoses of diabetes or leukemia can be—indeed, probably many of you believe something like this—only in totalitarian societies can one impose one's beliefs about psychopathology on an entire population by making the political system itself the agent of prevention and therapy. It may be useful to recall, in this connection, that while approximately one-half of American servicemen who received medical discharges during the Second World War were discharged for psychiatric reasons, there were no such discharges at all from the Russian armed forces. The Russians had no battle fatigue, no combat neurosis, no psychopathology of war at all. Of course, this was no great surprise for those who knew that already before the war the Soviets had managed to eradicate such troublesome civilian psychopathologies as alcoholism and crime. Today, China experts tell us that there are no neuroses in that country. Please do not scoff and say that these are ridiculous claims for which there is no evidence. What evidence is there for the claim that God gave the Jews the Promised Land, or that Jesus was the son of God, or that psychoanalysis is a science? In our everyday life we are awash with claims of all sorts. Our moral, religious, and political character is thus shaped and defined in large part by the claims we accept as valid and reject as invalid. Let me illustrate this point by means of some brief remarks about ancient Judaism and early Christianity as codes of conduct resting, ultimately, on certain unproved and indeed unprovable claims (about gods and their desires).

To the Israelites of antiquity, the supreme value was procreation. Accordingly, marriage was, in effect, compulsory and heterosexual behavior between husband and wife was approved and even prescribed. Early Christianity was, in my opinion a sort of libertarian revolt against this form of mandatory matrimony and copulation. Instead of marriage and procreation, the supreme Christian values were celibacy and chastity. Clearly, each of these religions has had a powerful effect in shaping the behavior of its members. However, it would be awkward, and indeed self-stupefying, to view Judaism as a method for the "primary prevention" of celibacy, or Christianity as a method for the "primary prevention" of matrimony.

Let us now jump two thousand years and look at the spectacle of another great religious-political metamorphosis and the convulsions occurring at its inception. For the past quarter of a century, the Shah of Iran was supposedly engaged in trying to "Westernize" his country. What did he actually do? Did he encourage individual liberty and responsibility through a limited, constitutional government? Freedom of the press? The free market? Not exactly. He did encourage alcoholism, pornography, and the destruction of the nation's traditional religion. That is not merely my opinion, it is the way many Iranians see what happened. I mention this example of the religious-political nature of what is now often smugly called psychopathology because it struck me, a good many years ago, that one of the things the Shah was trying to do was to "alcoholize" his people. I have borrowed and modified this phrase from Krafft-Ebing who spoke of "civilization and syphilization" to describe, nearly a century ago, the cultural impact of western colonists on primitive people. In my book *Ceremonial Chemistry*, I give a detailed account of the Shah's veritable program against opium (Szasz, 1974, pp. 49–51). Briefly put, the story is that until the 1950s, the cultivation and use of opium were legal in Iran. There was a special lounge in the Iranian Parliament set aside for the deputies to smoke opium. With the stroke of a pen, the Shah declared opium smoking an illness as well as a crime, and introduced draconian punishments for the cultivation, sale, and use of opium. At the same time the Shah permitted, and indeed tacitly promoted, the use of alcohol, which is prohibited by the Koran. One writer put it this way: "Prohibition [of opium] was motivated largely by prestige reasons. At a time of modernization, which in most developing countries means imitation of Western models, the use of opium was considered a shameful hangover of a dark Oriental past. It did not fit with the image of an awakening, Westernizing Iran that the Shah was creating" (Szasz, 1974, p. 51). As a result of such "reforms," swinging Iranian youngsters took to proving their westernization by drinking whisky and soda, forbidden by the Koran. During the riots in Iran in December, 1978, the protestors singled out movie theaters, symbols of Western decadence, as their special targets. After a few days of disturbances, all but 8 of nearly 200 theaters in Teheran lay in ruins. Evidently, the revolt was fanned, at least in part, by the fact that to many people the Shah's meat was poison, and his poison was meat: in other words, many people— even well-educated people—saw virtue in traditional Moslem dogma, and wickedness in modern Western doctrines. In Teheran, it was reported that "where most females wear Western dress, many college women these days are donning the chador, a traditional all-enveloping robe, as a gesture of defiance and explaining their actions in words that to some Western ears sound quaint." Their words may sound quaint to the reporters, but they do not sound quaint to me:

Nahid, a sociology major at Pahlavi University who wears slacks and drapes her head in a brown scarf so that no skin shows except for her face and hands, recalled: "When I first started college, my professors were telling us that we should kiss a boy if we like him, even sleep with a man if we wanted to. But inside we were confused. We knew that it was spiritual love that matters. Now we feel more secure because Islam tells us that it is the right way to feel. It tells us how to live." (Gage, 1978, p. 2)

Precisely!

The Koran tells people how to live.

The Bible tells people how to live.

Moses, Jesus, Marx, Lenin, Hitler, Stalin, and the Reverend Jim Jones tell people how to live.

The idea of "preventing psychopathology" thus comes down to this. First, we must examine the contents of various moral codes and the specific behavioral repertoires they promote and prohibit. Second, we must decide whether or not using coercion to enforce such codes is desirable, and if so under what circumstances and in what ways. Each of these issues must be dealt with separately. I shall indicate, briefly, the principal options we have with respect to these complex, age-old problems—and my own preferences.

Let us first consider coercion. The three classic Western religions are— and I prefer to be clear and candid about such things—authoritarian systems. Each prescribes a particular code of conduct and compels adherence to it by means of various sanctions. It is precisely their demand for submission to authority, their moral certitudes, and their communalism that make such (and similar) religions appealing to some people and unappealing to others. I dislike such authoritarian systems of external controls, especially when they rest their legitimacy on their alleged familiarity with the desires of divinities. I prefer a moral order in which self-control is valued more highly than external coercion, which envisions the peaceful co-existence of a multiplicity of legitimate human life styles rather than the eventual triumph and universality of a single—theologically or scientifically rationalized—code of conduct.

Turning to the behavioral content of various moral codes or "life styles," I would stress that this subject does not lend itself to summary analysis. The only generalization I would hazard is that such systems display an ends-means character, making efforts to alter the means without attending to the ends inefficient or worse. Furthermore, behind all such systems lurks the question of the ultimate aim of life, now often concealed or repressed by concentrating on the "technical fixing" or "problems." Matrimony versus celibacy, heterosexuality versus homosexuality, drinking alcohol versus smoking opium, and countless other human options are now promoted or prohibited without any effort to fit the option into the means-ends context of the individuals (or the society) for whom such behaviors are advocated.

The implications of this analysis for the prevention of psychopathology are obvious. I shall use a single example—the problem of what is now called "drug abuse"—as an illustration. Scrutinizing the pertinent behavioral repertoire, we might ask: Is smoking marijuana better or worse than smoking cigarettes? Is chewing coca leaves better or worse than drinking coffee or alcohol? Such questions imply, of course, the further necessity of choosing between making truthful statements about the chemical effects of certain substances or lying about them for the sake of one cause or another. Next, we must consider the question of coercion: Should we use politically legitimized coercion to prohibit (or promote) this or that substance, depending on its effect (or regardless of its effect)?

My own preferences are these. I would rather know the truth than be beguiled by lies. I would rather know that penicillin is more effective against pneumonia than prayer, that heroin is a better pain-killer than aspirin. And I would rather let people make their own decisions about matters that do not injure others than coerce them by means of religious, penal, or psychiatric sanctions. It is obvious, however, that adherence to these principles would require scuttling the vast majority of present-day programs devoted to preventing psychopathology.

References

Freud, E. L. (Ed.). *The letters of Sigmund Freud and Arnold Zweig*, trans. by E. and W. Robson-Scott. New York: Harcourt, Brace, Jovanovich, 1970.
Gage, N. Many Iran women seek return to Islam practice. *The International Herald Tribune*, December 19, 1978.

Szasz, T. S. *The myth of mental illness: Foundations of a theory of personal conduct.* New York: Harper & Row, 1961.

Szasz, T. S. *Ceremonial chemistry: The ritual persecution of drugs, addicts, and pushers.* Garden City, N.Y.: Doubleday, 1974.

Szasz, T. S. *Karl Kraus and the soul-doctors: A pioneer critic and his criticism of psychiatry and psychoanalysis.* Baton Rouge, La.: Louisiana State University Press, 1976.

Szasz, T. S. *The myth of psychotherapy: Mental healing as religion, rhetoric and repression.* Garden City, N.Y.: Doubleday Anchor, 1978.

Response to Szasz

Justin M. Joffe and George W. Albee

❖ In the course of examining alternatives, Albee discusses Rawls's analysis of social justice and also touches on the themes of liberty and coercion that are discussed by Thomas Szasz in his midwinter lecture.* In examining the links between the nature of mental illness and the nature of liberty, Szasz poses the question of the individual's right to behave "undesirably." His concern with the issue of *who is to decide* what constitutes undesirable behavior parallels Albee's. If "mental illness" is indeed only undesirable behavior, can it be prevented without destroying liberty? Szasz's discussion of this issue is complex and provocative.

On an initial reading, both authors appear to agree in arguing against coercion and for individual liberty. Clearly Albee and Szasz are at one in opposing involuntary hospitalization and/or treatment in the cause of mental health and in their belief that the psychiatric notion of mental illness is inextricably linked with coercion. But at another level there are profound differences in their views. Can power be redistributed equitably in a Jeffersonian framework of individual liberties? Is it sufficient to provide free individuals with accurate information on dangers (of drugs, or pollution, or racism), or is it necessary somehow to control people's access or exposure to dangerous substances or the dangerous behavior of others toward them? To protect individuals from the consequences of abuses of power, do we have to infringe on their liberties? Must society set limits on the damaging uses of power? To ameliorate the social factors implicated in producing psychopathology do we have the right to use coercion? From their papers it seems likely that Albee and Szasz would give very different answers to these questions and to others of a similar sort—and in these different answers is reflected one of the dilemmas of

---

*Szasz gave the midwinter Waters' Lecture; he was invited to talk on the theme of the forthcoming Fifth Conference—prevention through political action and social change. His talk was recorded (he spoke from notes); we transcribed it, and sent it to him for editing. He has kindly agreed to it being included in this volume.

those who would set about preventing psychopathology by political action and social change.

Most of the papers in this volume do not call for extensive comment. Szasz's paper is an exception, principally because he comes to a conclusion more or less opposite to everyone else's represented at the conference. The Szaszian reasoning goes something like this: There can be no such a thing as the prevention of mental illness because behavioral disturbances are not illnesses. Prevention programs can be shown to prevent genuine diseases, but since the conditions called "mental illnesses" are really moral and political judgments it is folly to talk about preventing them.

One can agree with Szasz that on the basis of present evidence the functional mental disorders are not real diseases. One can also agree that psychiatric coercion involving forced incarceration, forced treatment, and stigmatizing diagnoses is not justified and should be abandoned. But even if we agree with him on these issues, it does not follow that we must agree when he argues against programs to prevent psychopathology.

When these conferences began five years ago, we chose the term *psychopathology* because we wanted a neutral term that would avoid the use of the words "mental illness." *Psychopathology* means twisted, or disordered, mind. It does not require the discovery of any physical or organic causation. Perhaps the term has the disadvantage of possibly being associated with the medical specialty of pathology that studies tissues and other bodily components for evidence of disease. But the word also has other acceptable connotations—like the pathology of Nazism, the pathology of war, the pathology of prejudice—in which no organicity is suggested.

We would argue that behavioral abnormalities and serious emotional disturbances do exist, and that they often follow from pathological social experiences and dehumanizing conditions. Children of psychotic parents, for example, are at very high risk of becoming emotionally disturbed adults. Babies reared in orphanages very often grew up to be cold and affectionless adults. They have many of the same kind of social problems that Harry Harlow's motherless monkeys showed as adults. Babies born to very young unmarried women are at high risk. Marital disruption often leads to depression, suicide, and hypertension.

Szasz says that he prefers "to let people make their own decisions about matters that do not injure others rather than coerce them by means of religious, penal, or psychiatric sanctions." It is obvious, he concludes, that adherence to these libertarian principles would require "scuttling pathology." A key to his position is his statement that people should be left alone in "matters that do not injure others." But by saying this, Szasz undermines a significant part of his argument against attempts at the prevention of psychopathology. It is quite clear that large numbers of children and adults *are* victimized by a wide range of brutalizing, exploitative forces in society. It is also clear that such brutalization and exploitation produce serious emotional damage. Szasz does not consider the evidence that orphanages all but destroy warmth and spontaneity in children; that meaningless, underpaid, repetitive labor is dehumanizing; that physical and sexual abuse of children produces emotionally crippled adults; that the endless depiction by the mass media of women and minorities as inferior creatures and the disenfranchisement and enforced powerlessness of the elderly lead to higher risk of serious emotional distress.

Szasz picks his arguments carefully. People should have the right, he says, to smoke marijuana, to snort cocaine, and to kill themselves. But no libertarian, including Szasz, would support the freedom to kill, torture, or enslave others. Nor would Szasz be likely to defend the maiming of innocent children, the mutilation of women, the torment of the elderly. Yet all of these barbarisms exist in society and they result in serious psychological damage to the victims. John Stuart Mill argued that over one's own body one is sovereign—but *not* that one can be free to harm others. For twenty years Szasz has railed with passion and with reason against psychiatric coercion. To be consistent he should oppose with equal fervor the coercion of the weak and of the powerless by the powerful. Such is the key to the prevention of psychopathology.

We agree with Szasz when he argues against the medicalization of problems in living. The new Diagnostic and Statistical Manual of the American Psychiatric Association (DSM III) offers many examples of the nonsense of psychiatric "medical" diagnosis. But we disagree that human emotional distress ("the scope of psychopathology" Szasz calls it) would shrink to "near-nothingness" if psychiatric coercion were eliminated. We are far less concerned with the folly of the medical diagnosis of victims than with the prevention of victimization in the first place—the prevention of psychopathology.

The Argument for Primary Prevention

George W. Albee

I hope I'm not violating any debate rules by standing to speak. My daughter Sarah, the mathematician, once calculated that I have spent twenty-two thousand hours standing and talking in front of classes and groups. I can't really talk sitting down. So, with your indulgence, I will stand.

There's an old Vermont test of intelligence where you hand the subject a dipper and ask him or her to empty out a tub of water into which a tap is flowing. If the subject starts baling, without shutting off the tap, you consider him or her stupid. Those of you with a MAT score above a certain threshold will follow the argument. It was begun for me by John Gordon, a professor of epidemiology at Harvard, who in the late fifties sat me down and said: "No mass disorder afflicting humankind has ever been brought under control or eliminated by attempts at treating the afflicted individual nor by training large numbers of therapists." I never forgot his words, and I make my classes memorize them because this is the essence, the whole spirit of public health. One does not get rid of mass plagues afflicting humankind, including the plague of mental and emotional disorders, by attempts at treating the individual.

One of the arguments that we hear often from people on the political right is that there is no evidence to support primary prevention efforts. I have put out on the table, outside this room, brochures describing our series of seven books resulting from the seven annual conferences on primary prevention at the University of Vermont.

These books contain about a hundred and fifty chapters detailing effective prevention efforts. There also have been extensive reviews of primary prevention successes by Gerald Caplan (in a recent issue of a new journal, *The Journal of Primary Prevention*) by Mark Kessler and me, in *The Annual Review of Psychology,* 1975, and in a book by Steve Goldston and Donald Klein, *Primary Prevention: An Idea Whose Time has Come.* We have a lot of evidence of the effectiveness of primary prevention, and I'm not going to use my precious time tonight specifying and detailing all of this evidence, because it is available in the literature for all to read.

I am amused and intrigued by the proposition I am supposed to defend: that "Primary prevention is a valid and proven form of intervention." I am willing to defend that statement, but the curious thing is that psychiatry, for many, many years, has used interventions for which the research evidence is *far* from valid and *far* from proven. What is the valid and proven evidence, for example, that supported the use of megavitamin therapy, or lobotomy, or electric shock, or metrazol, or insulin coma, or all of the other periodic enthusiasms that have been seized, embraced, and used by psychiatry as intervention. Why should primary prevention by expected to have a much *higher* standard of validity for its research than the other research in the field. I am willing to defend the argument that we have it, but it's a kind of interesting commentary that the statement to be debated is framed in the way that it is.

A common objection to primary prevention says that we shouldn't be spending our money (this is really *the* key objection) on trying to prevent things when there are so many people lined up who need our treatment. The problem with this position is that we are only seeing a very, very small percentage of all the people who need treatment, and *not* those in greatest need. Dr. Klerman, who was head of the Alcohol, Drug Abuse and Mental Health Administration, has estimated that we have about 34-36 million "hard-core mentally ill" people (his phrase) in our society. And, he adds, in addition to that, there is a very large additional number of people (perhaps 50 million) with serious emotional distresses that are a result of the crises of daily life. But last year, in this country, we saw a total of only seven million people in *all* our mental health intervention programs put together! I want you to be sure to understand we are seeing a very, very small percentage of those needing help, and there is no prospect, no hope, that we will ever have the professional personnel required to do much more than we are doing at the present time. So to stress the importance of treatment, to say we can't spend any more money on prevention because we ought to be spending it on treatment, is really nonsense. Further, we are not treating the right people. In a book by the American Psychiatric Association, called *America's Psychiatrists,* it was shown that the average, the modal, psychiatric patient is a middle class, white, neurotic—sort of a Woody Allen type—who comes for frequent treatment which is psychotherapeutic and which is very expensive. So the disturbed people that we are *not* treating are children and adolescents, members of minority groups, the aged, people with real, genuine

psychotic disturbances, and those with real problems of senility involving brain degeneration. All of these true cases, that most need our
help, are *not* being seen because of the dedication of the interventionists to their private office psychotherapy.

In their famous, and widely-quoted article, Dr. Lamb and Dr.
Zusman (1979) said, "Mental illness is in large part probably
genetically determined and it is therefore not preventable, at most
only modifiable. Even that it can be modified is questioned by many
and there is little hard evidence one way or the other." Now, if their
statement is true, friends, we are in real trouble! If 34 million hard core
mentally ill people are the way they are because of genetic factors, we
have a real genetic disaster on our hands in this society! We really
don't know much of anything about genetic factors although there is a
lot of propaganda written about this. Leon Kamin, who did the mar-
velous expose of Sir Cyril Burt and all of the fakery that went on in the
studies in England Burt did on intelligence in twins, is about to come
out with an equally devastating paper on the defects in the studies involving the genetics of schizophrenia. I commend it to your reading
when it appears. I also recommend the book on schizophrenia by Sarbin and Mancuso as a serious criticism of the genetic research on
schizophrenia.

We have all been educated by the great popular medical journals
(like *Time, Newsweek,* the *Reader's Digest,* and the *New York Times
Sunday Magazine*), that periodically publish the same old article, and
I've got a huge collection of these. They go something like this:

> Behavioral and medical scientists today, at the University of Tasmania,
> have reported that there is a mysterious protein molecule in the spit of
> schizophrenics. They have been boiling schizophrenics' spit for the past
> five years and when they inject this substance into spiders, the spiders
> go and hide in corners. Dr. B. S. Pompous, director of the laboratory,
> has said, 'Send us more money because we are on the verge of
> disproving the nonsense that what happens to children affects their
> later lives.'

One of the serious problems I have had with Dr. Lamb's and
Zusman's papers, that I have quoted so frequently, is that they argue
that most mental disorders are genetic and therefore not preventable.
The problem is that the total number of mental disorders keeps expanding! And each time one of the *Diagnostic and Statistical Manuals*
of the American Psychiatric Association is published, we have many
new mental disorders! When DSM I was published in 1952, there were
60 mental disorders. In 1968 the number in DSM II had grown to 145.
By 1977 the latest DSM III contains 230 different forms of mental

illness! Now either new genetic mental defects are being discovered almost more rapidly than they can be printed. or there are *some* mental illnesses that are not genetic and not organically determined. If we can prevent some of the latter, then we have already won this debate! If we can prevent anything in DSM III, as there are the official diagnostic categories of mental illness of the American Psychiatric Association, we have succeeded!

I want you to know that I am cured of *my* former mental illness. I had a Tobacco Addiction Syndrome, and I quit smoking three years ago, just cold turkey. I have two daughters, however, that I am sorry to say are mentally ill because of the DSM III category of the *excessive use of any substance.* They are both yogurt addicts!

I don't want you to think that because Dr. Goldston and I are over here, and the psychiatrists are over there, that this is a psychology versus psychiatry debate. It is not. There are many distinguished psychiatrists who stand firmly for the truth, *for* primary prevention.

Leon Eisenberg, a distinguished professor of psychiatry at Harvard and past-President of the American Orthopsychiatric Association, some years ago said:

> As citizens we bear a moral responsibility, because of our specialized knowledge for political action to prevent socially induced psychiatric illness. This implies fighting for decent subsistance levels and public assistance programs, good housing, health care, education, and the right to work for all.

Another distinguished American psychiatrist, Harry Stack Sullivan (perhaps the greatest psychiatrist produced in America), says:

> Either you believe mental disorders are acts of God, predestined and inexorably fixed, arising from a constitutional or other irremediable substratum, the victims of which are to be helped through an innocuous life to a more or less euthanaistic exit, or you believe mental disorder is largely preventable and somewhat remedial by control of psychosociological factors.

That was Harry Stack Sullivan, and I'm glad to have him on my side. I could go on with Adolf Meyer, Freida Fromm Reichmann, Eric Lindemann, Gerald Caplan, and many other distinguished psychiatrists who support primary prevention efforts.

Another favorite argument of the anti-preventionists is that: "There is no evidence that poverty *causes* mental illness." Oh, yes, they admit there *is* a correlation between poverty and high rates of psychopathology, but this is a correlation only. Now I have to point out that medicine accepts correlation in other areas. There is a correlation between smoking and lung cancer. We are now in the process of trying to convince people not to smoke because of this correlational evidence. The "Downward Drift" theory, which is advocated by our distinguished opponents, says that, "It is not necessarily because poor people and people who are powerless have higher rates of disturbance; it is because middle-class people like us have drifted down to poverty levels because we were susceptible." This "Drift Down" hypothesis has been largely rejected in the literature. It really doesn't hold water when you examine the fact that people who *used* to be poor had high rates and now do not after their class level has improved. When the poor moved into the middle class, their rate of mental illness dropped. When the Irish moved up and out of poverty into the middle class, their rates of idiocy and lunacy, high in 1855, subsequently dropped. When the Swedes moved out of Class V and into the middle class, their rates dropped. The same thing was true of the Eastern European Jews, and the same thing was true of the Southern Italians. As each successive immigrant group moved up and out of poverty, their rate of psychopathology dropped. I don't know what happened to all those bad Irish and Swedish genes that accounted for their high rates of lunacy and idiocy, but whatever happened they have fallen to an average or middle class rate of distress.

Another kind of evidence against the "Downward Drift" hypothesis is the current high rate of psychopathology among the involuntarily unemployed. Today in many parts of the country, (i.e., Detroit, Michigan, Gary, Indiana, Youngstown, Ohio,) where there are high rates of involuntary unemployment, there are now also exceedingly high rates of admissions to mental institutions, hospitals, clinics, etc. There is also a dramatic increase, in those places, in child abuse and wife abuse, in the consumption of alcohol, and in alcohol-related deaths like cirrhosis of the liver, all as a consequence of unemployment. These people didn't "drift down" into these higher rates, but because of powerlessness and stress they have higher rates of disturbance.

Our clinical experience certainly ought to be enough to convince us that the consequences of childhood rejection, childhood emotional damage, inconsistent treatment of young children, all have devastating consequences for emotional disturbances in adult life. And this is an environmental approach.

Harry Harlow's studies on the effects of Monster Mothers and of social isolation on the development of baby monkeys are too well known to review here but they give us a perfect model of the damaging consequences of early pathological infant experience. A recent study in

Sweden, and another in Czechoslovakia, examined what happened to unwanted babies (where the mother had tried twice for an abortion and was turned down). These children were born, grew up, and were followed through high school. They had much higher rates of psychopathology than babies that were born to a control group of mothers who had *not* sought abortions. That is, unwanted children are at very high risk, and this is clearly not a "downward drift" but an environmental problem.

Another favorite argument of opponents of prevention goes something like this: "How can you prevent something if you don't know the cause?" This is probably the most frequent comment in the literature criticizing primary prevention. The answer to the question is: "Easy!" In the field of public health, when John Snow removed the handle from London's Broad Street pump and stopped a cholera epidemic, he didn't know what caused cholera. There are innumerable examples in the field of public health, involving miasma theory, for example, which resulted in effective reductions in disease without knowledge of cause.

I think the most important point I can make is that there is not a one-to-one correspondence between cause and effect for mental disorder. Virchow, a great medical expert back in the 1870s, contributed to medicine by announcing that every disease has a separate cause. This insight really put medicine into orbit because it led to the identification of specific diseases. It is *not* the case for psychiatric disorders, however, that each condition has a separate cause with a specific effect. For example, following the death or loss of a loved one (a cause) there can be any number of different consequent forms of psychopathology like depression, or alcoholism, or social withdrawal, or accident proneness. So if there isn't a one-to-one correspondence, this simply suggests that we ought to try to *reduce stress,* every kind of avoidable stress, including the stress of exploitation, the stress of powerlessness, the stress of discrimination, the stresses of sexism and racism and age prejudice. And as a consequence of the reduction of stress, we reduce the consequent distress. Another approach, of course, is to *strengthen the host.* (The typical public health model is either to remove the noxious agent, or to strengthen the resistance in the host. In our field this means competency building programs). In four of our published volumes, our concern is with competency building—building competencies in children, building self-esteem into children and adults, programs to help them resist stress.

The last thing I want to emphasize as a primary prevention technique, is the *building of support networks,* development of support groups. We have an abundance of evidence that people who belong to, or who can be encouraged to become, a part of strong networks and strong support systems, are very resistant not only to emotional and mental disorders, but to physical disorders also. If there is one overarching public health principle in this field, it is that being a part of a strong support network and support system is an effective form of primary prevention.

The Argument Against Primary Prevention

H. Richard Lamb

Tonight I'm departing from the cardinal rule that I have always set for myself in the conduct of my human interactions, and that is never to argue about religion. And here I am not only breaking that rule but I am debating with the Pope himself. I also want to thank Dr. Albee like my partner Dr. Zusman did this morning for doing his best to make us famous through frequent citations of our articles. I really appreciate that. I want to say that we are extremely pleased that Dr. Albee agrees with us in wholeheartedly supporting the eradication of poverty, racism, sexism, and other serious ills of our society. We are equally pleased that he supports programs which facilitate competency building—social, vocational, educational—and especially with those groups most in need of it, such as the disadvantaged and the chronically mentally ill. But we also feel as professionals, and as behavioral scientists, that it is crucial to clarify our thinking and our conceptualizations. For instance, it may be "common sense" that poverty causes mental illness, but where is the evidence? Why can we not be against poverty simply because it is bad and noxious, without making claims when we have no evidence? We need to resist the temptation of forgetting that we are behavioral scientists and leap to conclusions for which we have no proof.

The same holds true for efforts to build competence. Why can we not be for them simply because they are good for people, and not just to justify them by saying we are preventing mental illness.

To what extent is primary prevention a mental health activity? This is a more complex issue than it might superficially appear. For instance, to again use the example of poverty, even if it could be demonstrated that poverty is a causative agent of mental illness, this would not make it a condition to be dealt with by mental health professionals. To quote the eminent sociologist Elaine Cumming, "There is a certain arrogance in someone trained to heal the sick, imagining therefore that he therefore, has a certain expertise beyond that of any other thoughtful citizen in patching up the cracks in society." It would be more ap-

From H. Richard Lamb, "The Argument Against Primary Prevention," *Journal of Primary Prevention*, Vol. 5, pp. 220-224. Copyright © 1985 by Human Sciences Press. Reprinted by permission.

propriate for mental health professionals to emphasize the need for changes to professional and political groups with expertise and authority for implementing the changes.

Much of the confusion and debate over primary prevention is related to the fuzziness of the concepts and definitions underlying the issues. Unless care is taken to distinguish prevention of diagnosable mental illness from prevention of unhappiness, feelings of distress, or social incompetence, discussants will often be examining different phenomena while thinking they are focusing on a single phenomenon. Thus we need to be clear as to what we're trying to prevent.

Those concerned with primary prevention in the mental health field face a complex problem of definition in determining the boundaries of mental health. Public health practitioners almost always use the word prevention in regard to illness. Mental health services on the other hand usually deal with not only individuals that have a diagnosable illness, but also with those who have no recognized psychiatric illness but want help in interpersonal problems and concerns of everyday living that cause them distress and unhappiness. We feel that meaningful and reasonably objective exploration of prevention and mental illness require that the discussion be confined to diagnosable mental illness, including the neuroses of personality disorders.

Some mental health specialists seek to further expand the definition, believing that mental health services should be concerned with resolving basic social problems and improving the quality of life for everyone. Indeed, many advocates of community mental health feel its scope is and should remain without boundaries. However, the cause and effect relationship between most social conditions and mental illness is extremely questionable. It may well stretch both the definition of mental health and the public health concept of prevention beyond their useful limits to relate them to social problems. The concepts, techniques, and expertise necessary for effective resolution of social problems are in no way related to those used by clinicians. The resolution of social problems also requires a mandate to intervene, a mandate that mental health professionals have not been given.

Not that it is a simple matter to differentiate between mental illness, such as the adjustment disorders, emotional distress, and human suffering. While we are not defending the DSM-III with which there have been many problems, I would point out that I expect DSM-IV is about to come out soon. But nevertheless, I think that Dr. Albee misreads the DSM-III in many respects. For instance, using DSM-III, learning disorders are considered mental disorders, but the diagnosis can only be made when the learning environment is adequate. Also, there are many other problems in trying to distinguish mental disorder from many other disorders: incompetence, emotional disorder, stress, etc. For instance, we are aware what is day and what is night, but what about twilight? That often poses a problem. So, definition is not as easy a problem as it might appear.

Can investigators actually demonstrate that primary prevention is effective? There seems to be general agreement that research has only begun to reveal something about the causes of mental illness. Without knowledge of cause, primary prevention can only be shots in the dark. Of course, shots in the dark may occasionally hit the mark; but with the pressing demands, with scarce mental health dollars, how can we justify spending many millions on such long shots? Recent research has increasingly suggested the operation of genetic and biochemical factors in the causation of mental illness. And regardless of the criticism of these studies, we feel that the evidence is overwhelming.

The adoption studies of Kety and associates indicate that schizophrenia is in large part genetically determined. There is good evidence that the same is true for the major affective disorders and alcoholism. The effect of the genetic traits can be reduced, of course, through measures such as counseling and birth control, but that is not what most proponents of primary prevention seem to have in mind. It is also possible that the expression of genetic traits, the actual occurrence of the full-blown illness, may be related to environmental conditions. It is not yet clear what those environmental conditions are, nor is it clear that measures to prevent the expression of a genetic trait, for example a predisposition to schizophrenia, should be labeled primary prevention and directed at entire populations, rather than take the form of secondary prevention and be directed only toward mentally ill individuals who are either overtly ill or in remission.

I would like to say just a word or two about mental health promotion. Primary prevention has been subdivided into two categories, activities that promote health generally, and thereby increase resistance to disease, and activities that are aimed against the occurrence of specific illnesses. Promotion of general physical health is an easily understandable concept that seems valid in practice. Yet, in the area of mental health, most if not all, successful primary prevention activities have been aimed at specific diseases. In contrast to physical health there is no evidence that so called general mental health may be promoted or strengthened, and thus that resistance to mental illness can be increased by preventive activities. Despite massive efforts to combat poverty, to increase social welfare and social security benefits, and to change the educational systems and methods of childrearing, there is no indication that the incidence of any of the functional, and by that I mean nonorganic mental illnesses, has decreased. Nor is there evidence that other countries with stronger social welfare and different childrearing practices have different rates of mental illness. Thus, as far as we can see, the major functional mental illnesses, as well as the frequently occurring diagnosable minor illnesses, remain untouched by efforts to strengthen mental health. Nevertheless, mental health promotion has become one of the catch-phrases of the day.

Many programs that have been called preventive are geared towards the development of competence in individuals. Developing competence, interpersonally, vocationally, educationally, is a worthy goal in and of itself. There is no evidence, however, that such competence building prevents mental disorder. For instance, many mentally ill and emotionally disturbed persons are educationally incompetent, an observation that has led many researchers to believe that a cause and effect relationship exists (i.e., educational incompetence causes emotional disturbance). Reports have shown that various programs improve children's school achievement and social problem solving. Presumably this would in turn enhance self-esteem, although evidence is lacking, especially in the long term. However if it could be shown that confidence building prevents unpleasant stress-inducing problems, such as school failure and low self-esteem, there is still a need to distinguish such problems from mental illness.

There are primary prevention techniques in psychiatry that have been shown to be extremely effective. Psychiatric complications of syphilis and vitamin deficiency are seldom seen today in developed nations. Decreased rates of birth injury and improved prenatal care have lowered the incidence of major psychiatric problems that result from congenital brain damage. Elimination of lead from house paint has reduced the number of children suffering from organic brain syndrome. And control of industrial toxins have virtually eliminated madhatters and other such problems.

There are newer preventive programs that should also reduce problems and incidence of certain illnesses. For instance, counseling prospective mothers not to delay pregnancy until the latter childbearing years is likely to reduce the incidence of mongolism. Other programs show promise but await solid research findings demonstrating their effectiveness. Thus interventions directed toward abusing parents, such as Parents Anonymous, seem likely to prove effective in breaking the cycle of child abuse, which has been shown to be socially transmitted from generation to generation. Bolby, Provence, and Lipton have demonstrated the deleterious effects of raising infants in impersonal institutions or without a consistent mother figure over a long period of time. Programs to replace institutions for homeless children with long-term, high quality foster care or adoption should help to prevent personality disturbance.

In conclusion we have not yet developed techniques necessary to make true primary prevention a reality except in a few limited areas. When allocating funds for preventive activities therefore, we need to distinguish carefully among those programs that are proved, those that are not yet proved but seem well on the way to attaining this status, and those that are at best experimental. We must distinguish between programs aimed at preventing diagnosable mental illness, and those programs aimed at unhappiness or social incompetence where we can be certain of our objectives and make informed, intelligent judgments about our priorities. We must distinguish between programs for the primary prevention of mental illness and programs designed to alleviate broad, social, ethical problems which we believe are beyond the scope of mental health professionals per se.

One might well ask, why is there any need to be concerned with the definition of primary prevention and with the question of effectiveness of worthy social programs in preventing mental illness. If everyone agrees that a program to eliminate poverty, for example, can only lead to an improvement in the quality of life and is a good thing in and of itself, why raise these questions at all? Well why indeed? Mental health professionals are now operating in a world of shrinking resources. There is not enough money to support even basic mental health direct service programs that are fundamental and essential. Funding expensive programs that are unlikely to prevent mental illness with money allocated to mental health services seems to us a dangerously foolish gamble. Such programs should be supported from funds other than those allocated to mental health services.

Because of primary prevention's appeal, mental health professionals may use it as a glamorous rationalization for avoiding treatment of difficult patients such as the chronically psychotic, the alcoholic, and the addicted. This phenomenon has helped tarnish the image of community mental health in the eyes of many legislators, administrators, clinicians, and the general public. Sound, well conceived research and prevention based on controlled studies is sorely needed. But this research ought to be funded separately from direct treatment programs. The prevention of mental illness is a vitally important goal and we fully support generous funding of research to reach it. We do advocate, however, that applied programs, except on a pilot basis, await the outcome of further research.

Finally, there is as yet no easy solution, such as primary prevention, to solve the problems faced by professionals who serve the mentally ill. Our difficult patients will not magically go away. We will have to struggle with the discouraging and overwhelming obstacles to overcoming mental illness and resist the temptation of uncritically and perhaps emotionally embracing simple solutions offered to us.

Reaction

Stephen Goldston

Virtually every morning for the past seventeen years someone greets me either in the parking lot, an elevator or a hallway at the Parklawn Building in Rockville with the comment, "What are you going to prevent today, Goldston?" At the close of the day the question would be, "What have you prevented today?" Beyond the attempts at humor, such questions reflected the low status of and limited concern about prevention in the bureaucracy. Those disparaging questions characterized discussions of prevention within the bureaucracy until about six years ago. Fortunately, times have changed and prevention is taken seriously within the bureaucracy, as is in evidence with both prevention budgets and organizational units for prevention at NIMH.

I serve as guardian of some of your public monies and one of my tasks is to ensure that those public monies are not being used frivolously. Regretfully, the total sum of this allotment is small, but I predict that over time there will be considerably more public money allocated for prevention.

My ten minutes of comments will address the bureaucratic concerns relevant to this debate as viewed from the Federal perspective, which is a very different vantage point when compared to that of states, localities, and academic centers. At the outset, let me assure you, if preventive interventions were not valid mental health activities, Federal dollars would not be invested in this area.

I believe it is essential to differentiate clearly between prevention activities and mandates at the Federal level and those activities conducted in the name of prevention that may go on at the local operating level. I neither assume responsibility nor do I defend some of the so-called prevention efforts performed at the local level. Some local prevention activities may sometimes appear bizarre, or wild, making all kinds of claims for prevention, but this is not prevention at the Federal level. At the Federal level, our primary responsibilities are for the support of research and research utilization, or what is bureaucratically called "knowledge transfer." At the local level the primary responsibility is the provision of services, based on the research knowledge available.

In the last six years or so a very broad constituency of national mental health organizations, all part of the mental health establishment, has become involved in prevention through task forces, standing or ad hoc committees and the like. Every mental health organization is involved in prevention. Prevention is a national health and mental health priority. Prevention has been institutionalized at NIMH with the establishment of the Office of Prevention in 1979 and the Prevention Research Branch, which was formed in 1982. There is a law originally called Section 325 of the Mental Health Systems Act, which is now Section 455 of the Public Health Service Act, that says that the director of the NIMH shall establish an administrative unit for prevention at NIMH, and that administrative unit shall be charged with establishing national goals and priorities for the prevention of mental illness and the promotion of mental health. That law provides both a legislative mandate and a social mandate for prevention.

Presently, we are in the process of carrying out that mandate and formulating national goals and priorities for prevention and promotion. None of the advances which I've just cited would have occurred if we were selling snake oil. These advances have occurred because there are guidelines that have governed all our program developments: (1) We only advocate prevention activities based on solid research; (2) We make no wild promises or exaggerated claims for prevention; (3) We advocate preventive interventions to reduce the incidence of psychopathology and psychological dysfunction, including reducing the incidence of diagnosable mental illness; (4) We don't focus on activities that skeptics would label "happiness, quality of life" or other such vague entities. Promotion activities lag behind prevention, awaiting their time on center stage at the Federal level; the accelerated activity over the past three years has been solely in the area of prevention.

Many myths have been associated with prevention. A recurring charge, without any substance, which I have seen in print over the last dozen years, is that significant sums of Federal dollars were being used for prevention, specifically primary prevention. How odd, when one considers that there was no prevention budget at NIMH until fiscal year 1980 (which began in October 1979). Not one Federal dollar was specifically mandated and designated for prevention until October 1979, and yet the argument has existed for over a decade that monies earmarked for care of the chronically mental ill were being diverted into primary prevention.

Another myth is that mental health workers have been hopping on the prevention band-wagon, thereby abandoning the care, treatment and rehabilitation of the mentally ill. Absurd!

Then there is the myth that there is no knowledge base for preventive interventions. Twenty years ago the American Public Health Association published a document called *Mental Disorders—A guide to control methods,* which identified primary preventive interventions to reduce the incidence of mental disorders. Early last year, *The American Journal of Community Psychology,* in a special issue, reported on nine primary prevention studies with outcomes that included a reduction in the incidence of diagnosable mental disorders.

Now, a few words about NIMH prevention activities. One research grant program is focused on the impact of marital disruption on children. A second research grant program is concerned with the effects on children of having a severely disturbed, psychiatrically ill parent. A third research grant program deals with preventive interventions in infant psychiatry. A program notice was issued in May 1982 inviting applications for preventive intervention research centers, a new base for advancing prevention research. Last December a program notice was issued on investigator-initiated early preventive intervention research. We are supplementing the NIMH Epidemiological Catchment Area program to utilize the basic incidence and prevalence data on diagnosable mental disorders which are being collected, and to design preventive interventions so we will be able to demonstrate in those five communities around the country that these interventions are preventive.

There are two additional contract studies I want to mention. One study is being conducted by the Institute of Medicine and is looking at the health consequences of the stress of bereavement, identifying the research base and proposing intervention research directed at bereaved people in order to prevent deleterious outcomes, including pathological grief reactions. The second study deals with the mental health aspects of pediatric settings, including concerns about children hospitalized for medical and surgical conditions, post-hospital trauma and the involvement of parents in the care of their children.

We've conducted a number of research planning workshops in order to assess the state of research knowledge in a specific area. We do not invest money in grants until the scientists say an area is ready for preventive interventions. During the past year we have consulted with groups of scientists in research planning workshops on the following subject areas:

- use of the media to prevent and reduce stress and anxiety;
- preventive interventions to reduce the harmful consequences of severe and persistent loneliness;
- psychiatric epidemiology and primary prevention;

- preventive intervention programs for family units with a mentally ill relative;
- research issues in preventive psychiatry;
- research on preventive child psychiatry and chronic childhood illness;
- prevention research on the assessment of disabling anger;
- preventive aspects of suicide and affective disorders among adolescents and young adults.

Before tonight I'd never been in a debate. Rather, during the past twenty years I've been active in what I characterize as a struggle. Present company excluded, I have witnessed many professional mental health workers who remain uninformed about prevention but still continue to comment negatively about prevention and it's advocates. I believe that we are in a new era, where resources are being provided to conduct good scientific research on prevention. I think Dr. Lamb will feel quite differently three or five years from now when the journals that he reads and edits and those that the rest of us read and edit will report credible evidence, additional evidence I might add, about primary preventive interventions to reduce the incidence of diagnosable mental disorder and psychological dysfunction.

Reaction

Jack Zusman

I'm very impressed with the arguments of our opponents, but a little concerned. What concerns me is that I know Steve very well and George less well, but I know his writings very well and I respect them both as reasonable people. Yet I do believe that some of the things they've said tonight are clearly unreasonable. I can't really accept that they believe some of the things they have said. I don't have enough time to deal with every one of the issues but I'll cover a few.

For example, Steve referred to the pamphlet published by the American Public Health Association (APHA) on control of mental disorders. He did not have time to read to you from that pamphlet but if he had, you would have found that many of the mental disorders discussed there are the ones Dick Lamb mentioned as already being under control. We know how to control vitamin deficiencies and lead poisoning. There is no argument about them. The problems that we're concerned with now are the tough ones like schizophrenia, and manic depressive psychosis. The APHA pamphlet doesn't tell you how to prevent them nor does any other scientific publication except perhaps a handbook on genetic counseling.

Another example of unreasonable argument is the way George and Steve use terms very loosely. They slip terms by us so quickly that, for example, we tend to forget the major differences between "stress" and "mental illness."

Stress has many meanings. In one meaning, it is something we all experience in the normal course of life. Whether you define stress as the difficult unpleasant events which befall all of us or as the physiological and emotional changes which such events produce in us, the implications are the same. Stress is unavoidable, and, in moderate amounts, probably essential for growth into maturity. In large amounts, stress is certainly temporarily disruptive and if possible, to be avoided.

But stress is not mental illness and the connection between stress and mental illness is at best uncertain. Quite possibly there is no relation except in those people who already have such a strong tendency toward mental illness that almost anything will push them over.

When we prevent stress, as most primary prevention programs aim to do, we are not preventing mental illness. That is what George and Steve try to slip past you.

I like to think of the results of *stress* as *distress*. Distress is primarily a feeling—an unpleasant one. Distress and mental illness sometimes superficially appear to be the same. A bereaved person shows many of the same reactions as the pathologically depressed person. But there is a major difference between them—one has an illness, the other is exhibiting a normal response to an unpleasant situation. Indeed, the bereaved persons who did not cry, lose sleep and suffer from energy loss could be considered pathological.

Distress prevention is a worthy end—who would not want to live in the land of milk and honey—but is it a proper objective for the mental health service system? After all, are we prepared to make every resident of the U.S. a client or patient of ours? Who will pay for that? Who will take care of the real mentally ill?

Furthermore, we know that a distressed person, if left alone for awhile in a setting where stress has ceased, is going to feel better. In a few days or weeks, the person will usually be back to normal.

Many unemployed people are feeling distress right now. That shows—to use a technical term—good reality testing. If you are unemployed, you should get upset. You should be sleepless, you should be worried. You do need help. But that does not mean you're mentally ill. That does not mean you need a psychologist or a psychiatrist or you need medication. If you are feeling sad about not being able to feed your family, that does not mean you need antidepressant medication.

George and Steve also talk about psychopathology as if that is the same as mental illness. I'm not sure in what way they mean the term when they use it, but it sounds to me, particularly when George uses it, that he's talking about symptoms. I've just illustrated that sometimes symptoms are perfectly normal, if we use the term symptoms broadly. Someone who is sleepless, who is crying, who is sad, may have reason to be that way. These reactions can be perfectly normal and not something that we want to treat.

When George talks about the studies on schizophrenic spit, his general point is absolutely right. There have been many claims of discovery of the biochemical basis of schizophrenia, usually in blood, urine or spinal fluid. Typically, two months or six months later someone repeats the study and either discovers that the substance is there because patients in mental hospitals drink a lot of coffee and it is a metabolite of coffee; or the substance can not be found at all. The fact that the biochemical basis of schizophrenia hasn't been found doesn't mean that schizophrenia doesn't exist or even that the biochemical basis doesn't exist.

On the other hand, consider the genetic studies of schizophrenia which have been done in Scandinavia. The best are studies where twins have been separated at birth or shortly after birth and raised in different families. Those studies show very clearly that if there is a schizophrenic genetic background, regardless of how different and how positive the two twins' separate families are, both have a high probability of being schizophrenic. If they are identical twins, the probability is much higher than if they are fraternal twins. There are many other genetic studies which are very clear about the influence of inheritance of susceptibility to mental illness. I don't know of any reputable scientist who now doubts that there is some inheritable tendency for most of the major mental disorders, such as schizophrenia or manic depressive psychosis. Since such is the case, what can we do to prevent mental illness. Obviously genetic counseling is one action. Yet prevention proponents ignore that and concentrate on programs whose value is, at best, uncertain.

Another thing that George and Steve have done is to accuse us of all of the sins of psychiatry and ask you to assume that because psychiatry has committed some errors this strengthens the case for primary prevention.

Psychiatry, like most other scientific fields, has had many problems and made many errors over the years of its existence. The DSM III, the American Psychiatric Association Diagnostic and Statistical Manual, is indeed prepared by a committee as a result of compromise. As soon as DSM III came out it was recognized that there were problems in it. Furthermore, DSM III is not scientific law, it is not the bible of psychiatrists; it is a naming and classification system they use for the sake of convenience and by convention. The weaknesses in DSM III do not undercut the scientific underpinning of psychiatry. The fact that there are weaknesses in DSM III doesn't relieve all of us, including prevention proponents, of the obligation to do careful studies of the various projects which we want to undertake.

Now the final thing which George and Steve have done, is something of which George has accused psychiatrists in a number of his articles. That is to concentrate on the "sexy" problems rather than on the difficult ones. The "sexy" problems these days, the ones which make the headlines, earn the private practice dollars and are fun to work on, are such problems as not feeling "at one with yourself," not being able to communicate freely with those around you, not being able to control your kids and so forth. These are the problems which people want to talk about and if you are a therapist you can make a lot of money while doing that. What we on this side of the table are saying is let's act like professionals. Let's deal with the difficult problems before the "fun" ones. Our targets should be the people who have schizophrenia, the people who have manic depressive psychosis, the people who are wandering around downtown homeless in the rain because they have an illness that can't be prevented and can't even be treated very well.

Instead, mental health professionals, people who are trained often at society's expense to work with the seriously mentally ill, are out making money leading encounter groups and lecturing on how to bring up kids. They are charging high prices for dealing with problems that don't need professional help at all. Instead of encouraging distressed people to use a little bit of common sense and the advice that most grandmothers will provide at no cost, many primary prevention proponents have complicated and professionalized the most fundamental aspects of human interaction. In a manner analogous to taking your computer with you when you go grocery shopping instead of a handwritten list on a scrap of paper, they ask us to divert talent and money to activities which are simple and natural for most of us if we just go ahead and do them. At the same time they ask us to forget our responsibility to the mentally ill whose problems remain complex and unsolved.

Response to
Drs. Lamb and Zusman

George W. Albee

Jack, I *don't* believe that you believe that we don't believe what we say! I would really love to spend my allotted five minutes talking about schizophrenia because, as I told Jack this afternoon when we taped the TV interview, I spent ten years of my life doing research on schizophrenia. I am now convinced that there is no such thing as schizophrenia! I have been reading avidly reports of the cross-cultural study in which psychiatrists in England were compared with psychiatrists in the United States in terms of their diagnostic habits. It's interesting that in the United States there has been an enormous increase in the diagnosis of schizophrenia over the past forty years while in England it has leveled off and declined. When you show taped interviews of the same disturbed people to British psychiatrists and American psychiatrists, the British psychiatrists tend to call these people depressives, manics, personality disorders, borderlines, etc., while the American psychiatrists routinely call them schizophrenics. In preparing for this debate I summarized evidence of the unreliability of the diagnosis of schizophrenia, prepared by people who believe in schizophrenia!

The following quotes are from an article appearing in the *Schizophrenic Bulletin* published by NIMH! Among other things, experts say, "Given that hospital statistics reported in one region have a higher rate of schizophrenia than statistics reported in another region and across cultures this observation no longer justifies pursuing the hypothesis that there really are consistent diagnostic patterns and consistent rates of schizophrenia." And another quote, "The criteria applied to patient populations may even vary among wards of the same hospital and between different time periods within the same ward."

I went back and looked at the Kallmann studies. I read the Sarbin and Mancuso book that shows up the weaknesses of the genetic research in schizophrenia. And I am really sorry that Leon Kamin isn't here. He is coming to Vermont to talk on March 17 (Ed.: 1983), and if you have the time I hope you'll all come up and listen to him, because

From George W. Albee, "Response to Drs. Lamb and Zusman," *Journal of Primary Prevention*, Vol. 5, pp. 233-235. Copyright © 1985 by Human Sciences Press. Reprinted by permission.

he is going to be one careful scientist, Jack, who looks with great care at the inadequacy of the research data on the genetics of schizophrenia. In my heart of hearts, I believe that in the twin studies the data on the inheritance of schizophrenia are at least as fallacious as the data that Sir Cyril Burt invented on the genetics of the intelligence of identical twins reared apart which, as you know, we no longer accept, no longer believe. A final point: the bottom line of this entire argument is that the genetic studies of schizophrenia can only be as valid as the reliability of the diagnosis of schizophrenia. If the diagnosis is unreliable, then the genetic studies cannot be reliable. If the criterion is unreliable, the correlations can't be reliable. In short, we know nothing about the genetics of schizophrenia.

When you really listen to what all the enemies of prevention have to say, the argument (and maybe we can come back next year and debate this), is that there is a difference between *real* mental illness and disturbed interpersonal relationships. I teach my classes that *all* mental illnesses are difficulties in interpersonal and intrapersonal relationships. That is, people don't get psychotic about tables and chairs and horses; rather they get psychotic about their human relationships, or neurotic about their relationships with other *people*. This is a learned phenomenon, I think. There is a vast literature that suggests that these conditions are learned, not caused by defective genes or bad biochemistry. Now, Harry Haslow's infant monkey raised on "wire mothers" did develop biochemical abnormalities as adults. But we know that this was a consequence of the unfortunate infant experiences that they had. Surely, people trained in psychiatry and in psychoanalysis ought to be ready to accept a hundred years of clinical experience that says that what happens to infants and young children has important consequences for their adult behavior. Are we to believe that these eminent psychiatrists, with training in psychoanalysis, don't accept the Freudian, the psychoanalytic position that devastating experiences in early childhood, traumatic experiences in early childhood, won't have consequences in adulthood, that such experiences just make people nervous or anxious and *not* mentally disordered? In a very famous essay Jerome Bruner talked about the impact of Freud, about Freud's basic message. He compared Freud with Darwin, two of the greatest minds that have ever contributed to our understanding of nature. Darwin said that there is a *con-*

tinuity between lower animals and higher forms that make man (he used the word "man"), human beings, *not* creations a little lower than the angels, but actually a form evolved out of lower forms, and that was Darwin's message, accept it or not. Freud's message was also a message of *continuity*. What Freud said is that there is not a difference in kind, but only in degree, between the mind of the sane person and the mind of the insane person. And if you read and understand Freud, he is saying it is a continuous process. Sometimes we are all a little crazy, sometimes crazy people are quite normal, the *continuity* is the important consideration, so I would argue that there really isn't a distinction between mental illness and emotional distress, that we are really talking about a continuous process.

Response to
Drs. Albee and Goldston

H. Richard Lamb

Well, first of all, I hope I can get all my dos and don'ts right. I do believe that Dr. Zusman does believe that our opponents do not believe everything that they are saying. Also, I just can't resist saying to Steve that if they really are as confident about their proposed research in prevention as they say they are, I'd like to ask him why they haven't asked two, as he says, reasonable and, I assume, objective people like Jack and myself who are knowledgeable in this area, to sit on the study committee that determines who gets these grants. I would also just like to say that we think Dr. Albee sets up a straw man by calling us antipreventionists, I don't think we are. I think we wish that we could prevent mental illness, but simply wishing does not make it so. Now, I also think it's important in terms of how one looks at these things. Dr. Albee was talking about the genetic evidence for and against schizophrenia and I would just like to point out that with my strong psychoanalytic background, I have become convinced by the various adoption studies that have filled the literature in the last ten or fifteen years. I would hope that our opponents would read these studies very carefully and change their minds as I did.

I also think that probably nowhere in the mental health field is clarity of thinking more important than in the conceptualization of primary prevention. That is why clarity regarding some of the things that we have been talking about, such as the differences between mental illness, diagnosable mental illness and emotional distress, are really crucial. We feel that meaningful and reasonably objective exploration of primary prevention requires that the discussion be confined to diagnosable mental illness to the extent that that can be done. Now with the exception of such mental disorders as syphilis, vitamin deficiency, child abuse and the others that I have mentioned earlier, where is the evidence that we can prevent mental illness? I do not really think that when we talk about diagnosable mental illness that the evidence is there. When we have so many unmet needs for the treatment of the mentally ill, how can we justify spending millions of mental health dollars on programs whose effectiveness has not been

From H. Richard Lamb, "Response to Drs. Albee and Goldston," *Journal of Primary Prevention*, Vol. 5, pp. 236-237. Copyright © 1985 by Human Sciences Press. Reprinted by permission.

proven. And even if it can be shown that social factors are causative factors, we do not see mental health professionals as being effective in changing broad social factors. They certainly should make recommendations, but I certainly don't think of ourselves as the change agents. And if we try to be something that we are not trained to be, in the meantime, who will treat and rehabilitate the mentally ill? And that is the question with which I'd like to leave you.

VII. Last Words

We end our volume on social change and political action with two essays, one by someone who has spent her life attempting to combine individual social work practice with effective efforts at social change (Konopka). The other is a recent essay (Albee) that attempts to summarize the relationship between efforts at prevention and the need to build a more just and equitable society.

Social Change, Social Action as Prevention

Gisela Konopka

The subject, when I heard about it a year ago, made me jump. Here it was, the opportunity to talk about the effort of a lifetime: the combination of concern and work for the well-being of each individual that helps create societies which make possible full development of capacities, which enhance the beauty of interdependence, which help develop whatever it is we call "mental health." I thought it would be easy to express and share with you a lifetime as an old fighter for what I call "Social Justice with a Heart."

But when I sat down to write this paper it became a nightmare—more questions than answers sprang up—a cacophony of voices (was my mental health threatened?). Listen.

A letter from a friend in Germany:

The interrelatedness of social work and politics becomes very clear theoretically, without having an answer for the practical consequences. The more we strive for the betterment of social conditions in our own countries the less we have for the real needy in this world, or is the first the precondition for the latter? Who is your neighbor—in this last part of the twentieth century? (Schiller, 1979)

—A colleague coming from China: "I don't care about 'freedom of choice.' At least people have enough to eat." And another: "Did we ever realize the terror of the group? Nobody in China can be him- or herself. One *must* conform."

—A friend: "Rights of youth, you say? Okay, but what about my daughter spitting at me. What about *me*?"

—"The psychiatrist thought my depression is related to my not caring about clothes. What has that got to do with it?"

—"Poverty makes for unhappiness? I worked my head off to get out of it. My kids who have money now spend theirs on the 'shrinks.'"

—"We spent a lifetime to develop juvenile courts to get young people

From Gisela Konopka, "Social Change, Social Action as Prevention: The Role of the Professional," in Justin M. Joffe and George W. Albee (eds.) *Prevention Through Political Action and Social Change.* Copyright © 1981 by the Vermont Conference on the Primary Prevention of Psychopathology. Reprinted by permission.

out of the clutches of the adult court system. Now the 'rights movement' brings them back in."

—"You fought so hard for right for education for everybody. Now we kids are forced to stay in school when we want to get out and work. We are bored."

I have to shut out the voices. Do they just mock or do they say something that makes sense? They do!

I think those partially depressing, confusing voices convey some basic insights we must be aware of:

(1) Mental health concepts are related to value judgments and we must admit this and make them explicit. Maxwell Anderson (1947) said it better than I can say it:

> If you live you have to be going somewhere. You have to choose a direction. And science is completely impartial. It doesn't give a damn which way you go. It can invent the atom bomb but it can't tell you whether to use it or not. Science is like—well, it's like a flashlight in a totally dark room measuring two billion light-years across . . . the flash can show you where your feet are on the floor; it can show you the furniture or the people close by; but as for which direction you should take in that endless room it can tell you nothing. (p. 91)

(2) The public health model does not work too well with mental health because cause and effect are a myth. Yet there are factors that show a relationship between certain environmental (human and otherwise) influences and a person's reaction to them. And we must be aware of the infinite variety among people.

(3) In time—historically—a cultural environment changes, and that may change needs and demand new systems. Child labor laws and juvenile courts are recent examples of this.

(4) Perhaps the most important quality of the professional who genuinely wants to be of help to mankind is an inquiring, flexible mind combined with an almost searing honesty and courage to stand up against comfortable dogmas within and fashionable ones without.

With those premises in mind I will trace some of my own attempts at bringing about cultural change, share the underlying philosophy, and draw the lessons the professional may learn from them.

Let me take you back approximately 55 years. I quote from an article about a delinquency institution, called the *Lindenhof*, in the Germany of the 1920s, before the Holocaust:

> The Lindenhof was a beginning for the realization of human brotherhood, was a seedling toward a community of human beings, was a cell of a reborn human organism. . . . There was a strong belief that something different was possible,

that one could move into a new direction in delinquency treatment which is no more punishment or retribution, a poor substitution for school or a poor substitution for the parents or anything like that, but that it could be: a true school for life; an education that provides an opportunity for development of human potential.

Most significant to us, to my collaborators and myself, was the human being. The mutual relationship of man to man is one of the incredible miracles in the cosmos. (Konopka, 1971, p. 245)

A gaunt young man wrote this as he sat at his desk looking out of his open office door at a corridor freshly painted in bright colors. Sunshine flooded the end of the hallway. There were odd little stubs of iron at the bottom of the window sill, like decorations made by a modern artist. The young man smiled. He knew what those iron remnants were. Not so long ago there had been bars at all the windows. He, his staff, and the delinquents in his charge had sawed them off after several discussions of what it meant to be responsible for one's own limits (Konopka, 1971).

At the time when this happened, I belonged to a youth movement that fought the reactionary forces. Our philosophy clearly demanded a recognition of human dignity. There was never a question in our minds that direct work with individuals (we were influenced by Freud and Adler) and political action were both needed to make this a better world. I never understood the "either-or" positions. Years later, when I studied social work philosophy I again encountered the recurring question, "Is social work a palliative only or is it responsible also for changing institutions?" I found the same answer as in my adolescence and that answer covers all professions, not only social work:

The answer must be that social work is responsible for attempting both: to help individuals in the framework of existing conditions as well as to help change social institutions. When we recognize the multiple causation of problems and realize that the causes lie neither exclusively in the individual nor in the social structure, it becomes clear that a profession which works toward social justice in a wide sense must feel responsible for amelioration and social change. (Konopka, 1958, pp. 194–195)

How did we put this demand for concern for individuals as well as systems into action? Let me answer with examples.

In those times, youth groups consciously included individuals who were on probation or parole. We, 16–17 years old, would get a phone call and—as friends, not "helpers"—would visit the boy or girl, take him or her to our meetings or on adventurous hikes we all loved. They became part of our community.

Or, when brooding summer heat invaded the small stinking courtyards of the Berlin slums, where one overflowing toilet served a block with approximately 200 people, we would go—alone—into such a yard (our parents would have been horrified had they known about this) and start playing with children who sat listlessly and dejected on the stoops. I will never forget the thin arms around me, the white bloodless faces, occasionally rat-bitten or ravaged by illnesses I hardly understood. It was "individual" help to those children, but what it did for us! How we learned about other, painful worlds and how we learned to overcome horror and how it gave us a sense of self and a place in the universe, which is so hard to find as an adolescent. So, consciously, I decided to become a teacher to children who had no advantages.

Directly parallel to those individual approaches went conscious socio-political action. I worked for awhile as a steelworker in a factory, where I saw the plight of women who got up at 4 A.M. to bring their children to daycare centers, worked long hours of hard labor—at lower pay than men—picked up their children and started home for a day's work there. So, I joined labor unions, helped organize women, became part of the social reform movement. Again, individual effort and socio-political group action were not perceived as contrasts.

Then—the advent of the Nazis. We had fought them in debates, in writing literature, but still they came to power. Besides the terror, the killing, the torture, you should know that all the social reforms of human services were destroyed. Women were reduced again to an inferior position. (I heard a Nazi boast that he would have thrown out his wife had she borne a girl!) Homes for children or delinquency institutions returned to authoritarian practices. When I revisited such places after the war under the auspices of the American High Commissioner, I saw only the raw and demeaning treatment that is based on the widespread theory that "badness is inborn, is hereditary" and as a result authorities had to "train" them, beat them into obedience. All this after the efforts of Karl Wilker and August Aichhorn and many others. Nothing was left of mental health concepts.

We learned—the hard way.

Lesson No. 1: Social change cannot be taken for granted.

One has to remember that things have to be done over and over again. The task is never finished. The words on the Supreme Court Building in Washington, "Eternal vigilance is the price of liberty," surely apply to any effort human beings make.

In the years of Nazi terror, I, as most of us, became very conscious of the fact that one cannot do any significant and positive personal service when the total system does not allow for human dignity. Therefore, political action became far more important than anything else. There were underground movements in Germany that tried to fight an inhuman system damaging to young and old. Those who participated could not expect glory, recognition, or even much mutual support. What one could expect was not just death, but painful torture, ridicule, and abandonment.

It is out of such experiences that I totally reject the theory and practice of behavior modification. Not only is the idea of the "all-knowing" treatment person repulsive to me, but I wonder what kind of people we are educating who expect that life will justly distribute punishment and awards. No award could be expected by anybody who got actively involved in political action to destroy the Nazis. I have never forgotten the feeling I had several times when I was in solitary in a cell in the concentration camp. I was sure that I never would leave that place alive. What especially bothered me—and I was young and healthy and ambitious—was that nobody ever would know what wonderful thoughts I had, how much I wanted to love people, how much I had to say. I was very aware of the fact that dying for a cause was not glamorous, as it is so often portrayed in songs and stories and drama, but that it was just dying, just not existing anymore, and that it meant being forgotten. We have to remember that there are thousands who did not come out of this like me, alive, but did die after very courageously fighting the disastrous system. But nobody will ever talk about them, write about them, and thank them. I resented at that time, and still resent deeply today, those people—and they are very often professionals and intellectuals—who shout "social change" and exhort people into action, when they themselves sit in comfortable offices, draw good salaries, gain admiration for what they are doing, but do not face unemployment or persecution as do those whom they exhort to act.

Lesson No. 2: In regard to social action: Do not take the glory if you cannot take the pain.

If there is any danger in the way the political action develops, you have to take the risk of this danger. You must have more than the courage of your convictions, you must back it up with your own possessions, or yourself. If somebody really considers technical development dangerous to human mental health (and I do not) then this person cannot use all the advantages of technical development to spread his or her own ideas. They have to renounce cars and radio and television, and the (to me) extraordinary invention of the telephone, and must live that life they advocate. I say this earnestly because I do think that the greatest temptation for professionals lies in their beautiful gift to reason, to speak, to write, and they can easily fool themselves into believing that they are working for a cause when in reality they only serve themselves. I have struggled with this myself.

Now let me share with you examples of my work toward social change within the United States. The way I see it, the system of this country not only permits, but requires, people to participate in social action. Without it, the Constitution, which is based on an affirmation of the dignity of each individual, cannot be kept alive. This actually imposes a severe demand on every citizen, and especially on those whose professions have as a goal the safeguard of mental health. A professional in our fields—psychology, social work, psychiatry, nursing, education— cannot dispassionately "view" human beings the way scientists do. It is true that with any attempt to change an individual, the first step is a "viewing" or, as we sometimes call it, understanding. This, in itself, is difficult because the total living web of human life is many sided. One must observe, feel with the other person; one must use knowledge derived from other sciences, which describe, probe, and try to explain human behavior.

One must also learn to look at oneself, to learn about one's own biases that may distort or color the "view." The most important point, as I said earlier, is that every practitioner working with people cannot merely "understand"; he or she is always confronted with evaluations of the facts and with active intervention. One is constantly confronted with the dilemma between acceptance of a given situation, people, attitudes, and the demand for a change in them. Every professional effort is pervaded by this consideration. And this makes the whole work of change in an individual or in a society so difficult. Where does one get the right to do this? When we adhered to the medical model and called certain behavior or problems "sick," it made it easier for us. Sickness has to be eliminated. But we do not deal always with problems that we can call simply "sick." We deal with problems of human relationships. For instance, we deal with the problem of what race discrimination does to individuals, communities, and the whole of society. We deal with hostile adolescents who hit out, withdraw, or use drugs because of a variety of problems they face within the family, as, for instance, authoritarian parents, or a noncaring attitude, or perhaps because the school weighs heavily on them. Those are not problems located within that particular individual but derive from systems, or relationships. One does not deal with illness.

For instance, we deal with the deep-seated rejection of the offender by the large majority of the population. We must change public attitudes; otherwise no individual can be helped. I have just come back from Australia where I encountered a society deeply committed to family life. Yet this same society has for decades removed aboriginal children from their families, placed them in large, impersonal institutions, because the families did not follow the Anglo-Saxon pattern. In our country there still exist large institutions for girls, filled with young people whose only offense is premarital sex relations (permissible to boys for centuries but not to girls). All these are examples of our having to work toward change because of reasons beyond "understanding." As I said earlier, there is absolutely no question that we have used value judgments in doing this. The answers will lie more in philosophical, ethical considerations than in scientific inquiry. The effort requires three considerations:

1. A clear distinction between primary and secondary values.
2. An investigation into the sources of value judgment.
3. An acceptance of the interrelatedness of ends and means, of goals and methods.

To enlarge on these three aspects: Eduard C. Lindeman helped make a distinction between primary and secondary values (Konopka, 1958, Chap. 5). The two primary values are the dignity of each human being and the interdependence of individuals. The first one establishes the right of each human being to full development of his or her capacities, while the second makes a demand on each human being to act responsibly toward others in the framework of his or her own capacities. Those are values without which no profession can operate. They are "absolute" in the sense that they become the basic criteria for the practitioner's actions. We may disagree on the origin of those values: the religiously oriented person sees it in divine command, the humanist in ethical law. Both, however, agree on the content.

The recognition of this "absolute" justifies the effort to affect certain cultural changes, if the given culture violates basic human rights—by disparaging individuals because of their origin, race, or religion, for instance, or by an authoritarian, dictatorial way of life, which does not allow for freedom of expression or thought. The code of ethics developed in most "applied" professions is an expression of the binding force of primary values. Standards for professional practice in social work accepted in 1951 by the American Association of Social Workers (then the representative organization of the social work profession) read:

1. Firm faith in the dignity, worth and creative power of the individual.
2. Complete belief in his right to hold and express his own opinions and to act upon them, so long as by so doing he does not infringe upon the rights of others.
3. Unswerving conviction of the inherent, inalienable rights of each human being to choose and achieve his own destiny in the framework of a progressive, yet stable society. (Standards for the Professional Practice of Social Work, 1951)

And the Society of Applied Anthropology (interestingly enough in the same year, 1951) also published its Code of Ethics. It asked for respect for the individual and for human rights and the promotion of human and social well-being. It says: "To advance those forms of human relationships which contribute to the integrity of the individual human being; to respect both human personality and cultural values . . ." (Code of Ethics of the Society for Applied Anthropology, 1951, p. 32).

Both professional groups not only *justified* culture change by the realization of those primary values, they both made it a task of the profession to *promote* them.

But more debatable is practice when it influences secondary values. Those are values in *use*, sometimes related to the moral-ethical realm, often to customs, mode of living, or even aesthetics.

Here work toward change must be exercised with great caution or not at all. We must scrutinize carefully the sources of those values, in ourselves as well as in clients, groups, or community. Only such honest self-insight can help us to determine whether we "impose" our own values arbitrarily or whether they have true importance to the other person or group.

Secondary values are strongly influenced by four factors:

1. Cultural background
2. The precepts and demands of groups that are significant to us (religious organizations, social groups, task groups)
3. Strong personal experiences, such as illness or the death of friends or family
4. Adherence to certain theories regarding human behavior and motivation

Professionals must periodically look at themselves and determine whether their own secondary values enter their work in such a way as to impose their own value system on others. By no means should professionals strip themselves of these values (they would be empty creatures without them) but they must check themselves and examine whether these values are helpful and applicable to others. They have a right to present them or to even promote them, as long as they allow others to take them or leave them—except when primary values are violated.

This means a disciplined and honest insight into oneself.

A final consideration lies in the interrelatedness of means and end. Gandhi said it best: "The means may be likened to a seed, the end to a tree; and there is just the same inviolable connection between the means and the end as there is between the seed and the tree" (in Flesch, 1957, p. 167).

If the goal of our efforts is enhancement of human dignity and mutual responsibility, the means to this end must be in accord with it, otherwise the end is defeated.

Out of these philosophical considerations come *Lessons 3 and 4.*

Lesson 3: Think through your philosophy, and
Lesson 4: Be honest with the means you use even in the political arena.

I had to think a great deal of this during the harsh days of the 1960s when students revolted at universities and when the most neglected minorities, Blacks, Indians, and Chicanos, stood up for their rights. It bothered me that many professionals who had professed their concern for human beings suddenly cringed, became afraid, or yelled twice as loudly as those who had been hurt, perhaps because of their own fear. It seems to me that people in the mental health profession should have learned a great deal about the roots of hostile behavior, should have an understanding of it, and should have stayed calm, though compassionate, in the face of it.

At that time I became involved again in the public arena. I accepted the position of special advisor to the vice president for student affairs at our large state university, to deal with the political movements of the young and the disadvantaged minorities. I felt I had to stand up for mutual respect and not allow any group to think that they could drag down another one. Important new programs grew out of that period: special help for students who had little intellectual stimulation at home; special courses for first year students of all colors and backgrounds, conducted by faculty and community people together to let them learn about the beautiful variety of people existing in our country, and also to gain a sometimes painful look into their own prejudices; university policies were changed in regard to dormitory living, with the acceptance of students as responsible adults instead of the university acting as "parent."

In the wider community new legislation has worked through in regard to employment of minorities. It was exciting to become one of the first faculty members to serve on the newly created Center for Urban and Regional Affairs at the university, and to help make the intellectual resources of the university far more available to the community.

We helped to develop special curricula for women on welfare so that they could get degrees and better opportunities for employment. We worked with housing projects and sent students directly into them to help children with their school work. The university supplied specialists to teach in a Black summer school that had been started by the Black citizens of one of our neighborhoods. I still think with real fondness of the day when I myself went into one of those classes, saw some of the sullen, hostile faces looking at my own not so dark one, and then felt the changed attitude when together we realized the beauty of poetry written by both Blacks and Whites who had been hurt by others. The professional community had not been the one most effective in *starting* the move toward social change, yet it became helpful in implementing it. We had to realize that we were not the "leaders," but that we could contribute to a development most important to general mental health.

Times changed again. The beautiful enthusiasm of the 60s (I call it beautiful though I do not agree with everything that was happening at that time), began to fade and reaction set in. I find this especially in a field I know, in youth services, and particularly among those who deal with delinquents. A harshness and a hardening towards the young is occurring today. Beautiful phrases like "a person must learn to take on responsibility," with which I agree, are turning into "There is absolutely no reason for your bad behavior. You are responsible, and we will punish you for it." I do believe in responsibility, but I also know about the complexity of human motivation.

I find it is time again to swim against the stream. Just recently I talked with a young woman working in probation services, who said to me after one of my talks, "When I am trying to help these young people, I am being made fun of. All they want ("they" being the authorities) is to place them away from the community and preferably in solitary confinement. What can I do?" My only answer continues to be, "You will never be able to stop the good fight. Don't expect this in life. You have to continue standing up for what you do. Do your best with the young people you work with, go on committees, testify before legislatures armed with *knowledge* you gained by working with people, and do this all your life."

I am involved at this time in a nationwide project called the National Youthworker Education Project, started after I published my survey of the needs of adolescent girls (Konopka, 1976). Every month we bring together 20 people who work with youth and who are partially responsible for the policies of their organizations—and we purposely mix professionals from community youth organizations with those from corrections. For about a week we discuss needs, concerns, philosophy of working with young people. We do not brainwash, but we hope to make people think and strengthen their backs so that a basic mental health concern gets translated into practice. We meet the same group again three months later after participants have tried out some new or cooperative work in their communities. We help them to keep in touch with each other.

Almost everywhere adolescents have been neglected and maligned—or ridiculously romanticized. Adolescents still do not have a place in most societies, and those who have offended the mores of a society are frequently treated like concentration camp inmates. I think I have helped to start a nationwide network of people who work with adolescents become a force to help our next generation. This alone will not change everything, but it is a beginning. In the delinquency field there is legislation to remove "the status offender" from institutionalization. It would be all wrong if we now say "we have achieved." Only recently I visited an institution full of girls that I would call "status offenders" but they are placed there under another label. They live with regimentation and with the constant threat of "the hole," the demeaning solitary confinement that everybody seems to think is so necessary to keep "discipline." What can I do? I can only try to speak, to write, to develop more and more people who take mental health seriously. They should not think that their major goal in life is to develop some cheap, quick technique that will change people's behavior and make a lot of money for themselves.

This is really *Lesson No. 5. In any kind of work with individuals or with communities, "empty techniques" do not work.*

We cannot give neat, surefire recipes for work with people which promise "instant" success.

We can only help to develop professionals who deal with humans, who have patience and an inquiring mind, who are flexible, and who have real compassion for others. The professional has a task of developing and using knowledge in addition to feelings of empathy. Out of their vast practice, they can bring to the public the reality of the problems that are often buried under bureaucratic procedures or statistics. They can become advocates, but even beyond advocacy, they have to become coworkers with others in the community. Their knowledge, especially in social action, needs to be fused with the knowledge coming from others. The Messiah complex is just as dangerous as the idea that one has nothing to contribute. Too great assurance easily turns people into dictators. I remember when I was a teenager, a teacher read the following quote by Lessing to us:

If God should hold enclosed in his right hand all truth and in his left hand only the ever active inquiry after truth, although with the condition that I must always and forever err, I would with humility turn on to his left hand and say, "Father, give me this, pure truth is for Thee alone." (Lessing, 1890; *Oxford Dictionary of Quotations*, p. 313)

At the time I was angry with the writer because I would have chosen the hand that held the "whole truth." It took a long life to recognize the wisdom of Lessing, and to accept the fact that there is only the one absolute, namely the recognition of the dignity of every person, and that we always have to live with a kind of uncertainty whether we have translated it into reality best.

To me, the most important quality for anyone involved in the serious business of change, individually or in the community, is to keep integrity and courage, whether one is laughed at, hurt, seems out of step, or perhaps even dies unknown and unrewarded. I would like to quote Morris West:

It costs so much to be a full human being that there are very few who have the enlightenment or the courage, to pay the price. . . . One has to abandon altogether the search for security, and reach out to the risk of living with both arms. One has to embrace the world like a lover, and yet demand no easy return of love. One has to accept pain as a condition of existence. One has to court doubt and darkness as the cost of knowing. One needs a will stubborn in conflict, but apt always to the total acceptance of every consequence of living and dying. (1963, p. 196)

The professional who can approach this kind of demand will help toward social change and better mental health for everyone.

References

Anderson, M. *Joan of Lorraine*. Menasha, Wis.: George Banta Publishing Co., 1947.

Code of ethics of the Society for Applied Anthropology. *Human Organization*, 1951, *10*, 32.

Flesch, R. *The book of unusual quotations*. New York: Harper and Row, 1957.

Konopka, G. *Edward C. Lindeman and social work philosophy*. Minneapolis: University of Minnesota Press, 1958.

Konopka, G. Reform in delinquency institutions in revolutionary times: The 1920's in Germany. *The Social Service Review*, 1971, *45*, 245–258.

Konopka, G. *Young girls: A portrait of adolescence*. Englewood Cliffs, N.J.: Prentice-Hall, 1976.

Lessing, G. E. *Wolfenbüttler Fragmente*, 1890. Quoted in *Oxford Dictionary of Quotations*. New York: Oxford University Press, 1953, p. 313. (Original not seen).

Schiller, H. Letter to the author, December 1979.

Standards for the professional practice of social work. New York: American Association of Social Workers, 1951.

West, M. *The shoes of the fisherman*. New York: Dell Publishing Co., 1963.

Toward a Just Society: Lessons from Observations on the Primary Prevention of Psychopathology

George W. Albee

ABSTRACT: *Prevention efforts to reduce psychopathology use strategies similar to public health measures for disease prevention. However, an important distinction to be maintained is that many mental conditions are not discrete diseases; they are often learned patterns of socially deviant behavior or idiosyncratic thought that result from stress, powerlessness, and exploitation. Prevention efforts aimed at reducing psychopathology will often require social change and a redistribution of power. Efforts to change the power structure and to reduce social class inequalities are opposed by persons who accept (a) the belief that class differences are natural and even desirable from a social Darwinian perspective, and (b) the "Just World" belief that says that people deserve whatever happens to them. Prevention workers are more likely to accept the fatalistic view that people, only through their own political efforts, can improve the quality of life for most of humankind if they accept the fact that there is no "divine plan" and that evolution has no goal.*

The field of primary prevention of psychopathology owes enormous intellectual and ideological debts to the field of public health. Both fields make proactive efforts with groups, often high-risk groups, to reduce the incidence rates of undesirable conditions. Both fields are less visible than the more glamorous and more publicized fields of individual treatment. But there is one problem in trying to follow public health strategy too closely in prevention efforts in psychopathology: There is an important difference in the nature of the conditions to be prevented.

Public health has long been concerned with preventing specific diseases or pathological organic conditions, most of which can be defined and identified fairly precisely and objectively. The history of public health involves, to cite a few examples, efforts to prevent plague, rabies, and tuberculosis and, more recently, polio and smallpox, black lung, brown lung, asbestos damage, and lead and mercury poisoning. Today the field of public health is increasingly concerned with the contribution of life-styles to disease: For example, tobacco and alcohol use is associated with diseases like lung cancer and cirrhosis, and improper nutrition, excess stress, obesity, and lack of exercise are associated with coronary artery disease and stroke. Although the shift of attention to behavioral causes is a significant change in focus, one required by changes in the leading causes of death, it is important to remember that the goal for public health is still disease prevention. Efforts at isolating the causes of Legionnaires' Disease, acquired immune deficiency syndrome (AIDS), and genital herpes are all oriented toward the eventual prevention of these real diseases.

The critical difference in the field of psychopathological conditions is the high probability that many of the behavioral patterns to be prevented are *not* diseases in the usual sense. With a few obvious exceptions, most of the conditions defined as psychopathological are disorders of behavior for which no laboratory or other objective tests are available. The identification of a so-called mental illness is usually a judgment based on an interview or other behavioral observation. Despite a major reorientation of American and Canadian psychiatry in recent years away from a concern with psychodynamics and the childhood origins of adult distress and toward a biological approach, with growing emphasis on the search for genetic and biochemical causation and drug treatment, the bedrock fact remains—most mental conditions are not identifiable by objective tests, and most have not been shown to be real organic diseases. Rather, epidemiological studies find clear correlations between most forms of psychopathology and one or more of the following: (a) emotionally damaging infant and childhood experiences; (b) poverty and degrading life experiences; (c) powerlessness and low self-esteem; and (d) loneliness, social isolation, and social marginality.

This distinction between physical diseases and the phenomena identified as psychopathology is important because it exposes the lack of validity in the argument often used as a delaying tactic: The argument that psychopathology cannot be prevented unless the specific organic cause of each mental disease is discovered and understood. Although public health experts increasingly understand the role of the social environment in disease causation, they are still accustomed to think of real disease that involves organic pathology and are tempted to listen to voices that reinforce that view.

Opposition to Prevention Through Social Change

Psychiatrists Lamb and Zusman (1979), for example, sharply attacked the growing interest in social change ef-

From George W. Albee, "Toward a Just Society: Lessons from Observations on the Primary Prevention of Psychopathology," *American Psychologist*, Vol. 41, pp. 891–898. Copyright © 1986 by the American Psychological Association. Reprinted by permission.

forts as methods of primary prevention of mental disorders. They criticized the "fuzziness of the concepts" and the "assumption—which is yet unproved—that difficult life circumstances lead to mental illness" (p. 12). They argued for the importance of maintaining a distinction between preventing "real" mental illness and preventing emotional distress, and they said that "the cause and effect relationship between social conditions and mental illness is extremely questionable" (p. 12). According to Lamb and Zusman, primary prevention is impossible without a knowledge of the specific causes of mental illnesses; they credited medical and biological research with making progress in discovering some of the specific genetic and biochemical factors responsible for mental diseases, but warned that prevention thinking today is largely espoused by those who advocate social change. They made the bald statement that "there is *no evidence* [emphasis added] that it is possible to strengthen 'mental health' and thereby increase resistance to mental illness by general preventive activities" (p. 13). Further on, they stated, "Mental illness is probably in large part genetically determined and it is probably therefore not preventable, at most only modifiable. Even that it can be modified is questioned by many and there is little hard evidence one way or the other" (p. 13). In their view, research studies that have found relationships between indices of social disintegration and high rates of psychopathology are unconvincing because such studies "fail to demonstrate that there is a *causal* relationship between the particular stressful environmental factors under consideration and the occurrence of mental illness" (p. 14).

It is instructive, in this context, to contemplate the dramatic increase in the number of new mental illnesses over recent years and the disappearance of other mental illnesses. The latest edition of the official *Diagnostic and Statistical Manual of Mental Disorders* (DSM-III) of the American Psychiatric Association (1980) contains 60% more separate mental conditions than the DSM-II (1968), which in turn included nearly twice as many mental conditions as the first DSM published in 1952. Obviously, if the number of separate patterns of mental disturbance has increased so dramatically, the number of persons categorized (or categorizable) as mentally ill may have increased as well. For example, by identifying Reading Disorders in Children as a new category of mental illness, DSM-III created some five million new cases in the general category of the mentally disordered. A new Tobacco Dependence Syndrome raised the total by many more millions. In contrast, the majority vote of psychiatrists in the United States to eliminate homosexuality as a form of mental illness has dramatically reduced the total prevalence of mental illness. When DSM-III eliminated "the

This paper was presented on January 15, 1985, as an Invited Address at a Conference on Primary Health Care Management in International Health Promotion and Disease Prevention, School of Public Health, University of Hawaii at Manoa, Honolulu, Hawaii.

Correspondence concerning this article should be sent to George W. Albee, Department of Psychology, John Dewey Hall, University of Vermont, Burlington, VT 05405.

neuroses," the contributions of the psychoanalysts and ego psychologists were abandoned.

Evidence Concerning the Social Origins of Psychopathology

One of the problems with attempting to demonstrate the social origins of psychopathology (findings that suggest that primary prevention programs may often require social change) is that many of the examples of social factors being associated with rises and falls in incidence of mental conditions involve correlational studies. Correlational findings have long been convincing—and useful—in medicine. For example, the rate of tuberculosis was very high during the 19th century, and Dubos (1965) attributed this high rate to the poor level of general health of industrial workers and to abysmally poor living conditions, long working hours, and the helplessness of the laboring classes during the Industrial Revolution (p. 169). He suggested that as nutrition and other living conditions of the poor and working classes improved, mortality from tuberculosis declined, long before any specific medications were available for treating this disease.

Dohrenwend (1975) confronted the question of a causal relationship between poverty and mental disorders. She spelled out the kind of evidence that would be needed to establish the link between a biased social system and rates of individual emotional distress. It would be necessary, she said, to show that a general relationship exists between stress and disturbance among individuals in the general population, then to show that varying amounts of stressful experiences might be expected to happen among classes with corresponding differences in rates of mental disorders, and finally, to show that stress is more common in the lives of lower class individuals. After a careful empirical study involving interviews with five groups from varying social class levels and ethnic origins, she concluded:

Members of the lower class and women were found to be exposed to a relatively high rate of change or instability in their lives, with evidence in each case that this instability was a factor producing a relatively high level of individual distress in lower status individuals. (pp. 233–234)

One of the leading American public health preventionists, John Cassel, demonstrated the critical link between (a) severe social–environmental stresses and (b) susceptibility to both physical illness and emotional disorders. He and his colleagues demonstrated that high risk for all kinds of pathology accompanied the experience of poverty, social estrangement, unemployment, low social status, and powerlessness. In his Wade Hampton Frost Lecture, Cassel (1976) spelled out "the contribution of the social environment to host resistance." He reviewed both animal and human studies showing that destructive changes in the social environment are associated with profound changes in endocrinological response. From these data he argued that it is most improbable that researchers will ever find one-to-one correspondence between a specific stressor and a specific disease. He showed how psychosocial stress increases the general susceptibility of people to illness and concluded:

A remarkably similar set of social circumstances characterizes people who develop tuberculosis and schizophrenia, become alcoholic, are victims of multiple accidents, or commit suicide. Common to all these people is a marginal status in society. They are individuals who for a variety of reasons . . . have been deprived of meaningful social contact. (p. 110)

Cassel (and others who have followed his lead) established the relationship between stress and both disease and mental disorder, and the mitigating and protective benefits of strong support systems. Clearly, the implication of this research is that prevention can be achieved through stress reduction, increased self-esteem, mutual support groups, and community organization (Albee, 1982b; Kessler & Albee, 1975).

To be sure, some disturbances in behavior can be caused by biochemical or other organic imbalances. It is also clear that certain drugs do diminish the severity of symptoms of certain mental conditions. There is also some evidence of a genetic factor in some mental conditions. However, these relationships often are overemphasized, overstated, and overpublicized, perhaps for political and ideological reasons. Less public attention is paid to the truly massive and widespread emotional damage produced by poverty, child abuse, sexual abuse, sexism, racism, ageism, discrimination, and involuntary unemployment. For example, nearly every state now requires that babies be tested for phenylketonuria (PKU), a condition affecting fewer than 250 new babies a year in the United States. Yet little attention is paid to the many thousands of high-risk babies who are born to women (especially younger teenagers) who have received no prenatal care and whose poor diets and poor life circumstances result in high rates of premature births. Even when carried to term, infants born to these mothers often have low birth weights. These young mothers and their infants are both at high risk for later psychopathology.

Another source of confusion about the importance of the role of social factors in psychopathology is the growing epidemiological evidence that many real diseases are caused, or exacerbated, by life-styles. There is a striking inconsistency between the arguments of those psychiatrists who assert that mental disorders result largely from genetic and biochemical factors, rather than life experiences and stresses, and the views of their medical colleagues who are discovering that many physical diseases are a result of life stresses and behavior (Rosen & Solomon, 1985). Rates of hypertension and stroke, heart disease, and cancer are associated with life-styles and personality patterns. These conflicting messages often create a double bind because the arguments contradict each other.

Priorities

The prevention of psychopathology has not enjoyed much attention from the public health field in the United States, and it is clearly not high on the public health agendas of many other countries, particularly those with more urgent health problems. In societies that have high rates of infant mortality, of maternal death, and of inadequate nourishment—in short, in the countries of the 65% of the world's people who are among the "have-nots"—there is not much demand for expertise in the prevention of phobias, depressions, alcoholism, or the sexual neuroses and existential perplexities!

In addition to being low priority because of the presence of far more pressing life-and-death issues, problems involving psychopathology are viewed with some uncertainty and even suspicion by public health authorities, even in the developed countries. One reason for this attitude is that it is difficult to do serious and reliable epidemiological studies of conditions that have no physical markers. How can phobias or schizoid delusions be counted and differentiated from nonpathological fears or suspicions? How should investigators rate moderate depression or the degree of seriousness of inability to achieve complete sexual fulfillment? None of these conditions is a cause of death, and public health experts are used to dealing with measurable and unambiguous diseases that usually cause either death or serious incapacity.

Even though at least 43 million American adults are reported by the National Institute of Mental Health (see Regier et al., 1984) to have a diagnosable mental illness, no national panic has ensued. Yet parents who refuse to send their children to a classroom where a child with AIDS is enrolled—even though AIDS affects only a very small percentage of the population—appear not to be concerned about their children's contact with emotionally disturbed children (estimated at 25% of the total school population).

Of those mental conditions that do attract the attention of public health programs in the developed nations, those most likely to be investigated are organic mental illnesses, such as brain syphilis, pellagral psychosis, Alzheimer's disease, Huntington's chorea, and Korsakoff's syndrome, because these can be measured.

It is difficult to imagine a Third World public health program concerning itself with bed-wetting or sibling rivalry, when the overall infant death rate is 10 times greater than in developed countries, partly as a result of conditions such as infant diarrhea, which is easily preventable and treatable with safe water, sugar, and salt. It is equally difficult to imagine a program for reducing the emotional consequences of marital disruption and divorce in impoverished societies where there is no adequate housing, sanitation, or prenatal medical care. In those parts of the world where 35,000 people a day starve to death, it is not likely that much public health concern will be expended on persons who are depressed over their mid-life crises!

Barriers to a Just Society and Primary Prevention of Psychopathology

With all these sources of ambivalence, what can be said about the current efforts directed toward the primary prevention of psychopathology? Elsewhere it has been argued (Albee, 1982a, 1982b, 1983) that the same forces that contribute to psychopathology in citizens of developed nations are responsible for many of the serious health problems of the underdeveloped world (see Joffe & Albee, 1981). These forces cause an unequal distribution of the world's resources with resulting exploitation, powerlessness, and distress for the majority and scarcely believable power and affluence for the few.

It is within the capability of humankind to end poverty and to prevent many of the diseases that devastate hundreds of millions of families throughout the world. Until endemic poverty, disease, and powerlessness are greatly reduced, there will be excessive amounts of psychopathology in the developed countries and other forms of human misery and disease in the rest of the world.

One of the great innovations in the history of public health was the provision of adequate sewer systems. Sewerage, safe water, inoculation against childhood diseases, production of fast-growing trees for firewood, better farming methods, and fairer food distribution are readily available if their costs can be met. With serious investment in research and its application, even the problem of overpopulation could be solved without the scourges of famine and disease.

What stops the world's people from building a more just, more equitable world—a world in which preventable stress has been reduced for the majority of people—as is envisioned as a major goal by the World Health Organization? The forces that are barriers to a just world are some of the same forces that block significant efforts at reducing psychopathology in our own society: exploitation, imperialism, excessive concentration of economic power, nationalism, institutions that perpetuate powerlessness, hopelessness, poverty, discrimination, sexism, racism, and ageism. These forces control or influence the world's communications systems, especially mass media and educational systems, and they deliberately distribute rewards for conformity and for the support of injustice. Rather than remain at this high level of abstraction, let us focus on some specific ideological correlates of support for, or opposition to, prevention efforts in general.

Certain fundamental assumptions about human beings, about their relationships with each other and with their environments, and about the meaning and purpose of life have a significant influence on the attitudes of support or resistance toward the primary prevention of psychopathology and disease. Among these assumptions are belief in a just world, belief in a fixed mechanistic process of societal evolution, and belief in fatalism.

Belief in a Just World

Social psychologists (see Heider, 1958; Lerner, 1970, 1971; Lerner & Simmons, 1966) have studied people who do and do not believe in a just world. Individuals differ greatly in the extent to which they believe that people get what they deserve in life, that virtue is rewarded, and that hard work and sacrifice lead to success, whereas sloth and self-indulgence lead to failure. Believers in a just world often go so far as to explain all human misfortune, handicap, disease, and poverty as God's judgment on sinners.

In order to try to explain the paradox of the seemingly good and pleasurable life of some sinners, or some heathen, they find it necessary to add the belief that these sybarites eventually will be punished, perhaps in everlasting hellfire. And to explain why righteous and religious persons suffer misfortune, God's testing of faith, with eventual heavenly reward, is posited to make things come out even (see Rubin & Peplau, 1973).

There are many inconsistencies in the attitudes of believers in a just world. They will sometimes attempt to alleviate the suffering of specific individuals if they think these people do not deserve their fate (e.g., victims of child abuse), but they usually will not try to assist people who are mentally ill or morally tainted. Believers in a just world generally find it hard to entertain the concept of "innocent victim" because this concept threatens their basic belief system. So they often find ways to conclude that persons who suffer hunger, disease, slavery, exploitation, and persecution indeed must be deserving of their fate. People who believe in a just world are likely to be prejudiced and to accept without question the inferiority of women and of persecuted racial, religious, and ethnic groups. Their tendency to "blame the victim" has been clearly described by Ryan (1971) as a way of justifying poverty and powerlessness.

Related to the belief in a just world is the belief that ours is the only world, that it has existed for only a short time, and that its purpose is to fulfill a divine plan. To maintain the illusion of an orderly religious system, the believer often sacrifices logic, knowledge, and evidence. One important example is found in the set of beliefs about the recent origin of the earth and the universe. Although science has produced good evidence that the universe has existed for many billions of years, that our own solar system is very old, and that life on earth has evolved slowly, many religions are determined to dispute this evidence in order to defend a belief system that limits human existence to a few thousand years and that insists on a set of mythological beliefs about miraculous events that explain away evidence for evolution, such as fossils, geological strata, and species change.

What has the belief in a just world to do with primary prevention? Basically, to accept the argument that prevention or reduction of human misery is possible, it is necessary to accept an ambiguous, open world view, to accept that social and political change is possible, that the fate of humans is not rigidly predetermined and fixed, and that existence does not follow some externally imposed divine plan leading to salvation for the elect and damnation for the rest. To try to prevent sexism and racism, poverty and powerlessness, it is necessary to challenge the authority of belief systems that say that these prejudices and conditions are justified by divine law, or biblical revelation, or by immutable class structure. Any system that proclaims the "natural" or divine right of one group to exploit another group helps perpetuate injustice and powerlessness, conditions that are at the heart of human hunger and disease, misery, low self-esteem, depression, and the several functional varieties of psychopathology.

A humanistic position (that cannot be considered to be a scientific position) attributes equal value to all individual human lives. If each human being is equally deserving of the opportunity to maximize his or her life experience, work toward primary prevention goals must involve attempts at empowering the powerless.

Belief in a Fixed Mechanistic Process of Societal Evolution

Social Darwinism is somewhat more sophisticated than the just world, but similar in consequences. This position holds that evolution is occurring not only in animals and plants but also in human societies. The most articulate spokesperson for this position was Herbert Spencer (see 1873–1881), whose writings were widely embraced as justification of laissez-faire capitalism and the inevitable inequality of the social class system. The Spencerian view held that "survival of the fittest" occurs not only in lower forms in nature but also in human societies, and that this process weeds out the unfit and results in the continuous improvement of the human species. To interfere with this process through the imposition of health care for the poor, welfare schemes, or social assistance programs is to interfere with natural selection to the eventual disadvantage of the human race.

This philosophical position substitutes a set of immutable natural laws for an external divine providence as the controlling force in human affairs. It relies heavily on the science of genetics to explain social class position—the elite upper classes are superior because of superior genes, and the disadvantaged are inferior because of genetic deficiencies. Blum (1978) wrote:

General acceptance of Darwin's controversial theory, however, undermined traditional religious beliefs and created a need for new legitimating explanations. Into this void stepped Spencer, Galton, and other theorists, who took the older religious idea of predestination and adorned it with a new, scientific vocabulary. No longer were economic successes or failures preordained by God; they were predestined by differences in the complexity of individuals' nervous systems. Thus, eugenics, being an offshoot of Social Darwinism, would occasionally be referred to as "scientific capitalism." (p. 35)

There is a long, sorry record of oppression of people, cultures, and nations by "superior races" and, often, of the acceptance by subjected peoples of an imposed definition of their inferiority. In recent centuries the British have provided a clear example of how ideology can serve power—acclaiming and honoring persons whose science and history have been most useful in defending their own upper class's innate right to colonize, to rule, and to exploit. In 1796 Edmund Burke showed the ideological way for Galton and his successors. Burke spoke, half a century before Marx, of "a vast, tremendous, unformed spectre," the spectre of possible revolt against the rights of the great exploiters (cited in O'Brien, 1967). Burke viewed political democracy with horror and appealed to a gentlemanly consensus—of those with property and a proper Christian education—to maintain the existing social order based on clear and sharp graduations in rank, historically determined to be right and just.

In the United States, William Graham Sumner, one of the founders of American sociology, taught social Darwinism and laissez-faire economics. Sumner's sociology (1913) convinced several generations of Yale men that they and their wealthy fathers were deserving of their place in society by reason of high genetic worth. Some of Sumner's "scientific conclusions" about the nature of society are worth noting:

Competition is a law of nature. Nature is entirely neutral; she submits to him who most energetically and resolutely assails her. She grants her rewards to the fittest, therefore, without regard to other considerations of any kind . . . such is the system of nature. If we do not like it, and if we try to amend it, there is only one way in which we can do it. We can take from the better and give to the worse . . . let it be understood that we cannot go outside the alternatives: liberty, inequality, survival of the fittest; nonliberty, equality, survival of the unfittest. The former carries society forward and favours all its best members; the latter carries society downwards and favours all its worst members. (p. 25)

Such views led to the growth in England and America of the eugenics movement, which strove to give natural selection some help by eliminating or reducing the breeding of the unfit and the mentally deficient. Although these latter groups were more likely than the affluent to have their numbers reduced by poor nutrition, disease, and atrocious living conditions, they still managed to breed frighteningly large numbers of "genetically handicapped" children, whereas the better endowed upper classes were said not to be reproducing enough. To correct this unfortunate imbalance, sterilization programs aimed at the unfit were proposed, and in England and America strong immigration barriers were erected against the admission of the "brunette races."

Because the poor within Western nations as well as the colonial peoples of the world were seen as naturally inferior, there was ample ideological justification for exploitation of industrial workers, including children and women, for colonialism, and for racist policies leading to genocide. In the case of the exploitation of women, "science," as defined by Galton (1869) and his successors, established that females were incapable of abstract intellectual thought and the artistic creativity required for genius. It was a man's world, so long as the man was Nordic and upper class.

One of the many startling facts about this whole ideology is that it was so widely accepted by its victims. Although occasional voices of protest were heard, it is clear that women and the colonized, the lower classes, and the rest largely accepted the view that they were, indeed, inferior. Clearly, to the extent that similar views are held today, primary prevention programs will be opposed by many people—both exploiters and the exploited—if they seek to empower the powerless, if they seek to eliminate racism and sexism, and if they work toward establishing social justice for all as a way of reducing psychopathology and disease.

The dynamics of any prejudice, including racism and sexism, require careful and dispassionate examination. As Flynn (1980) pointed out, the racists (and sexists) may fear, reject, or exploit a total group of people (blacks, Jews, Orientals, or women) simply because of their appearance, or they may decide that members of these groups merit rejection, exploitation, or fear because their appearance is highly correlated with undesirable personal traits or negative characteristics. Flynn argued that every racist ideology has had to defend the position that the targeted group possesses undesirable, dangerous, repulsive, or threatening characteristics. Because many racists are intelligent and logical, they recognize that they must produce convincing evidence of the high correlation between membership in the group and the negative qualities.

But there is still a problem for the racist. Unless the correlation is extremely high, there will be a significant number of exceptions to the view that all members of the targeted group deserve the discrimination and exclusion to which they are subjected. So racists occasionally make minor qualifying statements allowing for possible exceptions in certain areas and at certain times. But this does not prevent them from barring all Chinese, all Hawaiians, all Jews, all blacks, or all women from their clubs, their private schools, their executive suites, and their neighborhoods. The life of the racist or the sexist is full of cognitive dissonance because of the logical inconsistencies that must be accommodated.

There is a further requirement for the racist—a belief that the despised characteristics of the target group are inborn, genetic, and unchangeable, rather than environmental in origin. If the undesirable traits could be eliminated through education or other environmental and social change, then the logical racist would have to join efforts to bring about this change. Instead, the racist or sexist must see the target group as biologically flawed and incapable of significant improvement. Flynn examined all the current arguments of the group that seeks to ban the immigration of persons of color into Britain. He asked, quite reasonably, why if, as is alleged, the intelligence of the immigrants is the real concern, should immigrants not be ranked on the basis of intelligence rather than skin color, and selectively admitted on the basis of high IQs?

Because they feel so strongly about the unmodifiability of genetic defects in such matters as intelligence, racists argue strongly against the possibility of success of early remedial compensatory experiences, including early compensatory education. It is not surprising that contemporary American psychologists, who argue that intelligence and criminal tendencies are largely genetically determined, also argue against the preventive value of early compensatory education or social change for disadvantaged groups.

Thus, persons who believe in a just world, in social Darwinism, or in superior or inferior classes or races whose differences are rooted in immutable genetic quality are going to oppose efforts at social change to prevent psychopathology. Such people have been responsible for colonialism, exploitation, inequality, and injustice in the world.

A Fatalistic View

At the other ideological extreme are persons who see the world as frequently random and capricious in dealing out rewards and punishments and who believe that innocent persons and groups are often damaged, victimized, or exploited through no fault of their own. In this view there is no divine master plan or guarantee of justice beyond that designed and put into effect by people themselves. Such a position is consistent with attempts to help victims, to correct injustices, and to interfere deliberately with the freedom of certain powerful individuals and groups to exploit others. This egalitarian position, often called "secular humanism" by religious fundamentalists, is anathema to believers in a just world and to believers in the genetic superiority and inferiority of races and classes.

One of the most painful, even frightening, scientific insights—one that stands in opposition to the view that the human species is gradually improving and moving toward a better future—is that evolution has no goal. It is understandable that the theory of evolution, a product of human observation and human thought, long included some notion of gradual progress and the improvement of species, especially, of course, the human species. Indeed, science has often reported findings of primitive early humans who were less intelligent and more apelike than contemporary people. And a few scientists have long held that the presumed intellectual superiority and inferiority of existing races can be explained by their differential position along the evolutionary scale of progression toward superiority.

The compelling evidence supporting the view that evolution is simply a blind process of differential survival forces one to consider the possibility that the human species could disappear and go the way of the dinosaur, and that the world may experience the survival of the cockroach. Understandably, persons who hold this view are often perceived to be subversive and dangerous. To accept the view that evolution has no goal, and that there is no divine plan, is to accept the essential randomness or meaninglessness of existence, to accept that there is no purpose to be discovered outside the raw facts of existence and human consciousness. Two reactions to this cold, comfortless view are possible. One is a fatalistic reaction that leads to inaction; the other is a decision that we human beings must create our own meaning and decide how to react to each other without outside divine guidance, inspiration, or interference. A strong ethical case can be made for the view that we should act as though we are all responsible for each other and for future generations, and that we must find ways to create a just society in which everyone has the opportunity to maximize his or her potential as long as such behavior does not infringe on the rights of others.

Creating a Just Society

But how do we create a just society without any external guidance? How can people, reasoning together, arrive at a plan for achieving a society and a world dedicated to justice? What would such a society and world look like?

The first problem, of course, is that there would be strong resistance to any attempt to institute the social changes required to achieve broad social justice. Imagine the passionate resistance to the proposal that private ownership of property be ended or that inheritance of wealth be abolished!

Pascal (see Hutchins, 1952) spoke eloquently about the problem:

Justice is subject to disputes; might is easily recognized and is not disputed. So we cannot give might to justice, because might has gainsaid justice and has declared that it is she herself who is just. And thus, being unable to make what is just strong, we have made what is strong, just. (p. 227)

Let us consider what would be the characteristics of a just society in which basic human needs are met, unnecessary stress is reduced, the competence of each person is maximized, and psychopathology and disease are minimized. Philosopher John Rawls's views on justice have had a strong impact on both social philosophy and the law; he described a just society in *A Theory of Justice* (1971). In this book Rawls developed the fantasy that a small group of competent people, chosen more or less at random, seated around a table, could reach unanimity about what would be required to plan and create a just society. There was one important limiting consideration, however. None of the persons seated around the table knew whether he or she was rich or poor, male or female, black or white, brown or yellow, old or young. Members of the group had the use of all their faculties *except* their personal awareness of their own immediate identities. They sat behind a "veil of ignorance" about themselves, so they would not be biased by selfish considerations.

Rawls examined the kind of discourse that would be engaged in by such a group whose members had no selfish commitment to the outcome—the designing of a just society.

In Rawls's book, the group developed the concept of justice as fairness, and in a complex series of steps arrived at two basic principles that are essential to the existence of a just society. According to the first principle, each person is to have an equal right to the most extensive basic liberty compatible with a similar liberty for others. According to the second, social and economic inequalities are to be arranged so that they are both to the greatest benefit of the least advantaged and attached to offices and positions open to all, under conditions of fair and equal opportunity.

This formulation of a system of justice, if applied to contemporary society, would guarantee, according to Rawls, political liberty together with freedom of speech and assembly, liberty of conscience, freedom of thought, freedom of the person, along with the right to hold personal property, and freedom from arbitrary arrest and seizures, the whole defined by the concept of the rule of law. These universal liberties must be accessible to all, by Rawls's first principle, because in a just society everyone is to have the same basic rights. Rawls's second principle is in opposition to both the traditional conservative and liberal conceptions. Contemporary American capitalist ideology, which is rarely questioned, allows for status and income to be determined by individual abilities and talents, but Rawls argued: "There is no more reason to permit the distribution of income and wealth to be settled by the distribution of natural assets, than by historical and social fortune" (p. 74).

In Rawls's theory, to provide real equality of opportunity, society must make every attempt to redress all those social and economic inequalities that have led to disadvantage. This attempt means providing more attention and more effort to assist persons in less favorable social and economic positions. It means redistribution of power.

This view of responsibility for supporting each other and for controlling the arbitrary and excessive use of power must be at the heart of any serious long-range effort directed toward the primary prevention of psychopathology. This is not to say that no effective prevention program can be instituted before universal human justice is established! A great many successful, but limited, prevention programs have involved stress reduction and competence promotion (see Albee & Joffe, 1977; Bond & Joffe, 1982; Bond & Rosen, 1980; and Kent & Rolf, 1979). Modest progress has been made in such areas as health education (see Rosen & Solomon, 1985), sex education (see Albee, Gordon, & Leitenberg, 1983), human rights, and supportive networks. But somewhere on the long-range agenda for prevention must be the development of programs leading to an end to exploitation, colonialism, and imperialism. If professionals are ever to escape the rigid limits on thinking imposed by carefully controlled professional training and by reactionary views of society and of the world, they must squarely face and answer the questions raised by Rawls. Is an Ethopian child, a Bangladeshi child, a Mexican child, or the child of a migrant farm worker in America more deserving of preventive efforts than is a child of the affluent and the powerful?

Kenneth Clark (1974) asked social scientists to find ways to help control human exploitation and intergroup hostility, and at the same time to study ways to foster love and human empathy. Clark asked psychologists to do research on the effects of human institutions and social arrangements and to study issues of status and hierarchical distinctions as these relate to injustice and cruelty. Psychologists should listen. Psychologists must join with persons who reject racism, sexism, colonialism, and exploitation and must find ways to redistribute social power and to increase social justice. Primary prevention research inevitably will make clear the relationship between social pathology and psychopathology and then will work to change social and political structures in the interest of social justice. It is as simple and as difficult as that!

REFERENCES

Albee, G. W. (1982a). Preventing psychopathology and promoting human potential. *American Psychologist, 37,* 1043–1050.

Albee, G. W. (1982b). *What causes our problems? Am I sick or is my society sick? The social origins of psychopathology* [The Maurice Brown Oration]. Camberwell, Australia: Cairnmillar Institute.

Albee, G. W. (1983). Psychopathology, prevention, and the just society. *Journal of Primary Prevention, 4*(1), 5–36.

Albee, G. W., Gordon, S., & Leitenberg, H. (Eds.). (1983). *Fostering mature sexuality and preventing sexual problems.* Hanover, NH: University Press of New England.

Albee, G. W., & Joffe, J. M. (Eds.). (1977). *The primary prevention of psychopathology: The issues.* Hanover, NH: University Press of New England.

American Psychiatric Association. (1952). *Mental disorders: Diagnostic and statistical manual.* Washington, DC: Author.

American Psychiatric Association. (1968). *Diagnostic and statistical manual of mental disorders* (2nd ed.). Washington, DC: Author.

American Psychiatric Association. (1980). *Diagnostic and statistical manual of mental disorders* (3rd ed.). Washington, DC: Author.

Blum, J. M. (1978). *Pseudoscience and mental ability.* New York: Monthly Review Press.

Bond, L. A., & Joffe, J. M. (Eds.). (1982). *Facilitating infant and early childhood development.* Hanover, NH: University Press of New England.

Bond, L., & Rosen, J. (Eds.). (1980). *Competence and coping during adulthood.* Hanover, NH: University Press of New England.

Cassel, J. (1976). The contribution of the social environment to host resistance. *American Journal of Epidemiology, 104,* 107–123.

Clark, K. B. (1974). *The pathos of power.* New York: Harper & Row.

Dohrenwend, B. (1975). Sociocultural and social-psychological factors in the genesis of mental disorders. *Journal of Health and Human Behavior, 16,* 365–392.

Dubos, R. (1965). *Man adapting.* New Haven, CT: Yale University Press.

Flynn, J. R. (1980). *Race, IQ and Jensen.* London: Routledge & Kegan Paul.

Galton, F. (1869). *Hereditary genius.* London: Macmillan & Company.

Heider, F. (1958). *The psychology of interpersonal relations.* New York: Wiley.

Hutchins, R. M. (Ed.). (1952). *Great books of the Western World: Vol. 33. Pascal.* Chicago: University of Chicago Press.

Joffe, J. M., & Albee, G. W. (Eds.). (1981). *Prevention through political action and social change.* Hanover, NH: University Press of New England.

Kessler, M., & Albee, G. (1975). Primary prevention. *Annual Review of Psychology, 26,* 557–591.

Kent, M. W., & Rolf, J. E. (Eds.). (1979). *Social competence in children.* Hanover, NH: University Press of New England.

Lamb, H. R., & Zusman, J. (1979). Primary prevention in perspective. *American Journal of Psychiatry, 136,* 12–17.

Lerner, M. J. (1970). The desire for justice and reactions to victims. In J. Macauley & L. Berkowitz (Eds.), *Altruism and helping behavior* (pp. 205–209). New York: Academic Press.

Lerner, M. J. (1971, June). All the world loathes a loser. *Psychology Today,* pp. 51–54.

Lerner, M. J., & Simmons, C. H. (1966). Observer's reaction to the "innocent victim": Compassion or rejection? *Journal of Personality and Social Psychology, 4,* 203–210.

O'Brien, C. (1967). Burke and Marx. *New American Review, 1,* 243–258.

Rawls, J. (1971). *A theory of justice.* Cambridge, MA: Belknap.

Regier, D. A., Myers, J. K., Kramer, M., Robins, L. N., Blazer, D. G., Hough, R. L., Eaton, W. W., & Locke, B. Z. (1984). The NIMH epidemiologic catchment area program. *Archives of General Psychiatry, 41,* 934–941.

Rosen, J. C., & Solomon, L. J. (1985). *Prevention in health psychology.* Hanover, NH: University Press of New England.

Rubin, Z., & Peplau, A. (1973). Belief in a just world and reactions to another's lot: A study of participants in the national draft lottery. *Journal of Social Issues, 29*(4), 73–92.

Ryan, W. (1971). *Blaming the victim.* New York: Random House.

Spencer, H. (1873–1881). *Descriptive sociology.* New York: D. Appleton.

Sumner, W. G. (1913). *The challenge of facts and other essays.* New Haven, CT: Yale University Press.

About the Editors

George W. Albee is Professor of Psychology at the University of Vermont and President of the Vermont Conference on the Primary Prevention of Psychopathology (VCPPP). Each year since 1975, VCPPP has held a conference on some aspect of prevention of mental/emotional disorders and/or the enhancement of competence. The volumes based on these conference are a major compilation of the significant writings of leaders in the field of prevention. The present book of readings is drawn largely from these books. Albee has a long history of involvement in social and political issues affecting prevention. He wrote a book in 1959 reporting to the Joint Commission on Mental Illness and Health (appointed by President Eisenhower). The book deals with the inevitability of shortage of trained professionals to deliver one-on-one mental health services. In 1977-78 he was Director of the Task Panel on Prevention for President Carter's Commission on Mental Health. More recently, he was a member of the Commission on Prevention of the National Mental Health Association, which reported to the nation in the spring of 1986.

Justin M. Joffe is Professor of Psychology at the University of Vermont and Executive Vice President of VCPPP. He and George Albee are General Editors of the series of books on prevention that results from the annual VCPPP conferences. An internationally known scientist, Joffe currently is involved in ongoing research projects in London, at the National Institute of Hygiene in Budapest, Hungary, and at the Biological Institute in Zagreb, Yugoslavia. His research focuses on the prenatal determinants of behavior, developmental psychobiology, and a broad range of preventive interventions. His studies on paternal drug exposure effects on reproduction and on progeny have been widely reported as an important contribution in the emerging field of teratology.

Linda A. Dusenbury is Assistant Professor of Psychology in the Department of Public Health at Cornell University. She "discovered preventive psychology" as an undergraduate and has pursued her interest in this field since then. She completed her doctorate in 1984 at the University of Vermont in social-developmental psychology with a dissertation on the relation of political ideology to attitudes toward prevention and beliefs about causation of mental disorder. During her graduate study she took an active role in VCPPP and shared in the editing of an earlier book of readings in prevention. Her current research deals with health promotion and substance abuse prevention with urban minority youth.

557